Adrenaline and the Inner World

Adrenaline
and the Inner World

An Introduction to Scientific
Integrative Medicine

David S. Goldstein, M.D., Ph.D.

Attending Physician, Clinical Center,
The National Institutes of Health
Senior Investigator and Chief, Clinical Neurocardiology Section,
National Institute of Neurological Disorders and Stroke
Bethesda, Maryland

The Johns Hopkins University Press • *Baltimore*

© 2006 The Johns Hopkins University Press
All rights reserved. Published 2006
Printed in the United States of America on acid-free paper
9 8 7 6 5 4 3 2 1

The Johns Hopkins University Press
2715 North Charles Street
Baltimore, Maryland 21218-4363
www.press.jhu.edu

Library of Congress Cataloging-in-Publication Data

Goldstein, David S., 1948–
   Adrenaline and the inner world : an introduction to scientific integrative
medicine / David S. Goldstein.
       p. ; cm.
   Includes bibliographical references and index.
   ISBN 0-8018-8288-5 (hardcover : alk. paper) — ISBN 0-8018-8289-3 (pbk. :
alk. paper)
   1. Adrenaline—Physiological effect. 2. Stress (Physiology). 3. Autonomic
nervous system. 4. Integrative medicine. I. Title. [DNLM: 1. Epinephrine—
physiology. 2. Autonomic Nervous System—physiology. 3. Autonomic Nervous
System Diseases. 4. Stress—physiopathology. WK 725 G624a 2006]
QP572.A27.G65 2006
612.4'5—dc22   2005013358

A catalog record for this book is available from the British Library.

The value of a man is not measured by the truth he possesses, but rather by his sincere effort to discover truth . . . even though this search be fraught with constant and unremitting erring.

G. E. Lessing, 1729–1781

Contents

6. Distress   141

Characteristics of Distress 141, Biblical Lie Detection 148, Distress versus the General Adaptation Syndrome 150, Fight Isn't Flight 151, The Nose of God 158, StressToons 160

7. Stress in Evolutionary Perspective   164

Why Evolution Is a Worthwhile Theory and Creationism Isn't 164, Darwin and Ethology 169, The Price of Complexity Is Eternal Stress 172, Primitive Specificity 176

8. Dysautonomias   181

The "Mind-Body" Problem 182, Primary versus Secondary Dysautonomias 184, Secondary Dysautonomias 185, Primary Dysautonomias 194

9. Tests for Dysautonomias   207

Physiological Tests 209, Neuropharmacological Tests 215, Neurochemical Tests 220, Neuroimaging Tests 222

10. Treatments for Dysautonomias   224

Nondrug Treatments 224, Drug Treatments 229

11. Drugs and the Family   235

Catecholamines as Drugs 235, Legal Addictions 236, Cocaine 240, Speed Kills 240, Morphine 242, Barbs and Benzos 242, You Aren't What You Eat, Luckily 243

12. The Future: Scientific Integrative Medicine   247

Return of the Getaway Car 248, Allostatic Load for People Who Hate Snakes 250, The Dialectic 254, Darwinian Medicine 259, Tactics and Strategies of Scientific Integrative Medicine 263, What, How, and Why 266, Conclusion 269

Preface

This book tells a life story, but it isn't a biography. It paints a family portrait, but not of a human family. Instead, this book depicts the world's most famous hormone, adrenaline, and its chemical family, the catecholamines (pronounced cat-a-COLA-means, or, if you are British, cat-a-coal-AY-means). They are part of you. They have kept you alive and are keeping you alive now as you read this, just as they sustained your ancestors from the beginning of mammalian time. Through them I hope to teach you a bit about the "wisdom of the body," as the great American physiologist, Walter B. Cannon, titled his classic book about seventy-five years ago.

I use the term *life story* quite deliberately here. Adrenaline exemplifies a type of chemical called *biogenic*. The word *biogenic* has a double meaning. Biochemists use it to signify that living things make these chemicals. Another meaning—and a main message of this book—is that higher organisms depend crucially on these chemicals for life, because catecholamines enable regulation of the body's "inner world" by the brain.

The year 2001 marked the centennial of adrenaline's discovery. Adrenaline was first purified, its structure was deduced, and attempts to measure it began in the early twentieth century. Indeed, adrenaline was the first hormone ever to be identified and produced in a laboratory. During the decades that followed, adrenaline acquired a unique mystique and folklore, which, for reasons that were largely technical, outpaced its science. Injected as a drug, adrenaline potently produces obvious effects. The skin turns pale, the heart pounds, the blood pressure rises, and the individual feels energized. Because of this potency, however, the plasma of healthy humans at rest contains remarkably low levels of adrenaline—a few millionths of a millionth of a gram per milliliter—measurable only during the past thirty years or so, since the introduction of sufficiently sensitive, specific assay methods. Inferences from the indirect physiological evidence of the early twentieth century led to speculative notions, then to legends, and then to pulp myths.

The technical problem of actually measuring levels of adrenaline directly in the bloodstream, rather than indirectly via adrenaline's effects, had consequences beyond obtaining scientific understanding about this particular hormone. The coinage of science is discovery, and novelty makes for easy sales. After the measurement of adrenaline levels posed a seemingly insurmountable challenge, biomedical researchers turned to other, newly discovered compounds in a succession extending until the present—insulin, adrenocortical steroids, serotonin, vasopressin, the renin-angiotensin-aldosterone system, hypothalamic releasing factors, prostaglandins, kinins, neurotrophic factors, atriopeptins, endothelins, nitric oxide, leptin, orexins, aquaporins, and an imposing, expanding array of cytokines.

In doing so, researchers followed a long tradition of studying such compounds one at a time. Dwelling on the workings of single systems, using single effector chemicals, is always easier and cheaper than focusing on interactions among multiple systems that use different effector chemicals. The emphasis on single systems in medical science comes from the belief that one best acquires knowledge by dissecting a problem into its component parts; reassembling the parts presumably would solve the problem. This approach is called *reductionism*. The technical difficulty in measuring adrenaline levels, coupled with the reductionist tradition in medical science, retarded development of integrative approaches that have only recently begun to attract bioscientists.

Scientific integrative medicine is not a discipline, a group of disorders, or a method of treatment but an approach, a way of thinking. Scientific integrative medicine uses *systems* concepts to explain disease processes and develop strategies to treat, prevent, or palliate them. It emphasizes disorders of the multiple interacting systems that regulate the body's inner world. Scientific integrative medicine asks researchers and clinicians to consider more than one system at a time, as assessed by measuring levels of more than one chemical effector at a time. One of those chemical effectors—but a very important one—is adrenaline.

For more than a century, from the discovery of adrenaline as the active principle of the adrenal gland, to the identification of norepinephrine, adrenaline's chemical father, as the neurotransmitter of the sympathetic nervous system, to the elucidation of the role of dopamine, adrenaline's chemical grandfather, as a neurotransmitter in the brain, research based on the adrenaline family has proven remarkably consistently fruitful and led to many Nobel Prizes. I believe that the evolution of scientific integrative medicine will depend on even more refined understanding of adrenaline's family and its interactions with other families of chemical effectors in the systems that the brain uses to regulate the inner world of the body.

Everyone Knows about Adrenaline—Why a Book about It?

Everyone knows legends about adrenaline. Few know the facts. For a century researchers and laypeople alike have viewed adrenaline as the "fight or flight" hormone, important in primitive emergencies but not in everyday life. In fact, adrenaline and its family are essential not only in emergencies but also for the continual, rapid adjustments required to tolerate even mundane stresses, such as simply standing up or walking out into the chilly outdoors. In fact, changes in activities of internal body systems, mediated by members of the adrenaline family, accompany virtually every motivated behavior and every experienced emotion. Moreover, externally observable effects of the same chemicals serve highly important roles in instinctive communication, a fact recognized since antiquity, as you will learn.

Writers in psychology and psychosomatic medicine have taught that the faster pace of human cultural than of physical evolution has led to inappropriate expression of built-in, instinctive, primordial, unconscious, involuntary behaviors—that is, behaviors mediated by the "automatic" nervous system—and that this inappropriate expression causes or contributes to chronic diseases. People therefore have come to think of chronic stress and distress, by way of high adrenaline levels, as causes or contributors to the development of medical problems such as high blood pressure and coronary artery disease. In fact, researchers still don't know for sure about the correctness of this belief.

People think that, during exercise, an adrenaline "surge" increases the force and rate of the heartbeat and raises the blood pressure. Instead, these changes depend mainly on release of norepinephrine from nerves in the heart and blood vessel walls. As you will learn, this seemingly trivial misidentification probably cost a Nobel Prize for one of the most prominent physiologists of the twentieth century—the venerable Walter B. Cannon.

People think there is "good stress" and "bad stress" and that "too much" stress harms health. For this sort of notion, the issue is not truth but value. As you will learn, the notion of "good stress" and "bad stress" has little value as a scientific idea because of circular definitions and untestability.

The popular notion, that adrenaline plays a key role in the responses to and experience of distress, probably *is* correct. In the setting of an independent disease, such as coronary artery disease, adrenaline release can even kill; however, most researchers who study mechanisms by which stressors exert their effects have focused on a different system, the system involving steroids produced in the outer layer of the adrenal gland. Adrenaline, produced in the core of the adrenal gland, has been relatively ignored.

Adrenaline is important scientifically, as demonstrated by numerous Nobel Prizes for discoveries based on it and the other members of its chemical family. It is important medically because of its many contributions to manifestations of disease, as a basis for monitoring responses of the body to treatments, and in establishing a prognosis. It is important culturally because of its ubiquity in politics, sports, and entertainment. In this book you will read about why a former Attorney General with Parkinson disease has a tendency to faint; why young astronauts in excellent physical shape can not stand up when re-exposed to earth's gravity, why professional football players can collapse and die of heat shock during summer training camp, and why baseball players spit so much. Adrenaline is important legally because of worker's compensation claims for alleged job stress–induced, adrenaline-mediated heart attacks, the medical risk of standing trial, alleged effects of toxic exposures—even the meaning and significance of the "plaintive wail" of Nicole Brown Simpson's pet Akita in the timing of her murder. Adrenaline is important philosophically because it operates at exactly the border between the mind and body, the voluntary and involuntary, the creature and the human. Adrenaline is important aesthetically because artists and playwrights have always relied on its effects to depict emotional states that are communicated instinctively and that words cannot hide. It is even important religiously for correct understanding of biblical narrative about Jacob's "faint," Miriam's "leprosy," the only biblical example of trial by ordeal, and the nose as the organ of rage.

Is This Book for You?

I wrote this book to supplement academic coursework in several fields— psychology, philosophy, biblical studies, physiology, biochemistry, the history of medicine, psychiatry, endocrinology, cardiology, and complementary and alternative medicine. You might be a college student seeking a bachelor of arts degree, a graduate student in natural sciences, a medical student, a practicing physician, or an academician. Taking into account the obviously diverse abilities to digest the medical scientific information, I have included a large glossary. The figures and figure legends provide a kind of parallel text simpler than the main text. The book teaches by analogy, example, and anecdote, with the intention of drawing you, by sheer fascination, into the world that populates you.

I wrote this book also for patients and their families, caretakers, and support groups seeking a source of information about dysautonomias. Dysautonomias are conditions in which altered function of the "automatic nervous system" adversely affects health. Dysautonomias are ubiquitous in modern society, ranging from occasional annoying sensations in otherwise healthy people to progressive, debilitating, fatal diseases. They occur in all age groups. Some are established diseases, with changes in body tissues that a pathologist can see. Some are functional disorders, with chemical or biological changes that a clinical investigator can measure. Some are mysterious and controversial because of a lack of accepted objective tests and treatments. All involve multiple body functions, multiple internal effector systems, and multiple disciplines in medicine. These features render dysautonomias an ideal entrée to scientific integrative medicine, which I believe will be at the forefront of medical thought and practice in the postgenome era.

I dedicate this book to my family—particularly my partner in life, Minka—for their support and understanding in allowing me the time to write this book; to my colleagues and friends at the National Institutes of Health (NIH) for their devotion to our research mission and to me; and to the many patients who have put their trust in me and provided sparkles of insight about adrenaline and the body's automatic systems in regulation and dysregulation of the inner world. Patients serve as a unique scientific resource. They report what is wrong; we have to make sense of what they teach. They tell us the truth; we have to avoid dismissiveness as a defense of our own ignorance. They seek our help; we have to commiserate with their unintended, unwanted metamorphosis from independent, private, integrated personhood to dependent, exposed, disintegrated patienthood.

I thank Mr. Herbert Abramowitz and Dr. Melvin Plotinsky for reading the book in its entirety and conveying their points of view and their always constructive suggestions for improvement. Finally, I thank my mentor and colleague, Dr. Irwin J. Kopin, an example of intellectual rigor, productivity, perspective, and integrity, an inspiration throughout my career at the NIH. Irv, you paid a high compliment to me as a scientist when you told me, "You ask good questions."

Adrenaline and the Inner World

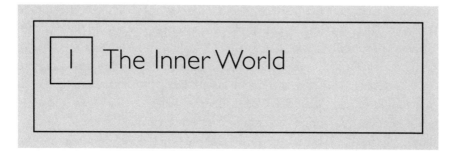

1 The Inner World

Inside you is an inner world, full of comings and goings and the beautiful paradox of seeming constancy despite continuous change. We are born, we develop and mature, we reproduce, we live out our lives, we get old, we get sick, and we die, yet for most of our existence we believe in our essential sameness day to day.

On average, human beings live longer than any other animals have ever lived. For most of this amazing longevity, we rarely notice the internal workings that constitute the political affairs of the inner world. Cells of the body "turn over"—you literally replace yourself over time—yet things inside seem to stay in a steady state so well, for so long. Body temperature, blood levels of key fuels, concentrations of red blood cells in the bloodstream, amounts of electrolytes, the rate of the heartbeat, blood flows to organs, and many more "variables" normally don't vary much. Even mood and personality remain about the same, characterizing us to others and to ourselves. When levels of these variables do change and you feel sick, you don't feel "like yourself."

These steady states do not happen by chance. In higher organisms, they depend on complex coordination by the brain. This chapter introduces a way of thinking about how the brain regulates the inner world, to maintain apparent constancy despite continual change. In a single word, the brain does so via *systems*. Just as the brain receives information from sense organs about and determines our interactions with the outside world, the brain also receives information from internal sensors and acts on that information to regulate the inner world. For most of our lives we can cling to our belief in sameness only because the brain tracks many monitored variables, by way of internal sensory information, and acts on this information to maintain levels of monitored variables at controlled, steady values by modulating numerous effectors that work simultaneously, in parallel.

A remarkable array of effectors, working largely unconsciously and automatically, maintain the stability of the inner world. For these effectors to work often depends on a small family of messenger chemicals, the catecholamines (pronounced cat-a-COLA-means). The most famous member of this chemical family is adrenaline. It is so famous that in this book I refer to the catecholamines as the adrenaline family. Keep in mind, though, that, as in actual families that achieve fame, the one that gives the family its name is not necessarily the one the family relies on to run the business. A major theme of this book is that the brain uses many effectors. You will have to learn about several to begin to acquire the knowledge necessary for thinking of diseases by using a systems approach.

"Systems biology" has gained cachet recently in academic medicine. Systems biology has been defined variously as an analytic approach to relationships of elements in a biological system to understand emergent properties of that system; the exploration of cell functions at the molecular level; the analysis of networks and interactions among genes, proteins, and other cellular chemicals; or the mathematical modeling of cellular control mechanisms to explain the functions of living things.

Scientific integrative medicine builds on systems biology, but it is also distinct in several ways. (1) Scientific integrative medicine recognizes that in higher organisms, including us humans, the brain dominates regulation of the inner world. The brain regulates the many internal monitored variables of the body in parallel—analogous to a computer's multitasking. (2) The brain has plasticity, which enables modifications in the step-by-step instructions for cellular, tissue, organ, and systemic processes—the algorithms of life. According to the concept of allostasis, about which you will learn later in this chapter, set points and other elements of these algorithms vary, depending on recollections, sensations, and anticipations by the brain. (3) Scientific integrative medicine is *medical*; its overall mission is to understand and rationally treat disorders and diseases. The systems that maintain the stability of the inner world eventually degenerate. Their efficiencies decline, and as they decline the likelihood of deleterious, self-reinforcing positive feedback loops increases, threatening organismic stability and survival. Clinicians rarely cure; they manage. They exploit negative feedback loops and attempt to forestall or counter positive feedback loops. (4) The medications and treatments clinicians prescribe interact with their patients' internal systems. Multiple, simultaneous degenerations, combined with multiple effects of multiple drugs and remedies and myriad interactions between the degenerations and the treatments, constitute the bulk of modern medical practice. The scientific integrative medicine approach provides a framework for understanding highly complex and dynamic challenges to our integrity as organisms.

A specific example may help make the point here. As we age, the efficiency of heart muscle function declines—in some sooner than in others, depending on hereditary predispositions and life exposures. As intrinsic heart muscle function declines, the brain senses the decreased pumping ability and directs a compensatory increase in nervous system outflow to the heart. This augments the delivery of norepinephrine (adrenaline's chemical father in the catecholamine family) to its receptors on heart muscle cells, keeping the cells' contractility and the heart's ejection of blood within normal limits. Bombardment of heart muscle cells by norepinephrine, however, decreases the threshold for the development of abnormal heart rhythms (arrhythmias). When an arrhythmia occurs, the heart instantaneously pumps less blood. The brain immediately directs a further increase in norepinephrine release from nerves in the heart, but this augments further the automaticity of the cells. When segments of heart muscle begin to contract autonomously, rather than synchronously, the heart ceases to function as a pump, and the patient suddenly, often unexpectedly, dies. A goal of scientific integrative medicine is to devise means to detect early or even prevent such a catastrophic positive feedback loop. Even after symptoms of heart failure develop, judicious treatment with drugs that modulate norepinephrine's effects could enhance survival.

Integrative medicine has also gained popularity recently. The word *integrative* has been used synonymously with *holistic, mind-body, complementary,* or *alternative*. The *scientific* integrative medicine approach, however, actually fits quite well with conventional, mainstream clinical medicine. Effective clinicians apply such an approach all the time. Observations over years and gleanings from course work and discussions with colleagues lead to inductions about disorders and predictions about what might help patients. Each patient is like an experiment, with the number of experimental subjects— the legendary *n* of statistics—being 1. The scientific integrative medicine approach provides a more formal framework, including controls and randomized placebo treatments, calculations of statistical parameters such as significance, power, sensitivity, specificity, and negative and positive predictive values, assessments of multiple, quantitative dependent measures, searching databases, cybernetic computer models, and so forth. The essence of the approach, however, the formulation of ideas and testing of predictions based on those ideas, is the same and is scientific. If anything, the intellectual challenge is greater for the practitioner who deals with patients as they come, with their multiple comorbidities, prescribed and unprescribed drugs, unidentified genetic predispositions, and subclinical pathophysiological processes not yet manifested as symptoms.

Scientific integrative medicine finds its roots in the seemingly simple, but actually enormously difficult, issue of how higher organisms maintain their integrity despite the vicissitudes of life. The great French physiologist of the mid-nineteenth century and prototypical experimentalist, Claude Bernard, propounded its founding concept.

The Seed and the Soil

Bernard introduced the idea of the inner world, when he theorized that body systems function as they do to maintain a constant internal environment—what he called the *milieu intérieur.* Bernard's conception evolved over several years. He taught that a fluid environment of nearly constant composition bathes and nourishes the cells. Near the end of his life, in about 1876, he postulated something more profound—that the body maintains the constant internal environment by myriad, continual, *compensatory* reactions. These compensatory reactions would tend to restore a state of equilibrium in response to any outside changes, enabling independence from the external environment. In response to perturbations of the inner world, body systems would react to counter those perturbations. Bernard therefore not only introduced the notion of an apparently constant inner world but also a purpose for body processes. His *Lectures on the Phenomena of Life Common to Animals and Vegetables* (Vol. 1, translated by Hoff HE, Guillemin R, Guillemin L. Springfield, IL: Charles C Thomas Publisher, 1974) contains one of the most famous passages in the history of physiology, "The constancy of the internal environment is the condition for free and independent life" (p. 84). "All the vital mechanisms, however varied they might be, always have one purpose, that of maintaining the integrity of the conditions of life within the internal environment" (p. 89). This view might seem straightforward or even simple minded today, but it was revolutionary in the history of medical ideas.

Bernard's views sometimes conflicted with those of his contemporary, Louis Pasteur, the father of microbiology and the germ theory of disease. The two argued over the cause of alcoholic fermentation, the basis for wine making. Pasteur claimed that fermentation required the presence of living organisms or germs. Bernard claimed that fermentation reflected a strictly chemical, intrinsic decomposition.

Students of Bernard and Pasteur came to argue analogously about the causes of diseases. According to Pasteur's followers, diseases would result mainly from external threats to the well-being of the organism, such as exposure to germs; the body's responses would be relatively unimportant. According to Bernard's followers, diseases would result from inappropriate or inadequate responses of the body; the actual threats would be relatively unimportant. To paraphrase the great American-Canadian-English physician, William Osler, the debate was over whether disease is caused by the "seed" or caused by the "soil."

During the era of ascendance of the germ theory of disease, at the end of the 1800s, the importance of the equilibrium of the organism receded. Now, in the era of molecular genetics, which views diseases as stemming from deleterious interactions between heredity and environment, or from genetic flaws outright, Bernard seems vindicated. Pasteur on his deathbed is said to have conceded, "Bernard was right. The microbe is nothing: the soil is everything."

The development and progression of diseases depend on genetic endowment and actual life experiences. Until relatively recently, however, biomedical researchers emphasized one or the other determinant almost to exclusion. Scientific integrative medicine provides a theoretical framework that gives these determinants appropriate weights. Pasteur and Bernard were probably both correct.

Cannon's Canons

Beginning about the turn of the twentieth century, the highly influential American physiologist, Walter B. Cannon, expanded on Bernard's theory of the *milieu intérieur*. Bernard's theory addressed the "why" of bodily processes by proposing that they help maintain a constant internal environment. Cannon's work and ideas began to flesh out the "how." In a series of magnificent experiments over about a quarter century, Cannon demonstrated for the first time the critical role that adrenaline plays in maintaining the constancy of the inner world.

Cannon introduced and popularized three ideas that by now are well known and widely accepted. Each of these merits discussion here, not only for their relevance to the themes of this book, which will become obvious, but also to teach about how scientists think and about how theories, just like organisms, must adapt or perish. Each of Cannon's canons has required modification to take into account experimental realities. The ideas are homeostasis, fight-or-flight responses, and the sympathoadrenal system.

Cannon invented the word *homeostasis*. By this term he referred to the stability of the inner world. The concept of homeostasis therefore was a direct extension from Bernard's of the *milieu intérieur*. According to Cannon, the brain would coordinate body systems, with the aim of maintaining a set of goal values for key internal variables. The core temperature would be kept at 98.6°F, the serum sodium level would be at 140 mEq/L, the blood glucose level would be at 90 mg/dL, and so forth. Internal or external disturbances threatening homeostasis, by causing large enough deviations from the goal values, would arouse internal nervous and hormone systems, induce emotional and motivational states, and generate externally observable behaviors, all of which would have the goal of reestablishing homeostasis. According to the more recent concept of allostasis, however, no single set of ideal values exists for levels of internal variables.

The brain would respond to all emergencies in the same way, by evoking increased secretion of adrenaline. How could the same response help maintain homeostasis in very different situations, such as too low a blood sugar level (hypoglycemia) and too high a blood sugar level, as in shock from uncontrolled diabetes mellitus? Surely some effects would work against rather than toward homeostasis for at least some body functions at least some of the time. Cannon's answer was that the body's response to emergencies, with adrenaline dominating that response, would, in general, enhance long-term survival, even if, in the short term, aspects of the response moved some of the levels for key variables from the ideal values. Accumulating experimental evidence has challenged Cannon's explanation by showing that there is no single response pattern for all threats to homeostasis.

Cannon also coined the phrase, "fight or flight." He asserted that not only physical emergencies, such as blood loss from trauma, but also psychological emergencies, such as antagonistic encounters between members of the same species, evoke release of adrenaline into the bloodstream. To Cannon, the body's responses to "fight" would be the same as those to "flight." Adrenaline exerts several important effects in different body organs, all of which, from Cannon's point of view, would maintain homeostasis in fight-or-flight situations. In the skeletal muscle of the limbs, adrenaline relaxes blood vessels, thereby increasing local blood flow. This would be important not only to provide metabolic fuels to exercising muscle but also to remove the waste products of metabolism that would otherwise accumulate in skeletal muscle and interfere with performance. Adrenaline constricts blood vessels in the skin and promotes clotting; both effects would minimize blood loss from physical trauma. Adrenaline releases the key metabolic fuel, glucose, by the liver into the bloodstream, via breakdown of the storage form of glucose, glycogen. (Claude Bernard discovered conversion of glycogen to glucose in the liver.) Adrenaline stimulates respiration, maximizing delivery of oxygen to the bloodstream via the lungs. Adrenaline removes the electrolyte, potassium ion, from the circulation, an effect that would also promote homeostasis, because trauma destroys cells, which contain high potassium ion concentrations, building up the potassium ion content in the surrounding fluid. From a psychological point of view, adrenaline intensifies emotional experiences and increases what Cannon called "reservoirs of power," exerting antifatigue and energizing effects.

The fact that aggressive attack and fearful escape both involve adrenaline release into the bloodstream does not imply an equivalence of "fight" with "flight" from a physiological or biochemical point of view. On the contrary, emotion-associated behaviors such as aggressive attack, fearful flight, immobile terror, hopeless defeat, emotional fainting, and sexual activity differ importantly in internal physiological and biochemical patterns, just as they do in external appearances and behaviors. Conversely, an increase in the level of adrenaline in the bloodstream does not imply that the individual is having a fight-or-flight experience. For instance, adrenaline levels approximately double just by a person's standing up, and even a mild fall in the blood glucose level stimulates adrenaline release. Because Cannon used only a single dependent variable, the adrenaline response, he could not appreciate the existence of the different physiological and biochemical patterns.

Cannon's third idea was the existence and functional unity of the sympathoadrenal (or "sympathoadrenomedullary" or "sympathicoadrenal") system. Cannon theorized that the sympathetic nervous system and the adrenal gland would work together as a unit to maintain homeostasis in emergencies. This probably was the first proposal of the existence of an integrated nervous-hormone, or neuroendocrine, system.

Cannon became so convinced that the sympathetic nervous system and adrenal gland functioned as a unit that in the 1930s he formally proposed that the sympathetic nervous system used the same chemical messenger—

adrenaline—as did the adrenal gland. He recognized that stimulation of sympathetic nerves produced effects somewhat different from those produced by injected adrenaline. After he obtained evidence for either release of a substance other than adrenaline during stimulation of sympathetic nerves, or else conversion of adrenaline to a different substance in the target cells, Cannon erroneously backed the latter view. He proposed two forms of the released chemical messenger, excitatory "sympathin E" and inhibitory "sympathin I." In 1939, he wrote that adrenaline was indeed the chemical messenger of the sympathetic nerves. Differences in organ responses to adrenaline and to "sympathin" would be due to conversion of the latter to another substance in the activated target cells.

This mistake probably cost Cannon a Nobel Prize. In 1946, a year after Cannon's death, the Swedish physiologist, U. S. von Euler, correctly identified the chemical messenger of the sympathetic nerves in mammals as not adrenaline but norepinephrine, adrenaline's chemical precursor, and for this discovery von Euler did share the Nobel Prize for Physiology or Medicine in 1970.

Cannon's notion of a unitary sympathoadrenal system persists to this day. Many situations, however, entail differential regulation of the sympathetic nervous system (SNS) and adrenomedullary hormonal system (AHS); and at least one clinical disorder—fainting—features a combination of shutdown of sympathetic nervous system outflows to the cardiovascular system yet marked stimulation of the adrenomedullary hormonal system. Researchers in the area have come to question the validity of the notion of a unitary sympathoadrenal system, although clinicians often continue to lump together the two components.

The Comfort Level in Building 10

I sit at a desk in an office in Building 10, the Clinical Center, of the National Institutes of Health—"the NIH"—in Bethesda, Maryland. Building 10 is the largest research hospital on earth. (It also happens to be the world's biggest red brick building.) Titans of academic medicine spent their formative years here.

Venerable as Building 10 is, it also contains a notoriously outdated heating, ventilation, and air-conditioning (HVAC) system. Suppose you had the task of reconstructing that system. Given Bethesda's steamy summer haze, you would certainly design in an air conditioner. If the outside temperature

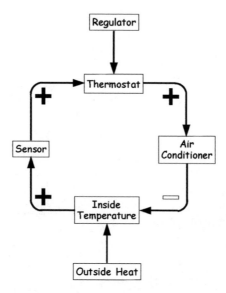

Fig. I. This temperature control system uses a negative feedback loop to regulate an air conditioner, thereby maintaining inside temperature despite outside heat.

became too hot, given the poor insulation of Building 10, the inside temperature would go up. You would include a thermostat to monitor the inside temperature. When the inside temperature exceeded a threshold, the thermostat would sense the discrepancy between the sensed temperature and the setting and turn on the air conditioner. When the inside temperature cooled sufficiently, the thermostat would no longer sense a large enough discrepancy between the sensed and set temperatures, and the air conditioner would turn off. In diagrammatic terms, the thermostat would maintain the internal temperature by a *negative feedback loop* (fig. 1).

A thermostat is in essence a *comparator*, a device that compares the temperature that is set with the temperature that is sensed. When the discrepancy is sufficiently large, the thermostat directs changes in activities of the effector, the air conditioner, reducing the discrepancy. It can be shown mathematically that in systems regulated by negative feedback, when the system is perturbed by a constant outside influence (e.g., outside heat), the level of the monitored variable, in this case the inside temperature, always eventually reaches a stable value, a steady state, which may not necessarily be the temperature actually set, because this would depend on factors such as the power of the air conditioner and efficiency of the insulation. Eventually, the inside temperature would be held somewhere between that out-

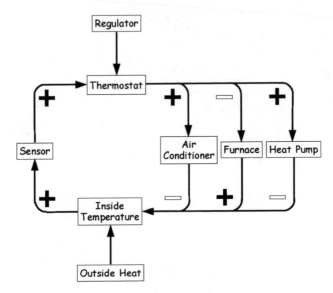

Fig. 2. This temperature control system includes multiple effectors. Having multiple effectors offers major advantages in cost-efficient regulation of inside temperature: greater range of control, compensatory activation, patterning, and minimized wear and tear.

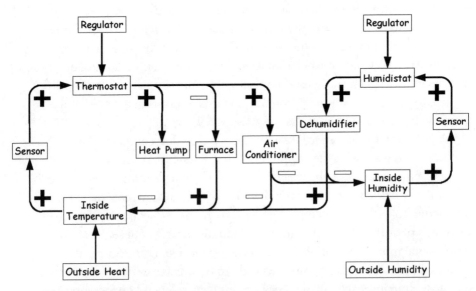

Fig. 3. In this model the systems for regulating temperature and humidity interact. The air conditioner cools the air but also dries it; the dehumidifier dries the air but also warms it. Both, therefore, operate as shared effectors.

side and that set. As long as the number of negative effects (denoted by minus signs) in the loop were odd, the level of the inside temperature, the monitored variable, would reach a stable value. It can also be shown mathematically that the more rapid, sensitive, and powerful the control by negative feedback, the smaller the fluctuations in levels of the monitored variable for a given acute perturbation. When a system regulated by negative feedback is exposed to a fluctuating outside influence, the swings in the levels of the monitored variable would be smaller than in the absence of negative feedback.

Imagine if the thermostat were programmed backward, so that an elevation of internal temperature turned on the furnace instead of the air conditioner. The inside temperature would increase, activating the furnace even more. Instead of the HVAC system maintaining inside temperature at a plateau value between the set and sensed temperatures, the inside temperature would increase at an accelerating rate. This situation corresponds to a *positive feedback loop*. In a positive feedback loop, all the relationships in the loop have plus signs. Positive feedback loops are inherently unstable.

In the winter you would use a furnace to regulate the inside temperature. In the spring and fall, you might open or close windows or operate a heat pump. You could also include ceiling fans, louver shades, or a choice of cool or hot lights in the HVAC system (fig. 2). The point is that you would use *multiple effectors*. Having multiple effectors offers several advantages. The multiplicity would extend the range of outside temperatures for which the inside temperature would be comfortable. If one effector failed, this would not eliminate the ability to regulate temperature; activities of the other effectors would change compensatorily. For instance, if the furnace failed on a cold day, the heat pump could still regulate the inside temperature. You could program the effectors so that they functioned in patterns, to maximize efficiency, minimize costs, and minimize wear and tear on the most expensive components. Finally, having multiple HVAC components would reduce use and therefore wear and tear on the individual components. Although the initial investment in multiple effectors might cost more, in the long run you would save money.

Anyone who has spent a summer in Bethesda knows that one's sense of comfort in hot weather depends not only on the temperature but also on the humidity. At the same hot temperature, high humidity makes you uncomfortable. This is why weather reports in the summer include calculations of the temperature-humidity index. In designing a comfort system for

Building 10, you would probably incorporate a dehumidifier. A dehumidifier, however, not only dries the air but also warms it, and an air conditioner not only cools the air but also dries it. This means that the systems for regulating temperature and for regulating humidity would *interact*. On a hot, muggy day, because of generation of heat by the dehumidifier, the air conditioner would be on more than if there were no dehumidifier; and because the air conditioner dries the air, the dehumidifier would be on less than if there were no air conditioner. Theoretically, you could use the air conditioner to cool the air, as an effector of the thermostatic system, or to dry the air, as an effector of the humidistatic system. In the language of scientific integrative medicine, the air conditioner and dehumidifier would be *shared effectors* (fig. 3).

An Amazing Cooking Experiment

Your body contains an HVAC system analogous to—but far more efficient than—the HVAC system in Building 10 or any other man-made structure. For the brain to operate effectively requires maintaining the blood temperature within a fairly narrow range. The brain in turn keeps the blood temperature, or core temperature, about the same, via regulating activities of multiple effectors.

In your brain you have a literal thermostat, which receives temperature information from two sources. The first source is temperature sensors in the skin, a key interface between the outside and the inner worlds. A second source is sensors within the substance of the brain itself, which monitor the temperature of the blood. This duality corresponds to the two main determinants of heat dissipation and heat generation in the body—evaporative loss of heat from the skin's surface and generation of heat by internal metabolic processes.

Losing body heat by evaporative sweat loss requires sweating, and stimulation of a particular component of the automatic nervous system, called the sympathetic cholinergic system (SCS), stimulates thermoregulatory sweating. Losing body heat by evaporative heat loss also requires delivering blood to the skin surface, so that the warm blood can equilibrate with the cool outside temperature. Inhibition of nerves supplying the skin in another component of the automatic nervous system, the sympathetic noradrenergic system (SNS), relaxes the local blood vessels, distributing the blood to the skin surface. All the multiple loops in a model describing normal responses

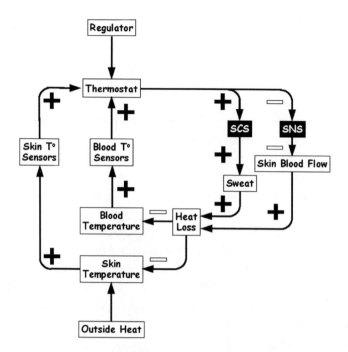

Fig. 4. The body has a remarkable ability to control blood temperature, despite exposure to extreme environmental heat. Two effectors—the sympathetic noradrenergic system (SNS) and the sympathetic cholinergic system (SCS)—normally work together to cool the blood via evaporative heat loss from the surface of the skin. Note that all the loops in the system involve an odd number of minus signs, a characteristic of negative feedback systems that maintain monitored variables at steady levels.

to heat exposure entail an odd number of "–" signs, a characteristic of a system that will maintain the monitored variables, in this case skin and blood temperatures, at steady levels (fig. 4).

On January 23, 1774, the almost incredible ability of the human body to maintain core temperature by evaporative heat loss was demonstrated experimentally for the first time. Five men, including Dr. Charles Blagden, 26 years old at the time, entered a room that was heated progressively with dry air. Eventually the temperature exceeded that of boiling water, so that an egg in the chamber roasted solid in 20 minutes. The temperature of Blagden's exhaled breath was relatively cool compared with the external temperature in the room, "the most striking effects proceeded from our power of preserving our natural temperature. . . . Whenever we breathed on a thermometer the quicksilver sank several degrees" (Blagden, *Philos. Trans. R. Soc.* 65:111–124, 1775). Three weeks later, Blagden reported his observations to the Royal Society of London, which published his report in its Proceedings in 1775.

In contrast with the marvelous ability of humans to adapt to alterations in external temperature, corals can survive only in water of a particular temperature, motion, and salinity. Corals do not possess means to regulate the temperature of their inner world via a negative feedback loop. As little as a 1°C increase in the water temperature will produce a loss of pigment, called bleaching, and organismic death. In 1998, reportedly the hottest year on average in at least six centuries, rising sea temperatures produced an extraordinary amount of bleaching and mortality in a huge band of coral reefs along the equator and into the southern hemisphere.

Llamas also have relatively little ability to adapt to external heat. These animals normally occupy chilly, mountainous regions of South America. A market had developed for them as pets and pack animals in the United States. As reported in a *New York Times* front-page story several years ago, a shipment of llamas and alpacas was held in quarantine on the tropical Caribbean island of Antigua. The animals apparently had never developed an instinct to seek shade in the heat, and their shaggy coats prevented evaporative heat loss from the skin. Large numbers died of heat stroke.

Death by Football

In the heat chamber Blagden eventually began to experience anxiety, his pulse rate increased excessively, and he decided to end the experiment. "[At 260°] I sweated, but not very profusely. For seven minutes my breathing continued perfectly good; but after that time I began to feel an oppression in my lungs, attended with a sense of anxiety; which gradually increasing for the space of a minute, I thought it most prudent to put an end to the experiment, and immediately left the room. My pulse, counted as soon as I came into the cool air, was found to beat at the rate of 144 pulsations in a minute, which is more than double its ordinary quickness" (Blagden, 1775).

Adrenaline, the main chemical messenger of the adrenomedullary hormonal system, potently constricts blood vessels in the skin and also increases the generation of metabolic heat. One may speculate that the amazing cooking experiment ended when the adrenaline level in Blagden's bloodstream reached a high enough value to constrict the blood vessels in his skin. Concomitantly increased heat production and decreased efficiency of evaporative cooling would have increased the core temperature, producing a conscious experience of distress and thereby further adrenaline release. In other words, the introduction of a positive feedback loop may have forced Blagden to call it quits.

The same explanation may apply to a modern, unusual, but highly publicized problem—the sudden development of heat exhaustion and shock, collapse, and death in seemingly vigorous and healthy football players while practicing in full gear in the heat. In such individuals, heat exposure leads to profuse sweating and markedly increased output of blood by the heart. As long as blood flow to the skin is high, the combination of perspiration and high skin blood flow enables sufficient evaporative heat loss to maintain core temperature, just as in Blagden's case. Over time, however, saturation of the uniform with moisture would limit further increases in evaporation. Moreover, exercise to above an anaerobic threshold stimulates the adrenomedullary hormonal system. Buildup of adrenaline in the bloodstream augments the output of blood by the heart, helping meet the high demand for blood flow to the exercising muscles; augments air exchange via the lungs, helping meet the high demand for oxygen; augments glucose entry into the bloodstream by the liver, helping meet the high demand for this key metabolic fuel; and augments muscular power and stamina, providing a crucial competitive edge.

These beneficial effects come at a cost, however. Adrenaline decreases the threshold for development of abnormal heart rhythms and can so potently contract heart muscle cells that the heart actually fails. Blood backs up into the lungs, decreasing oxygenation of the blood despite hyperventilation. These positive feedback loops could convert a seemingly stable situation—sustained exercise in a seasoned athlete—to collapse and sudden death (fig. 5).

Just as in the system controlling core temperature, all systems regulating the inner world of higher animals include at least one negative feedback loop. This is the key feature that results in maintaining stable levels of the monitored variable. Each system includes multiple effectors. Changes in the activities of the effectors lead to changes in levels of the monitored variable, closing the negative feedback loop. Each system also includes a "homeostat," a discrepancy sensor, able to detect when the level of the monitored variable deviates from the set level. Some homeostats of the body, such as the thermostat in the brain, are fairly well defined in terms of location, operation, and regulation. Others are less well identified, and some are little more than hypothetical.

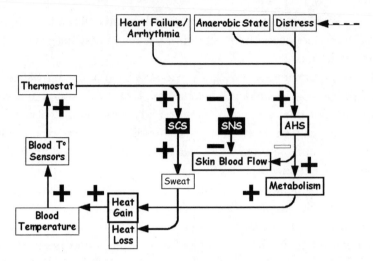

Fig. 5. A model to explain development of heat shock during sustained, severe exercise in the heat. Stimulation of the adrenomedullary hormonal system (AHS) increases circulating adrenaline levels. Adrenaline constricts skin blood vessels; this interferes with evaporative heat loss. Adrenaline also boosts metabolism; this generates metabolic heat. The diagram emphasizes a positive feedback loop, implying an unstable situation. Because of the positive feedback loop, blood temperature goes up uncontrollably.

The next section introduces a system that regulates a different monitored variable—blood flow to the brain. The brain does not actually monitor blood flow; instead, as a kind of proxy, the brain monitors the extent of stretching of blood vessel walls, which in turn depends on blood pressure.

The Sleeper Hold

My grandmother and I used to watch professional wrestling on TV. Propped in bed, she would cheer on her hero, Antonino Rocca, the barefoot master of the flying dropkick, and hiss at Skull Murphy, who was notorious for butting opponents with his shaved, vaselined head. In professional wrestling you could win by three smacks by the referee on the tarp, by disqualification, or by submission. In particular, in the "sleeper hold," the attacker unexpectedly would circle the victim and wrap his arms around the victim's neck, as if to choke him from behind; but instead of choking the victim he would massage both sides of the victim's neck vigorously below the angles of the jaw. After several seconds of this massaging, the opponent would slump to the mat unconscious, ending the bout.

I think there is a kernel of validity to the sleeper hold. Specialized distortion receptors, called baroreceptors, lie in the carotid sinus, in the crotch of the "Y" where the common carotid arteries, the main arteries delivering blood to the head, fork in the upper neck (fig. 6). When the blood pressure increases, the wall of the carotid sinus on each side expands, stimulating the baroreceptors in the artery wall. Nerve traffic to the brain increases in the carotid sinus nerve and reaches a particular cluster of cells in the lower brainstem (the nucleus of the solitary tract, or NTS). Activation of the NTS cells leads to a rapid, reflexive fall in pulse rate, relaxation of blood vessels, and weakened heartbeat. The blood pressure, and consequently the blood flow to the brainstem, plummets, and the victim loses consciousness and skeletal muscle tone—that is, the person faints.

The baroreceptor reflex, or baroreflex, is a classic, well-studied reflex that you will encounter repeatedly in this book. The baroreflex has all the components of a system for regulation of the inner world by the brain. As the name suggests, the baroreflex keeps the blood pressure relatively stable by a reflex. When the blood pressure increases, sensory information reaches a homeostat—the barostat—in the brain, the brain directs a decrease in

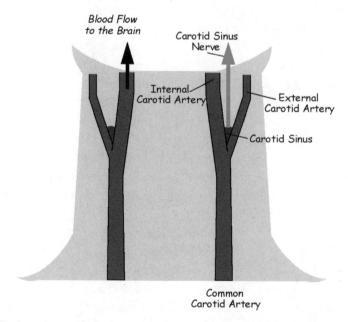

Fig. 6. The brain learns about the status of its own blood supply from stretch receptors in the walls of the carotid sinus.

the activity of the sympathetic nervous system, and the blood vessels relax. Also as part of the baroreflex, nerve traffic in the vagus nerve, a key nerve of the parasympathetic nervous system, increases, and the pulse rate drops. The baroreflex system therefore incorporates at least two negative feedback loops.

You might understand the baroreflex better by thinking about the water pressure in a garden hose. The pressure is determined by how much the faucet is turned on and by how much the nozzle is tightened. If you turned down the faucet, the pressure in the hose would decrease, but you could bring the pressure back up by tightening the nozzle. Baroreflexes control the amount of tightening of the blood vessels. When a person stands up, the blood vessels tighten reflexively, helping maintain the blood pressure. The main system responsible for reflexive tightening of the vascular nozzle is the sympathetic nervous system. Failure of the sympathetic nervous system, or of the baroreflex arc that regulates sympathetic nervous outflow to the blood vessels, causes orthostatic hypotension, a fall in blood pressure when the patient stands up, because the patient can't "tighten the nozzle."

Snakes That Faint?

In evolution, the more important and long standing the requirement for regulation of a particular monitored variable, the more likely that multiple effectors controlling levels of that monitored variable have evolved. This concept explains nicely why, in human beings and other higher organisms, many effectors contribute to regulation of blood levels of the key metabolic fuels, glucose and oxygen, for delivery of those fuels to vital organs via the heart and blood vessels, for maintaining the core temperature at which numerous enzymes function optimally, for breaking down toxins, and for excreting waste. The survival advantages of effector redundancy would far outweigh the costs in terms of the energy and other expenditures for maintaining the multiplicity of effectors.

In contrast, in evolutionary terms our ancestors began standing upright relatively recently. Standing erect afforded important survival advantages, such as freeing the hands to develop and use tools. To a large extent the ability to stand up enabled the evolution of the defining characteristics of us humans. Indeed, one prehistoric human species was *Homo erectus*. Adopting an upright posture, however, also posed a novel challenge—maintaining

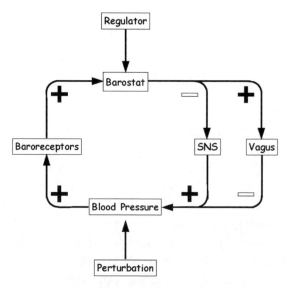

Fig. 7. The baroreflex, a system for keeping the blood pressure stable. Increased blood pressure stimulates the baroreceptors. The "barostat" in the brainstem receives the input. The sympathetic nervous system (SNS) is inhibited reflexively, relaxing blood vessels, and the vagus nerve is stimulated reflexively, decreasing the pulse rate. Notice the two negative feedback loops.

blood flow to the brain in the face of gravitational pooling of blood in the legs and pelvic organs and decreased venous return of blood to the heart. To redistribute blood rapidly and appropriately in this setting, a hormone system, in which the effector chemical would be released into the bloodstream and reach all cells at the same concentration, would not work as well as a nerve network, because a nerve network would enable differential regulation of the constrictor tone of blood vessels in different body regions by activation or inhibition of particular branches of the network.

In human evolution, only one such nerve network seems to have evolved—the sympathetic nervous system. Each time you stand up, this system becomes activated markedly, instantaneously, unconsciously, and automatically (fig. 7). By release of the chemical messenger, norepinephrine, from nerve terminals in the walls of blood vessels in the limbs, kidneys, and gut, blood vessels in these organs constrict, while blood vessels in the heart, lungs, and brain do not. Blood flows to the brain, heart, and lungs therefore are maintained during standing up, despite the fall in venous return to the heart.

When the sympathetic nervous system fails, norepinephrine release does not increase adequately when the patient stands up. Because of the novelty of the challenge in evolutionary terms, efficient compensatory activation via alternative effectors does not take place. The tone of blood vessels in the skeletal muscle, kidneys, and gut does not increase, and as the venous return to the heart falls, so does the blood pressure. This explains why orthostatic hypotension constitutes a cardinal manifestation of failure of the sympathetic nervous system.

Climbing snakes can wriggle up trees, but water snakes spend their lives horizontal, surrounded by about the same pressure from head to tail. Several years ago, Harvey Lillywhite, of the University of Florida at Gainesville, placed different types of snakes into a cylindrical plastic tube and then tilted them head-up. Among climbing snakes, nothing much happened, but among water snakes, during the tilting blood pooled in the tail end, the blood pressure at the midpoint of the body fell, and the heart rate increased compensatorily but inadequately to maintain the blood pressure at the level of the head. If kept in this situation, with a brain blood flow of zero, water snakes would have to lose consciousness eventually. Structural and functional differences between climbing and water snakes help explain the different abilities to maintain blood flow to the brain during head-up tilting. Climbing snakes have thin, tapered bodies, with the heart located relatively close to the brain. Water snakes have wider and more cylindrical bodies, with the heart close to the longitudinal center. Climbing snakes have higher blood pressure than water snakes, even when horizontal. Climbing snakes writhe when tilted, squeezing blood in the veins toward the heart like squeezing toothpaste up a tube. Analogously, in humans who are about to faint while standing up, voluntary muscle pumping, by curling the toes, twisting the legs, and tightening the buttocks, can deliver enough blood to the heart and brain to prevent loss of consciousness temporarily. Indeed, a patient with frequent fainting I evaluated several years ago obtained virtual cure of the problem by learning to contract her calf muscles isometrically.

Climbing snakes when tilted constrict blood vessels to organs and muscles in the lower half of the body but not to vital anterior organs such as the lung, brain, and heart. The blood vessels tailward of the heart in climbing snakes have a substantial nerve supply—presumably sympathetic nerves—consistent with the ability to constrict local blood vessels reflexively. In climbing snakes, as in humans, the sympathetic nervous system seems to have afforded a survival advantage, by helping counter effects of gravity on delivery of blood to vital organs and enabling occupation of a particular environmental niche. Considering that water snakes evolved from terrestrial snakes, in evolutionary history the ability to adapt to gravitational stress must have degenerated in the species that took to the water.

Some patients who have a long-term inability to tolerate prolonged standing (chronic orthostatic intolerance) appear to have a structural problem that predisposes them to fainting while upright. These patients can have evidence for increased flexibility of joints and of blood vessel walls, probably because of altered protein fibers. The blood vessels have increased "give." When the patient stands up, or blows against a resistance, or carries out any activity that impedes the return of blood to the heart, too much blood collects in the veins, decreasing delivery of blood to the brain.

Given the account of the climbing snakes and water snakes, maybe the greater prevalence of chronic orthostatic intolerance in women relates also to structural and functional gender differences—lower centers of gravity, lower blood pressure, less well developed skeletal muscle tailward of the heart, and greater inherent stretchability of blood vessels.

Rules of the Game

You have read about two monitored variables—temperature and blood pressure. The brain receives information about, and regulates levels of, a large number of monitored variables. For each monitored variable there is a corresponding literal or figurative homeostat and there are multiple effectors. This section presents formally the rules of the game of life in higher organisms.

A tremendous array of sensors detect changes in levels of monitored variables (fig. 8). Stretch receptors in the walls especially of the atria of the heart, the thin-walled chambers where the blood in the great veins enters the heart, provide information to the brain about cardiac filling and therefore about blood volume. Sensors for blood glucose levels exist in the "glucostat," in the hypothalamus at the top of the brainstem, and the main effectors for maintaining glucose levels are the hormones insulin, adrenaline, and glucagon. Also in the brain are sensors for serum osmolality, with arginine vasopressin (the antidiuretic hormone) the main effector. Chemoreceptors in the kidney monitor concentrations of the key element, sodium, and use

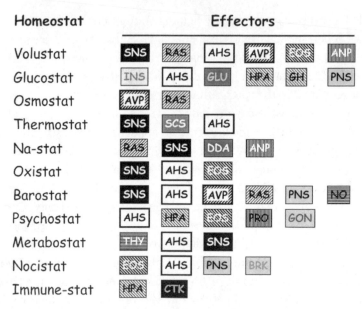

Homeostat	Effectors					
Volustat	SNS	RAS	AHS	AVP	EOS	ANP
Glucostat	INS	AHS	GLU	HPA	GH	PNS
Osmostat	AVP	RAS				
Thermostat	SNS	SCS	AHS			
Na-stat	RAS	SNS	DDA	ANP		
Oxistat	SNS	AHS	EOS			
Barostat	SNS	AHS	AVP	RAS	PNS	NO
Psychostat	AHS	HPA	EOS	PRO	GON	
Metabostat	THY	AHS	SNS			
Nocistat	EOS	AHS	PNS	BRK		
Immune-stat	HPA	CTK				

Fig. 8. Some homeostats and effectors. Effectors include the sympathetic noradrenergic system (SNS), renin-angiotensin-aldosterone (RAS), adrenomedullary hormonal system (AHS), vasopressin-aquaporin system (AVP), endogenous opiate system (EOS), atrial natriuretic peptide (ANP), insulin (INS), glucagon (GLU), hypothalamic-pituitary-adrenocortical axis (HPA), growth hormone (GH), parasympathetic nervous system (PNS), sympathetic cholinergic system (SCS), dopa-dopamine system (DDA), nitric oxide (NO), prolactin (PRO), gonadotropic-gonadal steroid system (GON), thyroid (THY), bradykinin (BRK), and cytokines (CTK).

the renin-angiotensin-aldosterone system (RAS) effector to regulate sodium and potassium balances in the body. Because of the close relationship between sodium (Na) balance and the volume of extracellular fluid (ECF), the total volume of the fluid environment surrounding cells of the body, the homeostat can be called the "Na-stat" or "ECF-stat." Chemoreceptors in the carotid body and lower brainstem sense concentrations of oxygen, the homeostat driving respiration and also the sympathetic nervous and adrenomedullary hormonal systems. The barostat, as already discussed, receives information from the baroreceptors, stretch receptors in the walls of major arteries, such as in the carotid sinus, keeping blood pressure stable by using the sympathetic nervous, adrenomedullary hormonal, vasopressin, and parasympathetic nervous effectors. Pain sensors—nociceptors—in the skin send information about pain up the spinal cord to the brain and elicit changes in activities of the endogenous opioid, sympathetic nervous, adrenomedullary hormonal, and pituitary-adrenocortical systems. Gastrointestinal distention by food stimulates local increases in blood flow, regional sympathetic nervous inhibition, and parasympathetic nervous activation. One can also conceptualize homeostats regulating the overall sense of emotional stability, total body metabolism, and immune surveillance.

Negative Feedback

Homeostatic systems of higher organisms always include regulation by negative feedback. Alterations in values of the monitored variable result in changes in effector activity that oppose and thereby "buffer" changes in that variable.

In homeostatic diagrams, the plus sign denotes a stimulatory relationship and the minus sign denotes an inhibitory relationship. Each minus changes the sign of the next relationship in the loop, whereas each plus does not affect the sign of the next relationship. In a stable system, that is, a system in which the monitored variable is maintained at a plateau level, all the loops involving that variable must have at least one plus and one minus, and all the loops must have an odd number of minus signs. For each perturbation of a monitored variable, the net effect of at least one effector must have a sign opposite to that of the perturbation.

If a loop has plus relationships and no minus relationships (a positive feedback loop), the system, if otherwise unchecked, will "explode," because levels of the monitored variable will increase or decrease exponentially. Positive feedback loops are inherently unstable. If a complex system includes both a positive feedback loop and a "nested" negative feedback loop, then the level of the monitored variable will change but to a stable plateau value.

Positive feedback loops do occur in clinical medicine. When they do, they always signify an unstable situation. For instance, positive feedback loops can explain the rapid decompensation in heat stroke, hypothermia, fainting, and sudden cardiac death.

Multiple Effectors

Homeostatic systems use more than one effector. This redundancy has several consequences.

—Multiple effectors extend the range of control of the monitored variable, in the face of swings in environmental conditions.

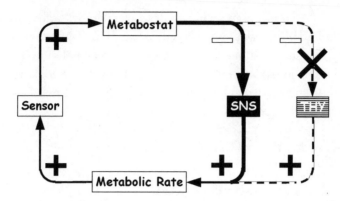

Fig. 9. An example of compensatory activation. Inactivation of the thyroid gland (THY) compensatorily activates the sympathetic nervous system (SNS), enabling at least partial maintenance of the total body metabolic rate. Compensatory activation is one beneficial consequence of having multiple effectors.

—Disabling an effector compensatorily activates the others, assuming no change in homeostat settings. This enables partial or even complete maintenance of the level of the monitored variable. The efficiency of the other effectors and algorithm used by the homeostat determine whether compensatory activation actually keeps normal the level of the monitored variable. For instance, exposure of a thyroidectomized animal to cold results in exaggerated increases in activities of the sympathetic nervous and adrenomedullary hormonal systems (fig. 9).

—Having multiple effectors enables patterning of effector responses. Patterning of hormonal, physiological, and behavioral effectors maximizes the likelihood of responses being appropriate for the particular threat to homeostasis. For instance, the body's responses to water deprivation are not the same as those to salt deprivation, which are not the same as to glucose deprivation. The responses associated with fight are not the same as those associated with flight, fright, or defeat. The different response patterns generally make sense in terms of the particular characteristics of the situation.

—Multiple effectors improve cost efficiency, which is measured by the energy used to maintain appropriate levels of the monitored variable.

—By decreasing wear and tear on effectors, having multiple effectors prolongs the average useful life of the entire system.

Effector Sharing

More than one homeostat can regulate activity of the same effector. An example involves sharing of the adrenomedullary hormonal system effector
by both the barostat and glucostat. This sharing helps explain a typical finding in emergency medicine, that is, when a patient with diabetes presents
with low blood pressure caused by a bleeding ulcer. The serum chemistries
come back from the lab showing a high blood glucose level. The doctor,
who is well experienced and expert, decides to treat the patient, not the
number. In a few days, after the gastroenterology consult has taken care of
the ulcer, and the patient has received a transfusion, the doctor orders a re-
peat set of serum chemistries, and the blood glucose level is now normal.

What about the emergency room setting would produce high glucose
levels? An answer (there probably would be several) is sharing of the adrenomedullary hormonal system effector by the barostat and glucostat. Because of the gastrointestinal bleeding, the patient would be in shock from
low blood volume. The volustat would direct release of adrenaline into the
bloodstream. Adrenaline exerts effects not only on the cardiovascular system but also on blood glucose levels. The adrenomedullary hormonal system is one of the body's three main effectors for regulating blood glucose
levels, the other two being the hormones insulin and glucagon. Adrenaline
releases glucose into the bloodstream and antagonizes insulin effects. The
net result, especially in a patient with diabetes, would be a high blood glucose level. A few days later, after restoration of cardiovascular homeostasis,
the volustat would no longer direct activation of the adrenomedullary hormonal system effector. Adrenaline levels in the bloodstream would return
toward baseline, and the stimulatory effect of adrenaline on blood glucose
levels would dissipate.

Examples of effector sharing abound in physiology (fig. 10). Both decreased blood pressure and decreased venous return to the heart stimulate
increases in sympathetic nervous system outflows. Both increased serum osmolality and decreased filling of the heart lead to increased vasopressin levels
(explaining why vasopressin, which is also known as the antidiuretic hormone,
dominates the body's response to water deprivation). Both exercise and low
blood glucose levels stimulate secretion of growth hormone by the pituitary
gland. Both decreased delivery of sodium to the kidneys and decreased blood
pressure stimulate increases in the activity of the renin-angiotensin-aldosterone

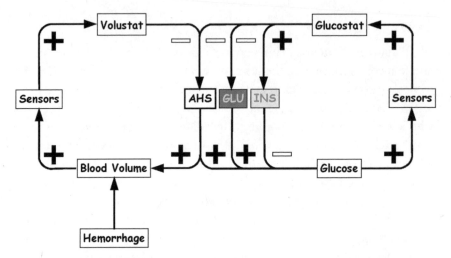

Fig. 10. An example of effector sharing. Both the "volustat" and "glucostat" share the adrenomedullary hormonal system (AHS) effector. Hemorrhage increases the circulating adrenaline level, which in turn increases the glucose level. The body's other main effectors for glucose regulation are glucagon (GLU) and insulin (INS).

system (explaining why the renin-angiotensin-aldosterone system dominates the body's response to salt deprivation).

Effector sharing also potentially can explain the syndromic nature of chronic degenerative diseases, as discussed in the chapter about scientific integrative medicine.

Effector Interactions

Effectors interact with each other indirectly, such as via compensatory activation, and also directly. Much of physiology research can be viewed as studying effector interactions. Examples are effects of adrenocortical steroids on adrenomedullary function and of angiotensin II on sympathetic nervous system outflows. The next chapter describes some interactions between effectors that use members of the adrenaline family and effectors that use other chemical messengers.

Variability from Homeostatic System Disruption

Disruption of a negative feedback loop, whether by blockade of afferent information, destruction of homeostats, or failure of effectors, increases variability of the monitored variable.

For example, irradiation of the neck accelerates stiffening of the carotid arteries. Because of this stiffening, the baroreceptors can become splinted in the rigidified carotid sinus. Normally when the blood pressure changes, expansion of the carotid sinus stimulates the baroreceptors; the brain acts on the afferent information by reflexively changing activities of several effectors, the net result being attenuation, or "buffering," the change in blood pressure. When the brain does not receive the information from the baroreceptors, because of splinting of the baroreceptors in the rigidified carotid sinus, changes in blood pressure do not elicit the reflexive buffering, and the patient develops symptoms and signs of labile blood pressure. Because of the typically long delay between the time of neck irradiation and the rigidification of the local arteries, researchers have only recently come to recognize the connection between blood pressure lability and therapeutic irradiation of the neck earlier in life.

Same Difference

Cannon's theory of homeostasis presumes ideal long-term goal levels of monitored variables of the inner world. Cannon did not consider the possibility that the goal levels might themselves change. In emergencies, activation of the sympathicoadrenal system would change the levels of some monitored variables, as an unavoidable, temporary by-product.

According to a newer concept, called *allostasis*, organisms maintain stability through change. Allostasis comes from two Greek words that mean "other sameness." This seems paradoxical. One way to grasp the meaning of the term is returning to the analogy of the HVAC system in Building 10. You would set the thermostat lower in the winter and higher in the summer, because this would save money and minimize wear and tear on the HVAC components. In addition, as noted previously, physical comfort depends not only on temperature but also on relative humidity, which changes seasonally. Moreover, people vary in individual metabolic rates, heat production, and toleration of increased or decreased environmental temperature. Some people simply like it hot, and some do not. You would change the thermostat setting, as appropriate for cost-efficiency, humidity, and characteristics of the patients; however, at any chosen temperature, the thermostat would keep the temperature at about the chosen level—"other sameness."

Just as the thermostat setting in Building 10 would depend on factors such as economy, relative humidity, air movement, and individual preferences, the allostatic approach as applied to regulation of the inner world of the body does not assume ideal single goals for individual variables monitored by the brain, such as core temperature, pulse rate, blood pressure, blood glucose, or blood oxygen. The settings can change.

Operation of an HVAC system entails immediate and long-term costs. One immediate cost is that of the energy used to run the HVAC components. Long-term costs include those of maintaining and repairing the components, related to factors such as wear and tear, latent manufacturing defects, and planned obsolescence. Different allostatic settings entail different amounts of energy expenditure acutely or wear and tear chronically.

Suppose you went on sabbatical for a year and when you left you forgot to close the windows. For the whole year, the temperature would be controlled at the programmed settings, but the air conditioner would be on more in the summer and the furnace would be on more in the winter. The extent of wear and tear on the HVAC components would be greater than had you shut the windows. In fact, when you returned, you might find that the entire HVAC system had failed, with the temperature inside the same as that outside. Even with the same amount of insulation, and even at the same thermostat setting, HVAC systems in different buildings could have different amounts of wear and tear, due to individual differences in HVAC system design or manufacturing, obsolescence, use history, and maintenance and repair.

According to the notion of allostatic load, it is by way of prolonged activation of effectors to maintain allostasis that chronic stress can contribute to the development of chronic degenerative diseases.

A company called Adrenaline Systems sells "overclocked" computer equipment to people who play video games. Overclocking makes a computer's processor run faster than originally intended. This speeds up system performance and improves the sense of reality of the game, without the high cost usually associated with such performance levels. Overclocking, however, also reduces the life expectancy of the processor. According to Adrenaline Systems, overclocking contributes "to stresses that will affect its life-cycle." The company also notes that in the computer field, system obsolescence occurs so quickly and predictably that reduced computer processor life may not be an important concern. Because of obsolescence, a computer would be replaced anyway before it would fail from overclocking. Instead of buying a more expensive computer chip, it might be preferable economically to overclock a cheaper one.

The notion of increased immediate gains of overclocking, at the cost of reduced life span, provides a useful analogy for the development of chronic diseases in people. Diseases involving degeneration of multiple systems in the elderly may be a predictable consequence of the evolutionary advantages of physiological overclocking in the reproductive years, an "evolutionary compromise," as discussed later in this book.

The All-Day Sucker

So far, the "regulator" in control systems has received little attention. For controlling the temperature in Building 10, you would be the regulator, via your proxy, the thermostat. For controlling the inner world in the body, the brain is the regulator.

As one moves upward from the level of the spinal cord in the central nervous system, and outward from the brain's core, one encounters layers of more and more subtle and complex regulation, in an arrangement like the layers in an all-day sucker. At the center of the brain is the brainstem, which along with the spinal cord is responsible for largely reflexive behaviors. At the top of the brainstem is the hypothalamus, responsible for expression of emotions and their automatic accompaniments. Higher, and further out from the center, is the "limbic system," responsible for processes like the memory of distressing events and learning of conditioned emotional responses. Highest, in the outermost layer, is the cortex, responsible for conscious, voluntary actions.

At each ascending (and centrifugal) level, the type of regulation changes. The higher, outer centers typically override and restrain the lower, inner centers. For instance, by using your cortex, you can decide to take an aspirin if you have a fever, or drink coffee if you want to stay alert, or lift a heavy weight if you want to increase your blood pressure. Yet input from lower centers can influence higher centers. For instance, stimulation of baroreceptors alters alertness, stretching of the urinary bladder elicits an urge to urinate, and adrenaline intensifies emotional experiences.

2 | The "Automatic Nervous System"

Some bodily activities, like standing up and moving legs to walk across a room, are voluntary, conscious, and observable from the outside. Others, like digesting, sweating, and tightening blood vessels, are unconscious, involuntary, and automatic, and they may or may not be observable from the outside. The brain uses different parts of the nervous system to regulate these activities.

The central nervous system consists of the brain and the spinal cord. The brain is a command and control center. The spinal cord is a rope of nerve bundles that runs from the base of the brain down the back inside the spinal column. Control signals travel from the brain to the limbs and organs by way of the peripheral nerves. The peripheral nerves are all the nerves that lie outside the brain and spinal cord.

The peripheral nervous system has two main divisions. The first is the somatic nervous system, which deals with the outside world. The second is designed to help regulate the inner world by making adjustments in the functions of a variety of organs inside the body. This is the autonomic nervous system. You can think of it as the "automatic nervous system."

In the late 1890s, the English physiologist John Newport Langley introduced the phrase "autonomic nervous system" to describe the nerves responsible for automatic regulation of the inner world. He found nerves that emanated from cell bodies located outside the central nervous system, in the walls of organs of the gastrointestinal tract and in clumps strung along each side of the spinal column. These nerves differed from those controlling movement by patterned contraction and relaxation of skeletal muscle of the limbs, because "somatic" nerves (nerves to the externally observable parts of the body, as opposed to the inner organs) travel directly from the spinal cord to the target organ.

Langley taught that the autonomic nervous system had three parts (fig.

11). Nerves in the gastrointestinal tract constituted the "enteric nervous system." He also conceptualized two functionally distinct systems of nerves in the clumps on each side of the spinal column. For one of these two systems, where the nerves derived from the brainstem at the top of the spinal cord and from the sacral tail of the spinal cord, he introduced the phrase, "parasympathetic nervous system." The prefix, "para," means "beside," "beyond," or "along with." Nerves of the sympathetic nervous system would emanate from the thoracic and lumbar midportions of the spinal cord, between the levels of origin of the parasympathetic nerves.

Langley did not invent the phrase, "sympathetic nervous system." The ancient Greek physician Galen is thought to have used this term. All the great academic physicians of the Middle Ages and Renaissance in Europe and the Middle East accepted Galen's teachings. Galen viewed the nerves as conduits for distributing the "animal spirit" in the body. By way of the nerves, the animal spirit would coordinate the activities of the body's organs, and so the organs would work in harmony with each other, in concert with each other—in "sympathy" with each other. The notion of the "spirits" was religious or philosophical, not scientific; however, Galen's teaching that the sympathetic nervous system plays an important role in regulation and coordination of the organs of the body was essentially, ironically correct.

Langley taught that the nerves of the enteric nervous system, parasympathetic nervous system, and sympathetic nervous system differed from the nerves of the somatic nervous system not only in terms of anatomic origins but also in terms of functions. The nerves of the enteric nervous system,

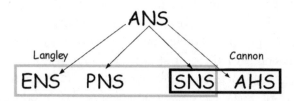

Fig. 11. Components of the autonomic nervous system, according to Langley and Cannon. Langley thought there were three components—the enteric nervous system (ENS), parasympathetic nervous system (PNS), and sympathetic nervous system (SNS). Cannon added a hormonal component, the adrenomedullary hormonal system (AHS), which he thought would work with the sympathetic nervous system as a functional unit to maintain homeostasis in emergencies. A fifth component, the sympathetic cholinergic system, plays a major role in sweating.

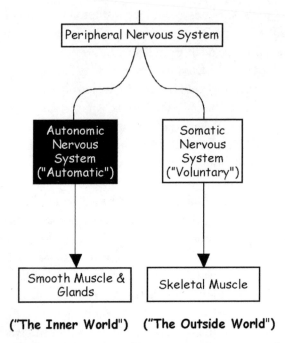

("The Inner World") ("The Outside World")

Fig. 12. The autonomic nervous system is the "automatic nervous system," the part of the peripheral nervous system that controls the inner world.

parasympathetic nervous system, and sympathetic nervous system would function independently, or autonomously, of the central nervous system. This is how Langley came to use the term, autonomic nervous system.

The distinction Langley drew between the somatic and autonomic nervous systems seems analogous to the distinction the philosopher, Descartes, drew between the "mind" and the "body." Neither distinction seems appropriate anymore. Langley's notion that the autonomic nervous system functions independently of the central nervous system was incorrect, because the brain directs the autonomic nervous system to regulate the inner world just as much as it directs the somatic nervous system to produce movements and thereby interact with the outside world. In fact, in every motion and emotion, the brain regulates these two great divisions of the peripheral nervous system, the somatic and the autonomic, together, in a highly integrated way (fig. 12). Voluntary, conscious behaviors and involuntary, autonomic changes are closely linked. For instance, standing up voluntarily, walking out into the cool air, and jogging around the block are associated with automatic adjustments that maintain appropriate blood flows to the brain, heart,

THE "AUTOMATIC NERVOUS SYSTEM"   33

and lungs. As you use up fuel, build up body heat, and produce metabolic by-products of the exercise, these automatic responses change dynamically. Alterations in involuntary or unconscious functions can in turn affect conscious experiences and voluntary behaviors. People become sleepy after eating a large meal, alert when enraged, and irritable when feverish; they sense pain less while exercising vigorously and lose their grip when scared. If you are a woman, you may avert your gaze and bat your eyelids when you talk with an unfamiliar attractive man; if you are a man, you may suck in your gut and stand more upright as an unfamiliar attractive woman passes by. It is no coincidence that the word "emotion" literally means "arising out of motion" and that we all get pleasure from the "uplifting" experience of being "moved." In my book, and for the rest of this book, "autonomic" and "automatic" are interchangeable. You will read later that the old distinction between the "mind" and "body" in medical research and practice has also lost its usefulness in the evaluation and management of patients with disorders of the autonomic nervous system and, more generally, in scientific integrative medicine.

Not only is the autonomic nervous system not really autonomic, it is also not only a nervous system. In the early twentieth century, Walter B. Cannon added a hormonal component when he showed that, as part of many key automatic responses, adrenaline is released into the bloodstream from the adrenal glands, the organs embedded in the fat at the top of the kidneys. Based on Cannon's influence, the combination of the sympathetic nervous system and adrenal glands came to be viewed as a single "emergency" system—the "sympathoadrenal" system, or "sympathicoadrenal" system. The notion of a unitary sympathoadrenal system that is important in emergencies but not in ordinary life persists to this day.

For the autonomic nervous system to maintain appropriate blood flows to vital organs, regulate body temperature, help deliver metabolic fuels and excrete waste, and elicit warning signs such as sweating, pallor, and trembling in dangerous situations, it regulates a particular type of muscle cells, called "smooth muscle" cells. Smooth muscle is found in organs such as the stomach, in blood vessel walls, and in glands such as the thyroid gland, adrenal gland, and sweat glands. Activation of the smooth muscle cells in the gut increases peristalsis, in blood vessel walls evokes constriction, and in glands elicits secretion. In contrast, when you move your head, trunk, and limbs voluntarily, you do so by way of coordinated contractions of "striated," or striped, skeletal muscle, the type of muscle that makes up chops

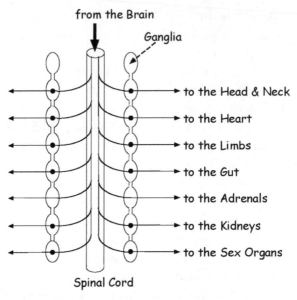

from the Brain

Ganglia

to the Head & Neck

to the Heart

to the Limbs

to the Gut

to the Adrenals

to the Kidneys

to the Sex Organs

Spinal Cord

Fig. 13. Ganglia are arranged like strands of pearls on each side of the spinal cord. Cells in ganglia relay control signals that regulate the inner world.

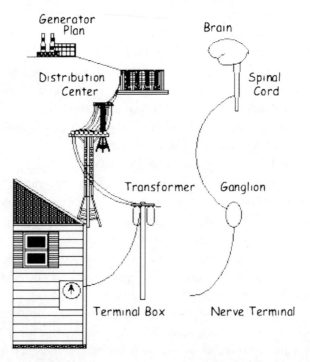

Generator Plan

Brain

Distribution Center

Spinal Cord

Transformer

Ganglion

Terminal Box

Nerve Terminal

Fig. 14. A ganglion is like the transformer on the utility pole outside a house.

of meat. Heart muscle cells are also striated but not subject to voluntary control.

Transformers

Whereas nerves to skeletal muscle travel to the target cells directly from the central nervous system, nerves of the autonomic nervous system travel indirectly, by way of clumps of cells called ganglia (fig. 13). Just as a transformer on a utility pole relays electricity from thick trunk lines to thin cables that deliver electricity to a house, cells in the ganglia relay signals from thick nerve trunks originating in the spinal cord to thin nerve fibers that travel to the target organs such as the heart (fig. 14).

The ganglia are arranged like pearls on a string on each side of the spinal column. It was partly because of this geographical separation from the central nervous system that Langley inferred that the nerve cells in the ganglia would have independent, or autonomous, functions.

As noted above, the idea of the sympathetic nervous system antedated the discovery of the circulation of the blood by fourteen centuries. In more modern times, the sympathetic nervous system reemerged in the early eighteenth century, referring specifically to the chains of ganglia and associated nerves on each side of the spinal column in the chest and abdomen. In contrast, adrenaline, the hormone of the adrenomedullary hormonal system, was not discovered until about a century ago.

Nerves from the spinal cord to the ganglia are called preganglionic, and nerves from the ganglia to the target organs are called postganglionic. The preganglionic nerves look pearly white, because a fatty sheath consisting of a chemical called myelin surrounds the nerve fibers. Myelinated fibers transmit nerve impulses relatively quickly. The postganglionic nerves, which are not myelinated, look dull gray, and they conduct nerve impulses relatively slowly. The difference in nerve conduction velocity, depending on whether a nerve has a myelin sheath or not, explains why if you touch a hot iron, you withdraw your finger reflexively and only later notice pain and throbbing.

Vegging

Cannon taught that the parasympathetic nervous system acts like the opposite of an emergency system and supports vegetative processes that pro-

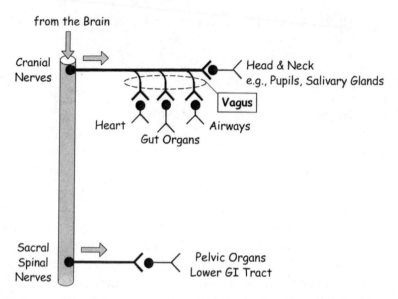

Fig. 15. The parasympathetic nervous system has two parts at opposite ends of the nervous system.

duce rather than use up energy. Vegetative activities include sleeping, eating, digesting, and excreting waste.

The parasympathetic nervous system has upper and lower divisions. The upper division consists of nerves that come from the innermost, lowest portion of the brain, the brainstem. The nerve fibers of the parasympathetic nervous system leave the brainstem in nerves from inside the skull; therefore, these nerves are called cranial nerves. The cranial nerves distribute parasympathetic nervous system fibers to many parts of the body, including the eyes, face, tongue, heart, and most of the gastrointestinal system.

The cranial nerves in which the parasympathetic nerve fibers travel have specific names. The oculomotor nerve connects to the eye, the facial nerve to the face, the glossopharyngeal nerve to the tongue and muscles involved with swallowing and talking, and the vagus nerve to the heart and most of the abdominal organs (fig. 15). Activation of the parasympathetic fibers to the eyes constricts the pupils, to the salivary glands increases production of watery saliva, to the stomach increases acid secretion, to the heart decreases the heart rate, and to the intestine increases gut motions.

Unlike ganglia of the sympathetic nervous system, which lie in chains on either side of the spinal column, parasympathetic ganglia are located very close to or even within the substance of the innervated organs. The postganglionic nerves therefore are short or nonexistent, and the vagus nerve contains preganglionic fibers.

The lower part of the parasympathetic nervous system consists of nerves that emanate from the bottom level of the spinal cord, which is called the sacral spinal cord. These nerves travel to the genital organs, urinary bladder, and lower gastrointestinal tract. Activation of the parasympathetic fibers to the urinary bladder promotes urination, to the large intestine defecation, and to the penis erection.

Beautiful but Deadly

Blockade of effects of the parasympathetic nervous system on the eyes causes the pupils to dilate. According to tradition, Italian women would instill into their eyes a product of the root of a plant in the genus *Atropa*, believing that the drug-induced dilation of the pupils would enhance attractiveness. The extract came to be called "belladonna," meaning "beautiful woman." The full taxonomic name of the plant is *Atropa belladonna*.

A less appealing appellation for the same plant is "deadly nightshade." Every part of the plant is poisonous, and an atropine overdose can be lethal. The word, *Atropa*, is derived from the Greek *Atropos*, one of the Fates. *Atropos* held the shears that could cut the thread of human life. As related by Plutarch, belladonna was used to poison the troops of Marcus Antonius in the Parthian Wars.

Cartoonists exploit effects of altered function of the autonomic nervous system on the pupils to convey the psychological state of their characters. Look at the four faces (fig. 16). One of them is neutral, one is cute and sweet, one is disoriented, and one is startled. Which is which? Doctors may not get it right, but laypeople usually do. The answer appears at the end of this chapter.

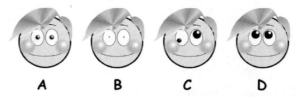

Fig. 16. Cartoonists use the pupils to convey the psychological state of the individual.

Spit   ·

The salivary glands possess a dual supply of "automatic" nerves. One supply, from the parasympathetic nervous system, is responsible for secretion of watery saliva. Think of sucking on a ripe, fragrant lemon. Such rumination evokes secretion of watery saliva because of the effects of the chemical messenger, acetylcholine, released from parasympathetic nerve terminals. Another nerve supply, from the sympathetic nervous system, is responsible for the secretion of saliva that is thicker and more mucoid because of its high protein content. Both nerve supplies participate in processing food for swallowing and digestion. The watery saliva lubricates the chewed food into a swallowable bolus. The proteinaceous saliva contains an enzyme that begins breaking down the carbohydrate in the food.

In the Bible, spitting is almost always used as a sign of contempt. For instance, according to biblical law, if a woman's husband had a brother, and her husband died, the brother-in-law would be obligated to marry the widow—a levirate marriage. If the brother-in-law refused to take on this responsibility, then as part of a public ritual to disgrace him, the widow would spit at his face.

Professional baseball players spit frequently. They chew bubble gum, gnaw on tobacco, or eat salted seeds. These all increase salivation. In baseball, as in the Bible, spitting is an instinctively communicated sign of aggressive disdain. In September 1996, a Baltimore Orioles baseball player, Roberto Alomar, in the heat of an argument with an umpire, spat into the umpire's face. Alomar immediately was ejected from the game, fined, and suspended.

In July 2003, John Carl Marquez, an Oklahoma man, was arrested for allegedly beating his wife. Marquez spat in the face of the police officer. For this act he was convicted of a felony and sentenced to life in prison.

Dry as a Bone, Red as a Beet, Mad as a Hatter

In medical school I learned the following mnemonic for the signs of atropine poisoning: "dry as a bone, red as a beet, mad as a hatter." Patients with atropine toxicity have dry skin, dry eyes, and dry mouths; they look flushed; and they act deliriously.

Just as stimulation of the parasympathetic nervous system evokes secretion of saliva, augments tear production, increases the motility of the gut, decreases the heart rate, and contracts the urinary bladder by way of the chemical messenger, acetylcholine, blockade by atropine of acetylcholine effects causes dry mouth, dry eyes, constipation, and urinary retention. The patient appears "dry as a bone." No one knows exactly why atropine poisoning produces flushing and thereby the appearance of being "red as a beet." One possibility is that the drug enters the brain and decreases sympathetic nervous system outflows, resulting in relaxation of blood vessels in the skin. Another is that atropine increases the core temperature because of the interference with thermoregulatory sweating; as a compensation, the brain might direct skin blood vessels to dilate, because this would augment loss of heat from the skin's surface. It is also possible that blockade of acetylcholine effects increases release of other chemicals that act locally to relax blood vessels in the skin.

The origin of the "madness" of hatters has nothing to do with atropine, but everything to do with mercury poisoning. In the hatting industry, an early step in preparation of cheap fur was to brush the pelt with a solution of a mercury compound, which would roughen the fibers and make them mat more easily. Mercury is poisonous to the kidneys and brain. Exactly why atropine poisoning causes delirium remains obscure.

The Sign of a Healthy Heart

The main nerve of the parasympathetic nervous system is the vagus nerve, so named because of its wandering course in the body. The vagus nerve emanates from the medulla of the brainstem, where it is the tenth cranial nerve, and it terminates in several target organs, including the heart, small airways, and gut.

Normally, when you take in a slow, deep breath, your pulse rate increases, and when you then breathe out, your pulse rate falls. These normal changes result mainly from modulation of vagus nerve traffic to the heart. The pulse rate, therefore, is not constant normally but changes with the breathing cycle. The wavelike rhythmic change in the heart rate due to breathing is called *respiratory sinus arrhythmia*. Despite the word *arrhythmia*, meaning "lacking rhythm," respiratory sinus arrhythmia is quite rhythmic and quite normal.

With aging and in many forms of heart disease, such as heart failure and pure autonomic failure, this modulation disappears, and the heart rate becomes constant. This phenomenon led its discoverer, the famous Dutch cardiologist Karel Frederik Wenckebach to write in the early 1900s that a variable pulse rate is the sign of a healthy heart.

Good Housekeeping

I think of the sympathetic nervous system as mainly a "housekeeping" system. Like a housekeeper, it performs numerous chores that keep things going, and it is underappreciated as human housekeepers often are. In a home, housekeeping chores include bringing in and putting away the groceries; making, serving, and cleaning up after meals; and taking out the trash. These tasks seem routine. Inside a living body, the sympathetic nervous system carries out many of the housekeeping chores of the inner world. When you stand up, the sympathetic nervous system keeps the blood from pooling in the legs and pelvis. When you exercise, the sympathetic nervous system prevents the core temperature from rising too high as you produce heat, and at the same time it maintains the blood flows to vital organs as you produce the by-products of metabolism, which relax blood vessels. When you go out into the cold, the sympathetic nervous system prevents the core temperature from falling. After you eat a large meal, the sympathetic nervous system maintains blood flows to the brain and heart, compensating for the concurrent shunting of blood to the gut.

Only when the housekeeper fails does the importance of the "routine" chores come to light, as the cupboard becomes bare, the meals are not made, the carpool does not run, and the trash accumulates. You can probably guess what the symptoms and signs might be if the sympathetic nervous system were to fail. When the patient stands, is exposed to moist heat, or eats a large meal, the blood pressure falls, sometimes to the extent that the patient faints. The patient cannot tolerate exposure to extremes of environmental temperature, has poor exercise tolerance, and develops shortness of breath on minimal exertion.

Heartstrings

The sympathetic nervous system consists of myriad, wispy fibers that travel to virtually all organs and tissues of the body (with the exception of the substance of the brain). Unlike in a hormone system, where the bloodstream delivers the chemical messenger to all the target tissues at the same concentration, in a nerve network system different tissues can be exposed to different concentrations of the chemical messenger by activation or inhibition of specific components of the network (fig. 17). For instance, activities of sweat glands and blood vessels in the skin change differentially when the body is exposed to heat. Increased traffic in sympathetic nerves to sweat glands

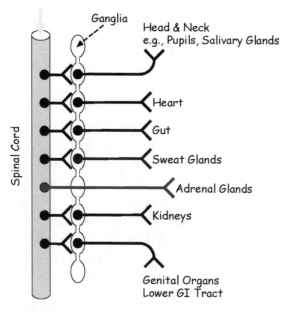

Fig. 17. The sympathetic nervous system is a key "housekeeping" system of the inner world. GI, gastrointestinal.

evokes sweating, while decreased traffic in sympathetic nerves to blood vessels produces flushing, even in the same limb.

The network arrangement of the sympathetic nervous system probably afforded important advantages in evolution by enabling localized, rapid, automatic changes in body functions in specific tissues in response to particular stressors. The advantages of a nerve network are perhaps best illustrated by regulation of the heart by the sympathetic nervous system—literally the body's "heartstrings." In mild heart failure, the sympathetic nervous system supply to the heart becomes activated relatively selectively, and this can maintain normal performance of the heart for many years. Stretching the wall of the left atrium, which delivers blood to the heart from the lungs, by inflating a balloon inside it, increases sympathetic nervous system outflow to the heart. This increases the force and rate of heart contraction, thereby compensating for what the brain senses as overfilling of the heart. Meanwhile, the brain also directs a decrease in the sympathetic nervous system outflow to the kidneys. This increases the filtration of the blood and "translates" blood volume into excreted urine.

The effects of altered activity of sympathetic nerves can be limited spatially because of the ability to send control signals to specific locations in the network, because of the several transporters and enzymes that inactivate the chemical messengers before those messengers reach the bloodstream, and because of the specific locations and types and subtypes of receptors for the messengers on the target cells.

Cannon did not think that the sympathetic nervous system plays much of a role in everyday life. He found that complete removal of the chain of sympathetic ganglia exerted no obvious long-term adverse effect, as long as the animals were kept in the controlled environment of the experimental laboratory and supplied with water and nutrition postoperatively. Cannon published a photograph of a cat that had successfully given birth to kittens, which were shown suckling at the dam. Above the mother cat, displayed affixed to a card, were the sympathetic chains that had been removed from the same cat before she had conceived. If a female cat could conceive, carry fetuses, deliver newborns, and suckle her young successfully, with her sympathetic nervous system completely gone from her body, then surely the sympathetic nervous system could not be necessary for ordinary life functions.

Nevertheless, Cannon's own observations, in his book, *Bodily Changes in Pain, Hunger, Fear, and Rage* (1929), might have convinced him that loss of the sympathetic nerves to the heart would limit cardiovascular responses to exercise: "[A dog], studied by Campos, Lundin, Walker and myself, had run 167 minutes . . . with the pulse rising from 96 to 156 beats per minute before showing signs of exhaustion. . . . The heart was denervated on November 1. Thereafter the greatest increase ever observed when the animal was induced to run was 12 beats per minute. The animal could not be made to run to an extent resulting in signs of being tired. She would travel for a relatively short time and then would brace all four feet and refuse to move" (p. 208).

Now we know that the body absolutely requires an intact and normally functioning sympathetic nervous system to tolerate even seemingly simple, mundane stressors, such as exercise, exposure to altered environmental temperature, and standing up. Because of Cannon's findings and viewpoint on this matter, about four decades passed after his death before the sympathetic nervous system began to gain recognition as a key effector for regulation of resting levels of body functions such as blood pressure and heart rate.

Cannon did not realize that multiple effectors determine blood pressure and that disruption of one effector activates others compensatorily (fig. 18).

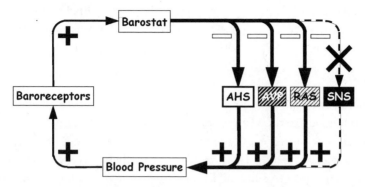

Fig. 18. Compensatory activation of alternative effectors, such as the adrenomedullary hormonal system (AHS), arginine vasopressin system (AVP), and renin-angiotensin-aldosterone system (RAS) explains why destruction of the sympathetic nervous system (SNS) produces only a relatively small influence on blood pressure. This misled Cannon into thinking that the sympathetic nervous system was unimportant in the regulation of blood pressure in organisms at rest.

Compensatory activation can obscure the contribution of any single effector to levels of the monitored variable. From the finding that removal of the sympathetic nerves did not affect blood pressure much, Cannon inferred that the sympathetic nervous system did not contribute to blood pressure in intact, undisturbed organisms. In the 1980s, however, several reports showed that sympathectomy compensatorily activates other effectors, such as the renin-angiotensin-aldosterone system, the vasopressin system, and the adrenal medulla, and compensatory activation of these effectors maintains blood pressure at approximately normal levels. In the setting of sympathectomy, interference with any of the other effectors evokes immediate, precipitous declines in blood pressure. Because Cannon was so firmly convinced of the functional unity of the sympathoadrenal system, which would be activated only in emergencies, he never considered adequately the possibility that the sympathetic nervous system might indeed contribute to levels of blood pressure and other monitored variables under resting conditions.

It also took decades after Cannon's death before researchers began to demonstrate effects of "nonemergency" stressors, such as mental challenge and exercise, on sympathetic nervous system outflow to the heart. One index of this outflow is the rate of entry of norepinephrine, the main neurotransmitter released by the sympathetic nerves, into the veins draining the heart (norepinephrine spillover). It has become clear that sympathetic nerves produce and release norepinephrine in the heart all the time, not just in emergencies. Only a few years ago was it shown for the first time that the pulse rate of people at rest is related to the rate of release of norepinephrine in the heart.

No Sweat

In general, sweating to control body temperature (thermoregulatory sweating), sweating evoked by eating spicy food (gustatory sweating), or sweating evoked by fear or anxiety (emotional sweating) is mediated by the sympathetic cholinergic system. The nerves are sympathetic nerves, and the chemical messenger is acetylcholine. Because the chemical messenger for sweating responses is acetylcholine, patients with an inability to manufacture norepinephrine have a fall in blood pressure when they stand up, but they sweat normally. And because sympathetic nerves mediate sweating, patients with severe palmar, armpit, or facial hyperhidrosis (excessive sweating) sometimes undergo surgical thoracic sympathectomies. The surgery usually alleviates the excessive perspiration, but it can also bring on a host of troublesome side effects, such as gustatory sweating (excessive facial sweating after eating food), increased pain sensitivity, decreased exercise tolerance, increased sweating of the feet, and even whitening of the hair above the level of the surgery.

Atropine poisoning produces skin that is "dry as a bone" by inhibiting the production of sweat. Atropine exerts this effect by blocking receptors for acetylcholine, the chemical messenger of the parasympathetic nervous system. The dry skin from atropine poisoning, however, comes not from blockade of the parasympathetic nervous system but from blockade of the portion of the sympathetic nervous system where acetylcholine is the main chemical messenger at the sweat glands.

Adrenaline and norepinephrine may play a role in the sweating attending distress. Unlike thermoregulatory sweating and sweating after eating spicy foods, in which the sweating is associated with flushing of the skin, sweating during distress is associated with pallor due to the constriction of blood vessels in the skin. Adrenaline evokes both watery sweat and a different type of sweat, which is thicker and has an odor due to secretion not only of sweat but also of some of the secreting cells. Frightened people break out in a "cold sweat" because of concurrent adrenaline-induced constriction of blood vessels in the skin. The skin becomes "clammy," referring to the damp, unpleasant chill. "Cold comfort" is no comfort at all. Perhaps dogs trained to recognize an incipient seizure in their epileptic masters do so by smelling the sweat of distress.

The Hot Line

The sympathetic nerves to most organs are postganglionic, because the nerve fibers originate from cell bodies in the ganglia. The sympathetic nerves that travel to the adrenal gland, the gland that sits on top of each kidney and releases adrenaline, constitute an exception, because they are preganglionic. The nerve fibers come directly from cell bodies in the spinal cord. The fibers pass through the ganglia and are delivered to the adrenal gland by way of the splanchnic nerves without relaying their signals via cells in the ganglia. It is like a direct wiring connection from the electrical distribution center to the terminal box affixed to a house, a direct "hot line" from the central nervous system to the adrenal gland. The speed of transmission is almost unbelievably fast, so fast that, for instance, if a rat is guillotined and blood obtained immediately from the headless trunk, the amount of adrenaline in the trunk blood already exceeds that in a conscious, undisturbed rat by about a hundredfold.

Whereas the sympathetic noradrenergic system determines unconscious "housekeeping" processes, mediated by the neurotransmitter, norepinephrine, the sympathetic adrenergic system, synonymous with the adrenomedullary hormonal system, plays a key role in "emergencies" and "distress," when all organs of the body are threatened, such as by low blood sugar (hypoglycemia), low blood temperature (hypothermia), asphyxiation, shock, or fear. Adrenaline increases blood glucose levels, increases pulse rate and blood pressure, stimulates metabolism, quiets the gut, and dilates blood vessels in skeletal muscle.

How Does the Autonomic Nervous System Work?

Chemical Messengers

The brain regulates the inner world by way of effectors, and the effectors work by way of chemical messengers. Different types of chemical messengers are released in the body (fig. 19).

The first chemical messenger to be identified were hormones, and the first hormone to be identified, in 1901, was adrenaline. Hormones are released directly into the bloodstream, which delivers them to target cells distant from the site of release. The discipline that focuses on regulation of the inner world by hormones is endocrinology, a specialty of internal medicine.

The second type of chemical messenger is released by nerves and acts on nearby target cells—a neurotransmitter. One of the most famous biomedical experiments of all time, which led to a Nobel Prize in 1936 for the investigator, Otto Loewi, demonstrated the existence of such a chemical messenger. The experimental setup consisted of the exposed, beating hearts of two frogs, a "donor" frog and a "recipient" frog. Loewi bathed the heart of the donor frog in a fluid and let the fluid drip onto the exposed, beating heart of the recipient frog. When he electrically stimulated the vagus nerve to the heart of the donor frog, the heart rate decreased. The stimulation also decreased the heart rate of the recipient frog, implying that the stimulation released something into the fluid that dripped from the donor heart onto the recipient heart. Loewi inferred that the nerve stimulation released a chemical substance that caused the recipient frog's heart to slow down too. He called that substance the "*Vagusstoff*," or "substance of the vagus." He then showed that the *Vagusstoff* produced a variety of responses in other tissues that were identical with those produced by a chemical, acetylcholine. In 1926 Loewi and a coworker identified the *Vagusstoff* as acetylcholine.

Loewi used virtually the same experimental setup to demonstrate that

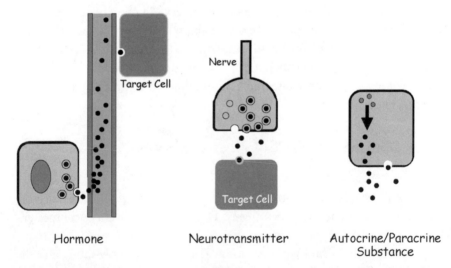

Hormone   Neurotransmitter   Autocrine/Paracrine
                                                        Substance

Fig. 19. The autonomic nervous system works by releasing chemical messengers. The chemicals are hormones, neurotransmitters, or autocrine/paracrine substances.

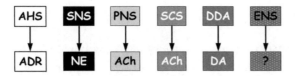

Fig. 20. Chemical messengers of the autonomic nervous system. Sympathetic nerves to the cardiovascular system release norepinephrine (NE). The main chemical messenger of the adrenomedullary hormonal system is adrenaline (ADR), and the main messenger of the DOPA/dopamine system (DDA) is dopamine (DA). Acetylcholine (ACh) is released by cells of the parasympathetic nervous system (PNS) and sympathetic cholinergic system (SCS). The messenger of the enteric nervous system (ENS) is unknown.

in frogs stimulation of the sympathetic nervous system supply to the heart releases adrenaline. This was in 1921, a few years before he identified the *Vagusstoff.* Now we know that in certain situations in humans, such as severe exercise, and in some disorders, such as panic disorder, adrenaline is indeed released by the heart; however, it is likely that the source of this adrenaline is that taken up as a hormone from the bloodstream by sympathetic nerves. Loewi's results might have helped convince Cannon to propose that in humans, as in frogs, adrenaline would be the neurotransmitter of the sympathetic nervous system. As noted previously, Cannon's misidentification of the neurotransmitter of the sympathetic nervous system probably cost him a Nobel Prize.

A third type of chemical messenger is an autocrine/paracrine substance. The messenger is produced in, released from, and acts on the same or nearby cells. Whereas adrenaline exemplifies a hormone and norepinephrine a neurotransmitter, dopamine, the third member of the small chemical family of catecholamines, seems to act as an autocrine/paracrine substance, at least in the kidneys.

The different components of the autonomic nervous system use different chemical messengers (fig. 20). Parasympathetic nerves release acetylcholine as the neurotransmitter. These nerves are "cholinergic." Norepinephrine is the main neurotransmitter used by the sympathetic nervous system (sympathetic "noradrenergic system") for regulation of the circulation. Acetylcholine is the neurotransmitter used by the "sympathetic cholinergic system," which is the main effector for regulation of sweating. Adrenaline is the main hormone released by the adrenal medulla. In the DOPA-dopamine autocrine/paracrine system, dopamine is produced within cells after uptake of DOPA from the bloodstream.

Receptors

Regardless of whether chemical messengers are hormones, neurotransmitters, or autocrine/paracrine substances, they all work by acting on receptors on or in the target cells (table 1).

Receptors are specialized proteins to which chemical messengers bind, like a key in the lock of your front door. Binding of chemical messengers to receptors changes the three-dimensional configuration of the receptors, initiating cascades of biochemical changes inside the cells that in turn alter the functional status of the cells. For instance, when you exercise on a hot day, an increased rate of nerve traffic in sympathetic nerves releases the neurotransmitter, acetylcholine, from the nerve terminals. The released acetylcholine binds to receptors on cells of the sweat glands, causing them to release sweat.

The chemical messengers binding to the receptors are called "first messengers," and those functioning within the cell after the receptors are occupied are called "second messengers."

Cells in different organs of the body possess hundreds of different types of receptors for scores of chemical messengers. To gain a hint about the resulting complexity, look at table 1, which summarizes the effects of receptors for catecholamines and acetylcholine, the main chemical messengers of the autonomic nervous system, and then multiply by about a hundred to take into account the other chemical messengers of the body's automatic systems.

The receptors for adrenaline, norepinephrine, and dopamine are discussed in the next chapter, which goes into some detail about the catecholamine systems of the body. The following discussion considers the receptors for acetylcholine.

Why Are Cigarettes Like Mushrooms?

Specific receptors mediate the effects of acetylcholine. Classically they have been divided into nicotinic and muscarinic.

Muscarinic receptors are named for the toxin, muscarine, in toadstools. Toadstools are of the species *Amanita muscaria*, a red mushroom with wool-like white spots on its top. The spots resemble the warts of a toad, explaining the designation, *toadstool.* The same species of mushroom contains muscimol and ibotenic acid, two other neurotoxins that affect other neurotransmitter systems. Stimulation of muscarinic receptors increases gut smooth muscle contraction and secretion by glands.

Table 1. Responses of target organs to autonomic nerve impulses

Organ	Receptor type	Responses to:	
		Adrenergic impulses	Cholinergic impulses
Eye			
Radial muscle, iris	α_1	Pupil dilation	—
Sphincter muscle, iris		—	Pupil constriction
Ciliary muscle	β	Relaxation for far vision	Contraction for near vision
Heart			
Sinoatrial node	β_1	Increased heart rate	Decrease in heart rate; sinus node arrest
Atria	β_1	Increased contractility and conduction velocity	Decrease in contractility and shortened action-potential duration
Atrioventricular node	β_1	Increased automaticity and conduction velocity	Decrease in conduction velocity; atrioventricular block
His-Purkinje system	β_1	Increased automaticity and conduction velocity	Little effect
Ventricles	β_1	Increased contractility, conduction velocity, automaticity, and rate of idioventricular pacemakers	Slight decrease in contractility claimed by some
Arterioles			
Coronary	$\alpha; \beta_2$	Little net effect	Dilation
Skin & mucosa	α	Constriction	Dilation
Skeletal muscle	$\alpha; \beta_2$	Dilation	Dilation
Cerebral	α	Little net effect	Dilation
Pulmonary	$\alpha; \beta_2$	Little net effect	Dilation
Abdominal viscera	$\alpha; \beta_2$	Constriction	—
Salivary glands	α	Constriction	Dilation
Renal	$\alpha_1; \beta_1; \beta_2$	Constriction	—
Veins (systemic)	$\alpha; \beta_2$	Constriction	—

(continued)

Table 1, continued

Organ	Receptor type	Responses to: Adrenergic impulses	Responses to: Cholinergic impulses
Lung			
Tracheal and bronchial	β_2	Relaxation	Contraction
Bronchial glands	$\alpha_1; \beta_2$	Decreased secretion; increased secretion	Stimulation
Stomach			
Motility and tone	$\alpha_2; \beta_2$	Decrease	Increase
Sphincters	α	Contraction (usually)	Relaxation
Secretion		Inhibition (?)	Stimulation
Intestine			
Motility and tone	$\alpha_1; \alpha_2; \beta_2$	Decrease	Increase
Sphincters	α	Contraction (usually)	Relaxation (usually)
Secretion		Inhibition (?)	Stimulation
Gallbladder	β_2	Relaxation	Contraction
Kidney	β_1	Renin secretion	—
Urinary bladder			
Detrusor	β	Relaxation (usually)	Contraction
Trigone and sphincter	β_1	Contraction	Relaxation
Ureter			
Motility and tone	α	Increase	Increase (?)
Uterus	$\alpha; \beta_2$	Pregnant: contraction (α); relaxation (β_2) Nonpregnant: relaxation (β_2)	Variable
Penis	α	Ejaculation	Erection
Skin			
Pilomotor muscles	α	Contraction	—
Sweat glands	α	Localized secretion	Generalized secretion

(continued)

Table I, continued

Organ	Receptor type	Responses to: Adrenergic impulses	Responses to: Cholinergic impulses
Spleen capsule	α; β_2	Contraction	—
Adrenal medulla		—	Secretion of adrenaline and norepinephrine (nicotinic effect)
Skeletal muscle	β_2	Increased contractility, glycogen breakdown, K^+ uptake	—
Liver	α; β_2	Glycogen breakdown, glucose synthesis	Glycogen synthesis
Pancreas			
Acini	α	Decreased secretion	Secretion
Islets (B cells)	α_2	Decreased secretion	—
	β_2	Increased secretion	—
Fat cells	α; β_1	Lipolysis	—
Salivary glands	α_1	K^+ and water secretion	K^+ and water secretion
	β	Amylase secretion	
Lacrimal glands		—	Secretion
Nasopharyngeal		—	Secretion
Pineal gland	β	Melatonin synthesis	—
Post.pituitary	β_1	Antidiuretic hormone secretion	—

Source: Adapted from Goodman LS, Gilman AG, eds. *The Pharmacologic Basis of Therapeutics,* 7th ed. New York: Macmillan, 1985.

People who try to get "high" by eating mushrooms can develop severe nausea, vomiting, and diarrhea because of the stimulation of muscarinic receptors. I remember well the scene in an emergency room when I was training in internal medicine, as a group of teenagers came in one night with mushroom poisoning. They had tried to get high by eating psychedelic psilocybin mushrooms, but instead they had ingested a species of the *Amanita* genus. They all vomited at about the same time. The vomit contained some of the undigested mushrooms, identified by an old botany professor whom we called in from home. This experience convinced me of the survival value of vomiting.

Acetylcholine is the main chemical messenger for relaying control signals in the ganglia, from the preganglionic to the postganglionic cells. Acetylcholine does so by binding to nicotinic receptors, which are present on the postganglionic cells and also on cells of the adrenal gland that secrete adrenaline. The rapid effects of nicotine in the body result from stimulation of these receptors. In people not already addicted to nicotine, the outpouring of adrenaline after smoking a cigar or cigarette probably accounts for the more rapid and forceful heartbeat and increased blood pressure. Nicotine-induced sweating probably reflects a combination of adrenaline effects and release of acetylcholine from sympathetic nerves supplying sweat glands. Nicotine also increases salivation, mainly from release of acetylcholine from parasympathetic nerves supplying the salivary glands. This is one reason why baseball players who chew tobacco spit so much.

In skeletal muscle, acetylcholine binds to nicotinic receptors that are distinct from those in the ganglia. Drugs such as curare, which block nicotinic receptors on skeletal muscle cells, cause paralysis of the limbs, decreased breathing, respiratory arrest, and death, as demonstrated by Claude Bernard. Other drugs, which block the nicotinic receptors in ganglia, cause paralysis of smooth muscle, such as in the gut and blood vessels, resulting in an inability to digest or to maintain blood pressure during standing.

The sympathetic nerves that trigger the release of adrenaline pass through the ganglia and directly supply the cells in the adrenal gland that produce and release adrenaline. Acetylcholine is released from the sympathetic nerve terminals in the center of the adrenal gland, the adrenal medulla. The acetylcholine then binds to nicotinic receptors on these cells, which causes them to release adrenaline into the bloodstream. The bloodstream delivers the adrenaline to organs throughout the body.

Acetylcholine itself is not used as a drug in clinical medicine, because it is broken down very rapidly by an enzyme, acetylcholinesterase. Drugs that act at nicotinic or muscarinic acetylcholine receptors are used widely to treat conditions as diverse as urinary incontinence, diarrhea, excessive sweating, dangerously fast or slow pulse rate, asthma, insomnia, peptic ulcer disease, mushroom poisoning, and even Parkinson disease. Drugs that inhibit the

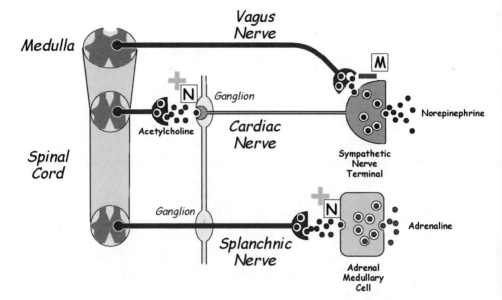

Fig. 21. Acetylcholine stimulates sympathetic nerve traffic and adrenaline release by occupying nicotinic receptors (N) in ganglia and in the adrenal medulla. Acetylcholine also inhibits release of norepinephrine from sympathetic nerve terminals by occupying muscarinic receptors (M).

enzyme that breaks down acetylcholine are mainstays in the treatment of myasthenia gravis, the disease that Aristotle Onassis had, and are often prescribed to treat patients with dementia.

Muscarinic receptors on sympathetic nerves inhibit norepinephrine release. A generalized increase in parasympathetic nervous system outflow, therefore, would be expected to stimulate adrenaline release via occupation of nicotinic receptors in the adrenal glands, while inhibiting norepinephrine release via occupation of muscarinic receptors on sympathetic nerves.

Yin and Yang

The parasympathetic nervous system regulates vegetative processes such as digestion and urination. Acetylcholine released from parasympathetic nerves acts to stimulate the gut, increase urinary bladder contractions, increase salivation, and decrease the pulse rate.

Cannon emphasized that the parasympathetic and sympathetic nervous systems generally oppose each other (fig. 21). Their effects would balance each other in the dynamic equilibrium of homeostasis. Activities spurred by the sympathetic nervous system do tend to expend energy during periods of movement, whereas activities spurred by the parasympathetic nervous system replenish energy stores during periods of quiescence. There are exceptions to this yin-yang rule, however. Because Cannon lumped together the sympathetic nervous system and adrenomedullary hormonal system in a single sympathoadrenal system, he never realized that in some situations activities of the sympathetic nervous system and adrenomedullary hormonal system change differentially. In these situations, parasympathetic nervous system and adrenomedullary hormonal system activities typically change in parallel.

Possibly the most glaring example of this phenomenon is in fainting. Three characteristic changes occur in the cardiovascular system when people faint. First, the skin turns pale, from constriction of local blood vessels, which can be explained by the high levels of adrenaline in the bloodstream. Second, the heart rate falls; sometimes, the heart stops completely for several seconds. The fall in heart rate results from activation of the vagus nerve supplying the heart. Third, the rate of blood flow in skeletal muscle of the limbs increases. The increase in blood flow results from relaxation of the blood vessels, which can be explained by a combination of high adrenaline levels in the bloodstream and simultaneous inhibition of norepinephrine release from sympathetic nerves: "sympathoadrenal imbalance."

Perhaps it would make more sense to view the parasympathetic nervous system as the "secretive" nervous system, to play a pun on the double meaning of the word, "secretive." "Secretive" can mean having the ability to secrete and also can mean hiding from view. Parasympathetic nervous system stimulation increases the secretion of saliva in the mouth, tears in the eyes, and fluid in the gut. Parasympathetic nervous system stimulation also promotes activities that are done in "secret," such as urination, defecation, sleep, and penile erection.

Acetylcholine usually relaxes blood vessel walls by a relatively recently discovered indirect mechanism. The relaxation depends on an intact inner layer of cells in the blood vessel wall, where acetylcholine increases the generation of a gas called nitric oxide (NO). NO potently inhibits the tone of nearby smooth muscle in the blood vessel wall. NO therefore acts as a gaseous autocrine/paracrine factor. In the penis, NO-induced venous engorgement is thought to play a major role in erection.

You now have a basic understanding of the autonomic nervous system. It plays critical roles both in emergencies and in our daily activities, working to keep us going and helping our bodies make adjustments throughout the day. Here is a summary of the functions of the different components of the "automatic" nervous system.

Parasympathetic Nervous System Effects
Constriction of the pupils
Decreased pulse rate
Increased gut activity
Increased salivation (watery)
Increased tear production
Increased urinary bladder tone
Penile erection

Sympathetic Cholinergic Nervous System Effects
Sweating from altered temperature (thermoregulatory sweating)
Sweating from eating spicy foods (gustatory sweating)
Sweating from emotional distress

Sympathetic Noradrenergic Nervous System Effects
Blood vessel constriction (skin, skeletal muscle, kidneys)
Dilation of the pupils
Ejaculation
Goosebumps and hair standing out
Increased force of the heartbeat
Increased pulse rate
Increased salivation (thick mucus)
Relaxation of the gut
Salt retention by the kidneys
Trembling

Adrenomedullary Hormonal System Effects
Antifatigue effect
Constriction of skin blood vessels (pallor)
Decreased serum potassium level
Dilation of the pupils
Emotional sweating
Increased blood sugar
Increased emotional intensity
Increased force of the heartbeat

(continued)

Increased pulse rate
Increased respiration
Relaxation of blood vessels in skeletal muscle
Relaxation of the gut
Trembling

DOPA-Dopamine Autocrine / Paracrine System Effects
Increased excretion of sodium
Inhibition of secretion of aldosterone by the adrenal cortex
Relaxation of blood vessels
Decreased acid production in the stomach

Enteric Nervous System
Gastrointestinal movements

About the cartoon faces: A is neutral, B is startled, C is disoriented, and D is cute and sweet. Cartoonists (and probably you) appreciate that pupil constriction instinctively conveys startle, inequality of the pupils conveys disorientation, and enlarged pupils convey cuteness (as in "belladonna," the drug used for centuries to enhance attractiveness by enlarging the pupils). Medical students are taught, incorrectly, that startle, a form of "stress response," should involve increased adrenaline levels and increased sympathetic nervous system outflows, and this would cause pupil dilation on both sides. They are also taught, in this case correctly, that a "blown," dilated pupil on one side and deviation of the eye on that side can disclose a catastrophe inside the head.

3 | The Arbiters of the Inner World

So much of the workings inside the body reflect the dynamic equilibria of production, release, recycling, and breakdown of catecholamines; so many researchers have spent so much of their careers learning about catecholamine systems and their intricacies; so much of importance to medicine and physiology is known about these systems; and so much of the history of the adrenaline family is just plain fascinating, that this chapter describes adrenaline and the other members of its small chemical family in some detail. Systems that use catecholamines are in many ways the arbiters in the political science of the inner world.

The Fat above the Kidneys

The Bible contains far more detailed and lengthy accounts about ritual animal sacrifice than about the entire history of the universe from the Creation to the ascent of man. In Exodus and Leviticus, the text lists the organs to be burnt by the priests. Of the remaining flesh the priests could and indeed were commanded to eat, but eating the organs specified for ritual burning was forbidden. One of these tissues was the "fat above the kidneys." The text mentions specifically—not once but nine times—that the fat above the kidneys was to be burnt. Eating the fat above the kidneys was proscribed not just for priests but for everyone.

Why was eating the fat above the kidneys disallowed? The fat above the kidneys is unique for its contents (fig. 22). Buried within it are the adrenal glands, which store the powerful hormones cortisol, aldosterone, adrenal androgens, and adrenaline. Depending on the efficiency of metabolic breakdown of these chemicals in the gut, eating adrenal gland tissue could result in entry of one or more physiologically active compounds into the bloodstream. Ingestion of adrenal gland tissue repeatedly by the priests over a long period could easily have made them ill.

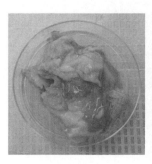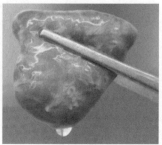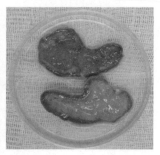

Fig. 22. The adrenal gland is embedded in the fat above the kidneys.

No one knew of the existence of the adrenal glands until Bartholomeo Eustachius (for whom the eustachian tube is named) described their anatomy in 1563; and the first discovery about the effects on the body of the chemicals within the adrenal glands did not take place until about a century ago. But perhaps there was an inkling, reflected in the ancient command to the priests to burn and not eat the fat above the kidneys.

On the Risk of Being a Physician's Son

Until about a century ago, no one had realized the contribution of the adrenal gland to regulation of the inner world. In the early 1890s, a physician and amateur inventor in Harrogate, England, Dr. George Oliver, tested one of his homemade devices on his son. The device was supposed to measure the caliber of arteries. To test the apparatus, Oliver applied it to his son's wrist at the radial artery, which carries blood to the hand. Oliver then administered an extract of adrenal gland to his son. The extract did appear to elicit constriction of the radial artery, as measured by Oliver's contraption. Meanwhile, in London, E. A. Schäfer, a renowned professor of physiology at the University College, was carrying out experiments on laboratory animals, involving measurement of blood pressure by the height of a column of mercury in a tube connected to an artery. Oliver visited Schäfer's laboratory and brought a vial of the adrenal extract. Schäfer allowed injection of the material into the vein of a dog. This set the stage for one of the epochal discoveries in medical history. The injection produced an immediate, startling increase in the animal's blood pressure, an increase so large that the column of mercury in the gauge actually overflowed the tube. In 1894 and 1895 Oliver and Schäfer published the first reports ever about the cardiovascular actions of a chemical extracted from a body organ.

About the exact mode of "administration" of the extract Oliver had given his son, versions of the story differ. At first glance this might appear to be a trivial historical detail. The answer actually is quite relevant to the subject matter of this book. According to Sir Henry Dale, an authority who shared (with Otto Loewi) the Nobel Prize for Physiology or Medicine in 1936, the extract had been injected. According to others, based on the writings of both Oliver and Schäfer themselves, the extract had been given orally. This disagreement relates to a concept about regulation of the inner world, that of an enzymatic "gut-blood barrier" for catecholamines. Considering humankind's omnivorous nature, the potency of adrenaline as a hormone, and the presence of high stored concentrations of adrenaline in the adrenal glands, out of evolutionary necessity one might expect that the gastrointestinal tract would possess impressively efficient means for detoxifying ingested catecholamines. The gut indeed does contain multiple, redundant enzymes that carry out this crucial task in helping maintain the constancy of the internal environment, despite the range of things we ingest. After swallowing an adrenaline solution, levels of adrenaline itself in the bloodstream hardly increase at all. This is one reason why today you can buy adrenal concentrate as a dietary supplement in health food stores. Oral ingestion of adrenal extract by Oliver's son probably would have elicited little if any constriction of blood vessels, because of the extremely efficient metabolic breakdown of adrenaline in the gastrointestinal tract and liver. If you lacked one or more of the gut enzymes that detoxify catecholamines, however, or were taking a medication that inhibited activities of the enzymes making up the "gut-blood barrier," then ingesting adrenal concentrate could cause illness, regardless of your having bought it at a "health" store. If Oliver had administered the extract directly by injection, he could well have killed his son.

What's in a Name?

The most famous member of the catecholamine family has two names—adrenaline and epinephrine. Its chemical father, the chemical messenger of the sympathetic nervous system, also has two names—noradrenaline and norepinephrine. Here is how this happened.

Beginning immediately after the reports by Oliver and Schäfer about the unexpected and profoundly powerful effects of injected extracts of the adrenal gland, researchers worldwide began a race to identify the "active principle." One of these was John Jacob Abel, of Johns Hopkins, who devoted about a decade of his life to this project. In 1897, Abel and Crawford reported partial purification of the compound. They isolated a benzoyl derivative of what Abel called epinephrin. This proved not to be epinephrine itself. The first person to isolate the active principle of the adrenal gland was a chemist in the laboratory of Jokichi Takamine. Takamine had visited Abel in 1900. In a 1927 lecture, Abel recalled the visit and its consequences:

> After I had completed the above described investigation and while I was still endeavoring to improve my processes, I was visited one day by the Japanese chemist, J. Takamine, who examined with great interest the various compounds and salts of epinephrine that were placed before him. He inquired particularly whether I did not think it possible that my salts of epinephrine could be prepared by a simpler process than mine, more especially without the trouble and in this case wasteful process of benzoylating extracts of an animal tissue. He remarked in this connection that he loved to plant a seed and see it grow in the technical field. I told Takamine that I was quite of his opinion and that the process could no doubt be improved and simplified. . . . Takamine prepared suprarenal extracts more concentrated than mine and without first attempting to separate the hormone for its numerous concomitants by benzoylating or otherwise, simply added ammonia—the reagent that I had so long employed—to his concentrated extracts, whereupon he immediately obtained the native base in the form of burr-like clusters of minute prisms in place of the amorphous base. I have often asked why I had not myself attempted to solve the problem in this very simple fashion. The truth is that I had tried to do so but always found that the dilute extract tested simply turned pink in a short time on the addition of ammonia without depositing the base either crystallized or amorphous. . . . Takamine's success was due to the employment of ammonia on very highly concentrated, though impure extracts. . . . The efforts of years on my part in this once mysterious field of suprarenal, medullary biochemistry, marred by blunders as they were, eventuated, then, in the isolation of the hormone not in the form of the free base but in that of its monobenzoyl derivative.

In the memorial appreciation for Abel from which I culled this quotation (located in the Abel Library of the Department of Pharmacology at Johns Hopkins), William MacNider, then dean of the medical school of the University of North Carolina at Chapel Hill, commented, "This extremely important and frank statement of the chemical birth of a new era in the understanding of tissue activity portrays as no words could the industry persisted in to the point of physical exhaustion, the frankness, the complete honesty untouched by jealousy or recrimination of a nobleman in the domain of science."

Takamine had set up a laboratory on East 103rd Street in New York City, under the patronage of Parke, Davis & Company. After Takamine's visit with Abel, Keizo Uenaka, whom Takamine had hired as a chemist, successfully crystallized, and therefore isolated in pure form, what Takamine called adrenaline. In 1901, Takamine reported this first successful crystallization of a hormone. Almost simultaneously, Thomas Aldrich, a colleague of Takamine at Parke-Davis (and, probably not coincidentally, a former assistant of Abel at Johns Hopkins), correctly deduced its chemical structure. Up to that point Abel had failed in his attempts to isolate the active principle of the adrenal gland, and he never published the correct chemical structure, so that medical historians gave Takamine and Aldrich the credit for one of the most important medical scientific feats ever—the first identification of a hormone. In 1904, Friedrich Stolz synthesized adrenaline entirely chemically; adrenaline therefore was also the first hormone to be produced artificially in a laboratory.

Takamine patented Adrenalin and became a millionaire. He had a mansion on Riverside Drive in Manhattan. He used the royalties to found three companies, Sankyo Pharmaceutical Company (one of the largest drug companies in Japan), the International Takamine Ferment Company in New York City, and the Takamine Laboratory in Clifton, New Jersey. Takamine funded the gift of cherry trees that have graced the Tidal Basin in Washington, D.C., to this day. For Takamine's scientific and entrepreneurial accomplishments, the emperor of Japan awarded Takamine with the Order of the Rising Sun, Fourth Class, and sent in his honor 15 cherry trees to Parke-Davis, where they remained planted in front of the administrative offices until World War II. Takamine's patron, Parke-Davis, retained the trademark for Adrenalin.

What about Abel? He continued to pursue his career goal of identifying, isolating, and purifying hormones. One of these was insulin, which he crystallized in 1926. Until his death in 1938 he ran a renowned laboratory and teaching program at Johns Hopkins. He helped found the American Society for Pharmacology and Experimental Therapeutics and served as editor of the society's official journal, the *Journal of Pharmacology and Experimental Therapeutics* (JPET), for 23 years. He also founded the *Journal of Biological Chemistry* (JBC). JPET and JBC remain among the most prestigious journals in pharmacology and biochemistry. Abel never rivaled Takamine in monetary success, but he did acquire the wealth of a good name. Scientific reports in American journals, such as the *Journal of Pharmacology and Experimental Therapeutics*, still use the word that Abel introduced, "epinephrine," whereas European journals use Takamine's "adrenaline." As an alumnus of The Johns Hopkins School of Medicine, I feel a sense of pride in the honesty, industry, and collegiality of John Jacob Abel, the father of American pharmacology. Partly from school ties, but mainly out of fairness, in this book I refer to the father in the catecholamine family as norepinephrine and the son as adrenaline.

Abel always maintained that Takamine's adrenaline had been impure. In this assertion he undoubtedly was correct. The drug Parke-Davis sold as Adrenalin, being an extract of adrenal gland tissue, must have contained not only adrenaline but a mixture of all three catecholamines of the body, adrenaline, norepinephrine (noradrenaline), and dopamine. Norepinephrine would have been the main contaminant. Under the brand name Arterenol, norepinephrine became available commercially in 1908, and it is still used clinically under the brand name, Levophed. Dopamine was first synthesized in 1910 but was not identified as a normal constituent of the adrenal gland until the early 1950s. Dopamine is present at only quite small concentrations in the adrenal gland, compared with the concentrations of adrenaline and norepinephrine, and so would not have contaminated Adrenalin noticeably.

Catecholamines Look Like Cats

Members of the adrenaline family are catecholamines, and catecholamines are catechols. The chemical, catechol, has a particular structure, consisting of a hexagon of carbon atoms with hydroxyl (—OH) groups attached to adjacent points of the hexagon. Catechol itself does not exist in the human body, but chemicals that contain catechol as part of their molecular structure are called catechols.

One way to remember what catechols look like is to picture their structure as the head of a cat (fig. 23). The hexagonal ring is the face. The two hydroxyl groups are the pointy ears.

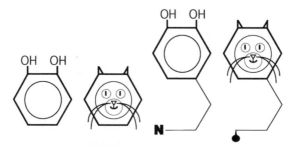

Fig. 23. Catechols look like the head of a cat. Catecholamines are catechols with a hydrocarbon tail ending in an amine group.

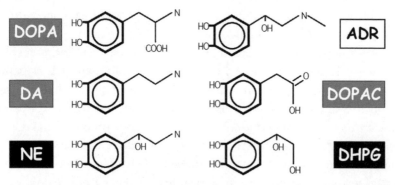

Fig. 24. Human plasma contains six catechols, including the three catecholamines, dopamine (DA), norepinephrine (NE), and adrenaline (ADR), the catecholamine precursor L-DOPA, the dopamine metabolite dihydroxyphenylacetic acid (DOPAC), and the norepinephrine metabolite dihydroxyphenylglycol (DHPG).

Human plasma contains six catechols (fig. 24). Three are the catecholamines, adrenaline, norepinephrine, and dopamine. Another catechol is L-DOPA, the same chemical that, as a drug, is used to treat Parkinson disease. Two other catechols are breakdown products—metabolites—of the catecholamines. Dihydroxyphenylglycol (DHPG) is a metabolite of norepinephrine and adrenaline, and dihydroxyphenylacetic acid (DOPAC) is a metabolite of dopamine.

Catecholamines look like the entire cat, including its tail. The tail of the cat is a short hydrocarbon strand, consisting of carbon and hydrogen atoms. At the end of the tail is an amine (ammonia) group. Think of a cat in its litter box, with the ammonia coming off the tail end producing a smell like urine.

The body's three catecholamines, dopamine, norepinephrine, and adrenaline, are like the grandfather, father, and son in a small chemical family. Adrenaline is derived from norepinephrine, and norepinephrine is derived from dopamine. The three catecholamines happen to represent the three different ways the body regulates the inner world. Adrenaline is a hormone, released from the adrenal gland into the bloodstream and then swept by the bloodstream to organs and tissues throughout the body, where adrenaline produces a large variety of effects. Norepinephrine is a neurotransmitter, released from nerves of the sympathetic nervous system and acting mainly locally on nearby target cells. Although a small proportion of the norepinephrine released from sympathetic nerves enters the bloodstream, norepinephrine in the bloodstream must reach relatively high concentrations before it exerts effects as a hormone.

Dopamine can be considered the "atavistic" catecholamine. Even invertebrates such as sea anemones produce dopamine. In mammals, dopamine in the central nervous system acts as a neurotransmitter, but in the periphery, such as in the gut, adrenal gland, and especially the kidneys, dopamine appears to be an autocrine/paracrine substance, produced in, released from, and acting locally on the same type of cells. Concentrations of dopamine in these organs seem to have little to do with local nerves. In evolutionary terms, dopamine systems appear to have dated from before the time of nerve networks or hormones.

Adrenaline's Effects on the Body

When injected into the bloodstream, all three catecholamines are potent drugs, but the most potent of the three by far is adrenaline. This seems to fit with its role as a hormone, whereas norepinephrine acts as a neurotransmitter and dopamine as an autocrine/paracrine substance. A hormone released from a particular gland would be diluted by manyfold in the blood coming from other organs, so that by the time the hormone reached the target cells via the blood pumped by the heart, usually at distant sites in the body, the concentration of the hormone would be quite low. For the chemical to work, it would have to be potent. Meanwhile, neurotransmitters and autocrine/paracrine substances work near their sites of release, before they enter the bloodstream.

Sticky Blood and Headless Rats

When Takamine patented Adrenalin, a major proposed use of the drug was for hemostasis, or slowing of bleeding. Adrenaline markedly decreases bleeding from trauma, by two self-reinforcing mechanisms. Adrenaline constricts blood vessels in the skin, and adrenaline promotes formation of platelet plugs in blood vessel walls. Platelets are tiny particles in the bloodstream that are fragments of particular cells made in the bone marrow. Platelets tend to clump into plugs when stimulated by certain chemicals, and one of these chemicals is adrenaline.

You probably have heard the phrase, "running around like a chicken with its head cut off." If you were to chop off a chicken's head, wouldn't the blood spurt out and the animal rapidly lose consciousness and become motionless? Actually, no. A remarkable amount of blood remains in the body, as the severed trunk oozes blood. If you guillotined a laboratory rat, it would shriek for several seconds. To obtain "trunk blood," you might have to squeeze it out! Adrenaline's actions promoting hemostasis explain this macabre scene. Chopping off an animal's head instantaneously evokes drastic release of catecholamines into the bloodstream by the adrenal gland. So much adrenaline pours out, so fast, that "trunk blood," even obtained immediately after decapitation, contains about a hundred times the resting concentration of adrenaline. The surge of adrenaline constricts blood vessels and promotes platelet plugging to such an extent that chickens actually do run around with their heads cut off.

Snow White and Cold Sweat

Pallor is probably the most obvious among the many effects of adrenaline as a hormone. The pallor results from constriction of blood vessels in the skin. Constriction of skin blood vessels minimizes blood loss from physical trauma and also promotes increased blood temperature by interfering with heat loss from the blood delivered to the skin's surface.

The blood vessel constricting action of adrenaline varies remarkably with the particular body organ. Just a few centimeters below the skin, in the skeletal muscle, adrenaline tends to dilate the blood vessels. This dilation redistributes blood toward the skeletal muscle, as would be appropriate in preparation for a "fight or flight" response. I carried out an experiment once that involved infusion of adrenaline into the brachial artery of normal volunteers. The brachial artery carries the blood to the forearm and hand. The infusion produced obvious pallor of the hands, yet total forearm blood flow, determined mainly by the blood vessels in skeletal muscle, actually increased in some people. Adrenaline also constricts blood vessels in the gut and kidneys. In contrast, adrenaline exerts relatively small direct effects on the blood vessels in the heart muscle, the lungs, and the brain. Adrenaline's net effect on the distribution of the blood ejected by the heart therefore is to shunt blood away from the skin and toward skeletal muscle, while maintaining blood flow to the three vital organs.

Adrenaline-induced pallor constitutes an instinctively communicated sign of terror. You turn "white with fright" and look "pale as a ghost." You seem "ashen," "wan," and "pallid," indicating not only pallor but also sickliness. Your skin becomes "pasty," and you "blanch" as the "color drains from your face." I think this is why waving a white flag is a universal sign of surrender. Terrorized people display their open palms to the adversary, as if submitting for inspection and confirmation physical evidence for the absence of aggressive intent. Although it is true that you can become "livid" with rage, more likely you "burn" or "seethe," the skin flushing hot rather than blanching cold. When enraged you "see red," not white. In Chinese, the calligraphic characters that together mean "fear" literally denote "white face."

In the Old Testament, Moses and Miriam, brother and sister, both turn "white as snow" in separate episodes when confronted directly by God. In Miriam's case,

> and the anger of the Lord was kindled against them; and he departed; and the cloud departed from off the tabernacle; and, behold, Miriam became leprous, white as snow: and Aaron looked upon Miriam, and, behold, she was leprous. and Aaron said unto Moses, Alas, my lord, I beseech thee, lay not the sin upon us, wherein we have done foolishly, and wherein we have sinned. Let her not be as one dead, of whom the flesh is half consumed when he cometh out of his mother's womb. and Moses cried unto the Lord, saying, Heal her now, O God, I beseech thee.

Miriam's sudden pallor could not have signified leprosy, in the modern medical sense of the term, because leprosy is a chronic infectious disease. Instead, the suddenness and the setting of emotional distress indicate an involuntary, automatic, instinctively communicated sign of terror. That sign would result from constriction of blood vessels in the skin, and the constriction would result from the local action of adrenaline.

At the same time and for the same reason that the skin becomes pale under the influence of adrenaline, the skin also turns cold. When the blood vessels in the skin constrict, delivery of blood to the skin decreases. Because the arteries carry blood to the skin, the largest organ of the body, at the core temperature, which typically exceeds the ambient temperature, the temperature of the skin falls toward that of the cooler environment. You develop "cold feet."

People withdrawing suddenly from an addictive drug go "cold turkey." The origin of this phrase is obscure. Perhaps it refers to simultaneous constriction of skin blood vessels and development of goose bumps, both of which are produced by adrenaline as a hormone and by locally released norepinephrine as a neurotransmitter.

Also related to withdrawal is "the shakes" (i.e., trembling). Tremulousness is another instinctively communicated sign of fear to the point of panic, appreciated by writers since ancient times. The Old Testament contains numerous references to trembling as a sign of emotional upset. For instance, Isaac trembles as an automatic, immediate response, when he realizes that he has been deceived into giving his paternal blessing to Jacob, not Esau.

Both adrenaline released from the adrenal gland and norepinephrine released from sympathetic nerves can produce this ineffectual, rhythmic skeletal muscle contraction. Terrorized people are "shaken." They "quake in their boots." To "shudder," "quiver," "quake," and "quail" mean not only to tremble but also to do so in fear or uncertainty. The terrorized person trembles as if "frozen." Indeed, I have observed that people receiving an infusion of yohimbine, which releases norepinephrine from sympathetic nerves and adrenaline from the adrenal gland, can have sufficient trembling of the jaw that the teeth chatter.

Trembling and shivering during distress both probably reflect activation of the sympathetic nervous system, since, as Cannon first showed, surgical inactivation of the adrenal glands augments, rather than prevents, shivering of animals exposed to cold. Perhaps predictably, patients with benign essential tremor can obtain relief by treatment with a beta-adrenoceptor blocker, which attenuates some of the effects of both norepinephrine and adrenaline. Musicians with stage fright or performance anxiety often take a beta-blocker before concerts. A friend of mine, a professional cellist, told me that not only did several of his colleagues take a beta-blocker prophylactically before a concert but also that he could tell when a musician had done so. The performance would be technically highly accurate but with a subtle emotional restraint. The performance would seem detached or cool.

StressDots

StressCards, StressDots, StressRulers, BioDots, StressPens, StressPoints, StressControl cards, and similar items all include a shiny black patch of plastic. You press a fingertip on the patch for a minute or so, and the color changes. Depending on the color, you are "stressed," neutral, or relaxed. You are supposed try to change the color to that corresponding to being relaxed.

StressDots and the like all work by the same principle. The key is the liquid crystal patch or dot, which changes color as the temperature changes. When you learn to control your "stress," you really learn to increase your skin temperature—a kind of biofeedback.

Why should skin temperature provide a gauge of stress? When you are in distress (later in this book I give quite a bit of attention to the distinction between stress and distress), you release adrenaline into the bloodstream. The bloodstream delivers adrenaline to all organs of the body, and, as noted previously, adrenaline tightens blood vessels in the skin. When the skin blood flow decreases due to blood vessel constriction, the skin temperature falls toward that of the usually much cooler room temperature. The StressCard reports that you are "stressed."

The Heart of the Bible

All emotions entail changes in heart functions, a fact recognized by one of the giants in the history of medicine and physiology, William Harvey—the same William Harvey who in 1628 described the circulation of the blood for the first time. In exactly the book in which he reported his monumental discovery, *On the Circulation of the Blood* (the English translation of the Latin title), he also promulgated one of the founding ideas of psychosomatic medicine and neurocardiology, "For every affection of the mind that is attended with either pain or pleasure, hope or fear, is the cause of an agitation whose influence extends to the heart" (Harvey, 1628).

The notion that the heart functions as a pump is new in medical history. For fourteen centuries, until Harvey's description of the circulation of the blood, practitioners following the teachings of Galen viewed the heart as a furnace, imbuing the blood with the "vital spirit," and not as a pump.

In the Bible, the Hebrew word for heart appears at least 776 times but virtually never as a physical organ in the body. Instead, the heart of the

Bible is essentially identical with the mind. Even today, in modern Hebrew, one way to describe paying attention is *sim lev*, or "Put forth the heart."

In Genesis 46, Jacob learns that his beloved son, Joseph, whom he had given up for dead, is not only alive but is a prince in Egypt: "and they went up out of Egypt, and came into the land of Canaan unto Jacob their father, and told him, saying, Joseph is yet alive, and he is governor over all the land of Egypt. and Jacob's heart fainted, for he believed them not. and they told him all the words of Joseph, which he had said unto them: and when he saw the wagons which Joseph had sent to carry him, the spirit of Jacob their father revived."

What does the text mean by Jacob's heart "fainting"? Jacob did not lose consciousness, because he was able to hear and see. Whatever the state he was in, it was reversed by the evidence provided by his senses about events in the outside world. His heart did not faint; rather, he became "disheartened."

In modern English we have many words and phrases that refer to the heart in the biblical sense—weak of heart, hard of heart, sick of heart, faint of heart, strong of heart, change of heart, heartfelt, take heart, take to heart, lay to heart, lose heart, have a heart, halfhearted, wholehearted, warm-hearted, coldhearted, lionhearted, tenderhearted, brokenhearted, with a heavy heart, heartfelt, heartless, heart-rending, hearten, heartwarming, dis-heartened, set one's heart on, and from the bottom of one's heart.

By now most people know that injected adrenaline increases the force and rate of the heartbeat. Every emergency that poses a global threat to the organism, from cold exposure to low blood sugar to low blood pressure from hemorrhage to emotional distress, leads to adrenaline release into the bloodstream. The concept that adrenaline functions as a powerful hor-mone in emergencies can be credited to one man—Walter B. Cannon. Many of his most important findings, including those demonstrating the role of adrenaline in the tachycardia (fast heart rate) attending emergencies, appeared in the *American Journal of Physiology* (AJP) in the 1920s. Indeed, his first article was published in the first issue of the AJP, in 1898, before he had obtained his medical degree. As Abel was the father of American pharma-cology, one can argue that Cannon was the father of American physiology.

To identify and quantify adrenaline release during stress, beginning in about 1919 Cannon developed and, over the next two decades, exploited an ingenious experimental setup. He would surgically excise the nerves supplying the heart of a laboratory animal such as a dog or cat. Then he would subject the animal to a stressor such as one of those listed above and record the heart rate response. With the nerves to the heart removed, he could deduce that if the heart rate increased in response to the perturbation, then the increase in heart rate must have resulted from the actions of a hormone. Finally, he would compare the results in an animal with intact adrenal glands with those in an animal from which he had removed the adrenal glands. From the difference in the heart rate between the two animals, he could infer further that the hormone responsible for the increase in heart rate came from the adrenal glands. Moreover, the amount of increase in the heart rate provided a measure of the amount of hormone released.

Because cutting the sympathetic nerves to the heart was an integral part of the experimental setup, Cannon could not appreciate the contribution of those nerves to regulation of the heart's functions. The experimental design also prevented him from recognizing that disabling one component of the sympathoadrenal system would activate the other compensatorily. The notion spread afterward that the sympathoadrenal system was active only in emergencies. In fact, the parasympathetic nervous system, by way of release of its neurotransmitter, acetylcholine, works in a dynamic balance with the sympathetic nervous system, by way of release of its neuro-transmitter, norepinephrine, to modulate the rate of the heartbeat, even in people at rest. Levels of adrenaline in the bloodstream, however, have not been found to correlate with resting heart rate.

The sympathetic nerve supply to the heart resembles a complex cat's cradle of strings, distributed in fibrils surrounding the heart muscle cells. Except for unusual situations such as severe exercise, in healthy people the main medium for regulation of the force and rate of the heartbeat is not adrenaline the hormone but norepinephrine and acetylcholine released from the body's "heartstrings."

At a lower blood level than that required to increase the force and rate of the heartbeat, adrenaline decreases the total peripheral resistance to blood flow in the body, mainly by relaxing blood vessels in skeletal muscle. Exactly how the same chemical, working via the same types of receptors and iden-tified intracellular mechanisms, relaxes smooth muscle in the walls of blood vessels in skeletal muscle while contracting smooth muscle in the heart remains unclear.

An overdose of adrenaline is, of course, highly dangerous. Animals given overdoses of adrenaline die of blood seeping into and clogging the air sacs in the lungs. At first, adrenaline drastically stimulates the heart, and the force and rate of the heartbeat increase remarkably. The heart muscle cells can actually rupture, just like overstrained skeletal muscle. A peculiar type of heart cell death, called contraction band necrosis, then develops. The blood backs up into the lungs because of failure of the heart to contract further— in essence, a form of overwhelming and rapidly fatal heart failure.

An Unusual Weight-lifting Feat

Several years ago, the *Guinness Book of World Records* section on weight lifting contained the following entry, "It was reported that a hysterical 123-lb. woman, Mrs. Maxwell Rogers, lifted one end of a 3,600-lb. car which, after the collapse of a jack, had fallen on top of her son at Tampa, Florida, on April 24, 1960. She cracked some vertebrae" (*Guinness Book of World Records,* 1976, 669). Apparently, Mrs. Rogers had tapped automatically into what Cannon would have called her "reservoirs of power."

Some of Cannon's papers described the direct effects of adrenaline in augmenting the force of skeletal muscle contraction or in antagonizing the fatigue effect of continual trains of electrical stimulation–induced excitation of skeletal muscle contraction. Researchers seem to have doubted and certainly subsequently lost interest in the direct effects of adrenaline in augmenting contraction of skeletal muscle and preventing skeletal muscle fatigue. But all would agree that emotionally distressing situations, such as that encountered by Mrs. Maxwell, temporarily enable people to perform extraordinary feats of strength and speed. Because these behaviors are automatic, involuntary, and unconscious, they probably importantly involve the autonomic nervous system. In his *Expression of the Emotions in Man and Animals,* originally published in 1872, Charles Darwin noted the self-reinforcing, energizing effect of some emotions. He wrote, "The excited brain gives strength to the muscles, and at the same time energy to the will" (p. 239). He also wrote: "Anger and joy are from the first exciting emotions, and they naturally lead, more especially the former, to energetic movements, which react on the heart and this again on the brain" (p. 79).

In the early 1960s, the psychologists Stanley Schachter and Jerome Singer, of Columbia University, studied effects of adrenaline on the intensity of emotional experiences. The investigators injected adrenaline into healthy subjects and either informed them correctly or misinformed them about what the side effects of the injected drug might be. Then they exposed the subjects to situations that would provoke annoyance or amusement. The subjects who had been informed correctly about the side effects of the adrenaline injection did not report feeling more emotional than the subjects who had received an injection of a placebo; however, the subjects who had been misinformed reported feeling more emotional, in terms of anger or elation depending on the cognitive circumstances, than did the subjects who had been informed correctly about what the drug would do. These findings supported the view that the intensity of emotional experience, whether negative or positive, is greater when people sense physiological activation and do not have an explanation for that activation besides the emotional experience. That is, both physiological arousal and cognitions consonant with an emotion determine together the intensity of experienced emotion.

It would not be a great leap to propose that the more intense an emotional experience, the greater the amount of involuntary, automatic, unconscious augmentation of the behavioral concomitants of that experience. If adrenaline amplified and prolonged rage, for instance, and rage involuntarily contracted skeletal muscle of the limbs, then adrenaline could augment skeletal muscle contraction and delay the onset of fatigue, even without a direct effect on the skeletal muscle.

People have an obvious capacity to regulate autonomic nervous system changes by exploiting the strong associations between autonomic and somatic activities, even if they can't regulate the autonomic nervous system effectors directly. For instance, I doubt you could raise your blood pressure by just thinking about it, but if you realized that clenching your fists tightly automatically increased blood pressure, by built-in associated increases in sympathetic nervous system outflows to blood vessels, you could easily exploit that knowledge and raise your blood pressure voluntarily by skeletal muscle contraction. Unfortunately, the opposite of this phenomenon, lowering blood pressure by skeletal muscle relaxation, has had only variable success as a treatment for hypertension. It is also true that you can use your cognitions about the force or rate of your heartbeat to gauge how emotional you are. This means that there is a potential for another positive feedback loop, which might explain why in some people, anxiety leads to fear and fear to panic, or anger leads to rage and rage to frenzy.

In modern vernacular, the word "adrenaline" connotes excitement, energy, and uncertainty, experiences that are accompanied by involuntary, unconscious, automatic, visible signs and by bodily sensations.

"Adrenaline rush" conveys these signs and sensations in a popular phrase. The cable television show "Adrenaline Rush Hour" claims to deliver 60 minutes of "hair-raising, heart pounding, nail-biting excitement." With expensive sporty cars, such as Cadillac Seville STS, Jaguar XJS, and Porsche Boxter S, "adrenaline rush comes standard." Adrenaline Rush is the official Web site of the Dax Rush Owners Club. The Dax Rush is a two-seater roadster produced by DJ Sportscars of Harlow, England. An ad for Adrenaline R/C Accessories, Ltd., which sells parts for radio-controlled model cars, asks, "Do you feel the rush?" Adrenaline Rush is also an organization that reviews and reports about roller coasters worldwide. The Adrenaline Rush 3 Pack includes three of the most "extreme" sports computer games. Adrenaline Rush is a brand of "maximum energy supplement" sold by SoBe. The drink contains taurine, D-ribose, L-carnitine, inositol, Siberian ginseng, guarana, vitamins, and caffeine, but not adrenaline itself.

The documentary movie *Adrenaline Rush: The Science of Risk* centers on the relationship of adrenaline to the thrill of risk taking. In 1485, Leonardo da Vinci sketched his idea for the world's first parachute. A half-millennium later, in the movie, a Norwegian husband-and-wife team of sports adventurers constructs a parachute according to da Vinci's design. They test it by actually jumping off the cliff of a fjord. According to the screenplay, exposing ourselves willingly to risk allows us to practice confronting fear and spurs us on to action. Risk taking therefore may have offered a survival advantage in human evolution. Of course, the movie might not have made such an assertion had da Vinci's parachute not opened.

Probably because injected adrenaline increases the force of the heartbeat, advertisements often refer to adrenaline "pumping." Adrenaline, a sports-betting Web site, caters to those for whom betting "gets your adrenaline pumping like a fearless linebacker." AdrenalineRadio offers "sports, music, and other things to get your adrenaline pumping." The Adrenaline Joe company sells sportswear for "the aggressive adrenaline pumped winners that want to wear their attitude." Rock bands such as Audio-Adrenaline, Genuine Adrenaline, Adrenaline Junkies, Adrenaline Flow, AdreNaLiNe-DJ, Bobot Adrenaline, and Philadelphia's and Fort Wayne, Indiana's Adrenaline bands have included adrenaline in their names, conveying rhythmic pumping action.

Descriptions of sports and games use adrenaline to imply an inherent thrill or risk. "24 Hours of Adrenaline" is the name of a mountain bicycle race held in the United States and Canada. Adrenaline Games runs paintball parks and advertises that it is the world's largest manufacturer of inflatable obstacles, which are used in paintball games. The Adrenaline Outdoor

Center, in Belgium, arranges aircraft events, archery, horse riding, climbing, helicopter rides, kayaking, mountain biking, paintball, obstacle courses, rafting, skiing, caving, crossbow archery, shooting, and airdrops. The Buck company makes an Adrenaline-Ti brand of titanium folding knife, Apex makes an Adrenaline bowling ball, Browning makes an Adrenaline SX 2003 twin cam bow, Jay Borderou makes an Adrenaline pro skateboard deck, and Brooks makes Adrenaline GTS sneakers. Adrenaline Junkies describes itself as a "diverse group of men and women who thrive on excitement and adventure. If you are the kind of person who would rather go whitewater rafting than lounge in the neighbors' pool or if the idea of a paintball game interests you, then you may be an Adrenaline Junkie." Adrenaline Air Sports of Blacksburg, Virginia, offers the thrill of free-fall skydiving. Adrenaline Zone operates video game parlors. Adrenaline Freaks Track Day Excursions, LLC, "allows licensed motorcycle riders and racers the opportunity to get out on a professional track without the worries of everyday street riding." Adrenaline also is a brand of football trading cards, and Pacific Adrenaline is a brand of hockey trading cards. Fleer prints Adrenaline trading cards as "the first trading cards to feature extreme athletes." They also print a line of Feminine Adrenaline cards featuring female professional basketball players. The American Adrenaline Company arranges rafting trips in the ominous sounding Frank Church River of No Return Wilderness, in Central Idaho.

Since adrenaline doesn't penetrate the blood-brain barrier, little of adrenaline in the bloodstream actually reaches most sites in the central nervous system. Then how can adrenaline produce such clear effects on the intensity of emotional experiences? One way may be via the cognitions people have about the state of their inner world, such as rapid pulse rate, increased force of the heartbeat, pallor, sweating, trembling, and increased ventilation. According to this view, treatment with a drug that blocks these effects, without altering adrenaline levels themselves, could prevent the emotional-physical positive feedback loop. As noted above, such treatment does seem to work, sometimes remarkably well, in people with performance anxiety or stage fright. It is also possible that high catecholamine levels could alter levels of chemicals that do penetrate the blood-brain barrier; or that circulating adrenaline can reach some central nervous system sites because of local deficiencies in the blood-brain barrier.

The 23rd Psalm

Psalm 23, a triumph of literature, has at its core the following passage.

> Yea, though I walk through the valley of the shadow of death, I fear no evil: for thou art with me; thy rod and thy staff they comfort me.
>
> Thou preparest a table before me in the presence of mine enemies: thou anointest my head with oil; my cup runneth over.

How would setting a table in the presence of enemies relate to the theme of the psalm? About a century ago, Walter B. Cannon drew blood from a cat exposed to a barking dog. This evoked release into the cat's blood of a substance that relaxed a strip of gut tissue but contracted a strip of blood vessel tissue. The pattern of relaxation of gut tissue but contraction of blood vessel tissue was the first experimental finding indicating adrenaline release by emotional distress. Because adrenaline decreases the ability of gut smooth muscle to contract, and given the inability to digest during distress, if you were able to eat in the presence of your enemies, you could not be distressed. The passage about setting a table in the presence of enemies therefore does indeed fit with the theme of the psalm: Because the "Lord is my shepherd . . . I fear no evil."

Several instances occur in the Old Testament narrative in which the distressed individual cannot eat. Aaron is unable to eat the sacrifice, his priestly duty, after his sons' death. You will read later about the swelling of the belly of the adulteress upon ingestion of the "water of bitterness," in the biblical trial by ordeal. Hannah cannot eat when tormented by Peninah, Jonathan eats no food after Saul obsesses about David, Ahab does not eat out of jealousy of Elijah, and Job in his suffering "abhorreth bread, and his soul dainty meat" (33:20).

A Little Pain Can't Hurt

At the beginning of the preceding section, in the anecdote about the mother who lifted a car off her child, the entry about this feat of weight lifting in the *Guinness Book of World Records* mentioned that as a consequence of extraordinary straining she had suffered several cracked vertebrae. We all know that emotion-related feats of strength and speed are associated with remarkable loss of the sensation of pain. In scientific jargon this has been called "stress-induced analgesia." This is why the woman didn't feel the pain, but how?

Pain causes adrenaline release from the adrenal gland, as Cannon showed about a century ago. A difficult issue—which remains incompletely understood—is what, if anything, adrenaline or other members of its chemical family have to do with the perception of pain.

For one thing, as noted above, little if any of adrenaline in the circulation enters the central nervous system, and yet injected adrenaline increases the intensity of any emotion. Some of this augmentation may result not from a direct effect of adrenaline on the brain but from indirect effects, such as the individual's sense of a thumping heartbeat, which could be interpreted as something having gone very awry in the inner world. The individual might then respond to that perception, such as in terms of the ability to cope.

In conscious people, pain has an affective component. That is, pain *hurts*. People don't want to be in pain. It interferes with daily activities and incites a worried search for the cause. Over time, chronic pain can become a pathophysiological entity itself, a disorder in its own right, almost regardless of the original source of the noxious stimulation. Another contribution of adrenaline release in the setting of painful stimulation might be to enhance the experience of distress.

Adrenaline, or members of its chemical family, may alter the experience of pain by occupying alpha-2 adrenoceptors in the spinal cord. These receptors appear to contribute to a "gate" for transmitting pain impulses up to the brain. The likely source of the chemical transmitter that would occupy these alpha-2 adrenoceptors would not be circulating adrenaline, or even norepinephrine released as a neurotransmitter from sympathetic nerves, but rather norepinephrine released from nerves that descend from locus ceruleus cells in the brainstem. As you will read later, the locus ceruleus, a small cluster of cells in the back of the pons, is the main source of norepinephrine in the brain. Locus ceruleus cells also send widely ramifying fibers throughout the brain, probably contributing to psychoemotional phenomena such as vigilance and the memory of distressing events.

The main known effectors for pain sensation are endogenous opioids. Behaviors such as exercise increase occupation of opioid receptors in the brain, explaining the sense of elation people feel after a workout. In response to painful stimuli, the brain releases opioids that apparently limit the severity of experienced pain, because blockade of opioid receptors augments the amount of pain for a given amount of stimulation. Because of the augmentation of pain, blockade of opioid receptors also augments the release of adrenaline. Finally, stimulation of the adrenal gland releases not only adrenaline but also endogenous painkiller opiates called enkephalins.

Before dental surgery, dentists often include adrenaline in the local anesthetic, not only because this decreases bleeding but also because it prolongs the anesthesia time. Injection of adrenaline with the local anesthetic always produces large, physiologically active increases in circulating adrenaline levels. Adrenaline injection actually inhibits, rather than augments, responses of circulating levels of the body's opioid, beta-endorphin, in the setting of wisdom tooth extraction. How and why injection of adrenaline would inhibit the opioid response is unknown.

Lose Weight Fast!

Injected adrenaline evokes several effects that, taken together, rapidly mobilize metabolic fuels from storage sites and burn calories. The rate of metabolism in the body as a whole increases; oxygen consumption by the heart increases; body temperature increases; stores of glycogen in the liver are broken down into the metabolic fuel, glucose; and fats are converted to free fatty acids, generating heat in the process.

Several effective weight loss drugs share the effect of augmenting occupation of receptors for catecholamines, both inside and outside the brain. Amphetamines such as phentermine increase release and inhibit reuptake of catecholamines, suppressing appetite and increasing metabolic rate. Phentermine, prescribed with fenfluramine, constituted the notorious "Phen-Fen," which, while effective in promoting weight loss in dieters, produced harmful heart and lung side effects. Phenylpropanolamine (PPE), another sympathomimetic amine, was the active ingredient in many over-the-counter weight loss drugs, until PPE also was removed from the market. Conversely, treatment with beta-adrenoceptor blockers, which inhibit adrenaline effects, may promote weight gain. Recent research has indicated a statistical association between polymorphisms of beta-adrenoceptor subtypes and obesity; and weight loss drugs are being tested now that work by stimulating particular beta-adrenoceptor subtypes.

Sweet Urine

The seventeenth-century English physician Thomas Willis may have been the first scientist to note that patients with diabetes excrete sweet urine. The sweetness results from high blood levels of glucose, which is a sugar. Adrenaline is one of the three main hormones that regulate blood glucose levels, the other two being insulin and glucagon. Injection of adrenaline increases the blood glucose level by accelerating the production of glucose from its storage form, glycogen, in the liver and by inhibiting the release and actions of insulin. It was Claude Bernard, the originator of the concept of the inner world, who first showed that glucose in the bloodstream is derived not from dietary intake of sugar but from its production within body organs. Bernard isolated glycogen from liver tissue and demonstrated its conversion to glucose in the liver (Bernard, 1957, 164).

Bernard wondered whether release of glucose from the liver into the bloodstream would depend on nerves supplying the liver. He tried stimulating the vagus nerve, but this produced no effect on blood glucose. In 1849 he conducted an experiment in which he punctured the spot in the brainstem from which the vagus nerve emanated. This produced hyperglycemia. Within an hour the urine contained abundant sugar. Diabetes by *piqûre*, or puncture, has been associated with Bernard's name ever since (Olmsted and Olmsted, 1952, 66–67). Bernard thought that he had discovered a neuronal cause of diabetes. To demonstrate that trauma to the floor of the fourth ventricle released glucose from the liver by way of the vagus nerves, he cut them before the puncture. To his dismay, the puncture still produced hyperglycemia. He had to reject the notion of diabetes from vagus nerve stimulation, and he inferred—correctly—that the nervous system contributed to the release of glucose by the liver. He then found that cutting the spinal cord just above the site of exit of the splanchnic nerves, which carry preganglionic fibers of the sympathetic nervous system, did abolish the increase in blood glucose levels consequent to puncturing the floor of the fourth ventricle. He reasoned that *piqûre* diabetes resulted from stimulation of sympathetic nerves supplying the liver. This was long before the discovery of the sympathetic nervous supply of fibers to the adrenal gland. Now we know that *piqûre* diabetes probably mainly results from the effects of adrenaline released into the bloodstream; however, sympathetic nerves to the liver probably also contribute.

Decades later, deficiency of insulin was shown to be the culprit in juvenile-onset diabetes; however, ironically, modern research about insulin resistance in adult-onset diabetes has returned to the concept, based on Bernard's experiment, that the brain does play a role.

Neuronal Soda Pop

This section describes the stations on the catecholamine assembly line—the steps in catecholamine biosynthesis—and the fate of catecholamines in the body.

Make Your Own DOPA

To people with Parkinson disease, DOPA (also called L-DOPA and levodopa), the key component of Sinemet, is a miracle drug. Within minutes, DOPA converts a shuffling, tremulous, slow-moving person with head bowed to a vigorous, upright, normally moving person with head held erect. I will never forget the first time I witnessed this phenomenon, while I was a medical student. At the beginning of the lecture, the professor introduced a patient with Parkinson disease who had not yet taken his DOPA that day. Slowly, unsteadily, and with help the patient made his way up the steps of the amphitheater and exited the doors at the top. He took his DOPA outside. At the end of the lecture the professor reintroduced him. The patient literally bounded down the steps, and when he reached the lectern he turned around swiftly to the assembled students, a broad grin on his face. The audience erupted in applause.

In the body, all the catecholamines come from DOPA, and the DOPA comes from tyrosine, an amino acid. Amino acids are the building blocks of proteins. Tyrosine is an amino acid that is not a catechol. (If you don't remember what catechols look like, see the previous section about catechols looking like the head of a cat.) Tyrosine is converted to DOPA by the actions of an enzyme, a protein that speeds up a particular chemical process. The enzyme that speeds up the conversion of tyrosine to DOPA is tyrosine hydroxylase (fig. 25).

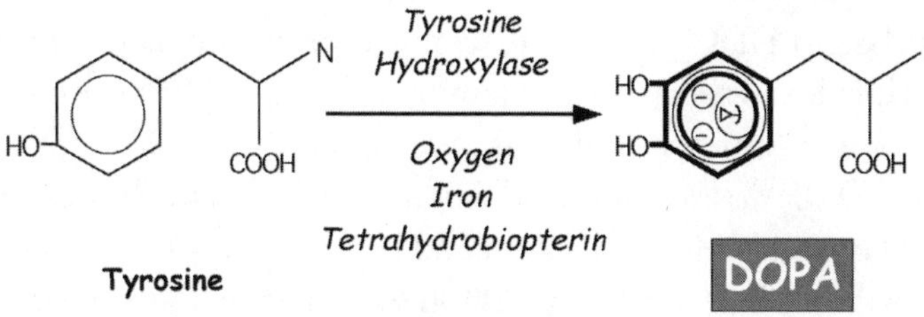

Fig. 25. The first step in production of adrenaline is conversion of tyrosine to DOPA, a catechol. See the cat's head?

For tyrosine hydroxylase to work requires cofactors. These are oxygen, iron, and tetrahydrobiopterin, abbreviated BH_4. BH_4 is a very important cofactor. If you can't make it or recycle it, you are doomed. If you have read the label on a can of diet soda pop that contains the sweetener, aspartame, you have noticed that people with a disease called phenylketonuria (PKU) should be careful drinking the soda. This is because people with classic PKU have a deficiency of phenylalanine hydroxylase, an enzyme that converts the amino acid phenylalanine to tyrosine. Because of this deficiency, ingesting foods rich in phenylalanine can lead to a buildup of phenylalanine, and too much of it is toxic, especially in infants and children. Aspartame is broken down to phenylalanine in the body, and so drinking the diet soda pop theoretically could cause damage. For phenylalanine hydroxylase to work requires exactly the same cofactor, BH_4, that tyrosine hydroxylase requires to work. An inability to recycle BH_4 causes an atypical form of PKU, in which even restricting phenylalanine does not protect the infant from developing a neurodegenerative disease, with death coming on in childhood. Deficiency of enzymes required to produce BH_4 also can produce a different pediatric neurodegenerative disease, or else a movement disorder called DOPA-responsive dystonia.

If you are a healthy adult, then you are making your own DOPA, all the time. The levels attained in the bloodstream, however, are about one-thousandth of those required to treat Parkinson disease.

Cat-a-COLA-means

The next step in producing adrenaline is the conversion of DOPA, which is a catechol but not a catecholamine, to dopamine, the grandfather in the catecholamine family. This step takes place in many types of cells, not just cells with the rest of the machinery required to store, release, and recycle catecholamines. To make dopamine from DOPA requires the enzyme, L-aromatic amino-acid decarboxylase (LAAAD, sometimes called DOPA decarboxylase, or DDC), and the cofactor pyridoxal phosphate, which is vitamin B_6. (Incidentally, the word "vitamin" comes from "vital amine," even though several vitamins, including B_6, are not amines at all.)

Because DOPA is an amino acid, it is taken up from the bloodstream by virtually all types of cells in the body, and because many cell types, such as kidney and liver cells, contain LAAAD, in several organs dopamine is made from the DOPA after uptake of the DOPA from the bloodstream. The same ability may hold true in cells of the brain. This may help explain how

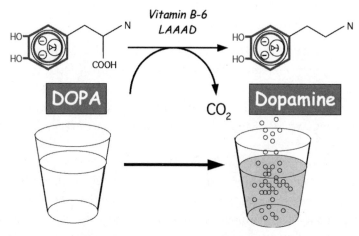

Fig. 26. The process of producing dopamine from DOPA results in formation of carbon dioxide, the bubbles in soda pop.

a patient with Parkinson disease, who has a severe loss of cells that store and release dopamine as a chemical messenger, can still have some benefit from taking levodopa.

A drug called carbidopa is a catechol that blocks LAAAD. Carbidopa in the bloodstream does not cross the blood-brain barrier. This means that if a patient were to take DOPA with carbidopa, the DOPA would not be converted as efficiently to dopamine by LAAAD outside the brain, whereas DOPA that entered the brain could be turned into dopamine by LAAAD in brain cells. The combination of DOPA with carbidopa therefore improves the efficiency of levodopa treatment for Parkinson disease, while decreasing the toxic effects from too much dopamine being made outside the brain. The main such toxic effect is vomiting. This explains the brand name for the levodopa-carbidopa combination to treat Parkinson disease, Sinemet, from the Latin words for "without vomiting."

The conversion of DOPA to dopamine involves cleaving off carbon dioxide from the molecule of DOPA. If you were to carry out this chemical reaction in a glass of water, the carbon dioxide gas would bubble up to the surface, like the effervescence in seltzer (fig. 26). Maybe this will help you remember that by this reaction, DOPA turns into a cat-a-COLA-mean. (Actually, because of the rapid oxidation of dopamine in solution to form a tan breakdown product, you might better think about ginger ale.)

The Case of the Depressed Dog

The third step in making adrenaline is the most complex, because it requires not only a specific enzyme and cofactors but also physical sequestration of dopamine into particular organelles, tiny bubbles called vesicles, within catecholamine-producing cells. It is only within vesicles that norepinephrine, the main chemical messenger of the sympathetic nervous system, is made in sympathetic nerves.

By the same mechanism, norepinephrine is produced in particular cells in the brain. This is how the story turns to the case of the depressed dog. I was testing whether a particular chemical our group had developed at the NIH, an analog of dopamine tagged with radioactivity, could successfully visualize sympathetic nerves by a special type of nuclear medicine scan called a PET scan. To test this idea, I ordered that a dog receive some reserpine. Reserpine exerts a highly specific effect in the body. It prevents uptake of amines, including catecholamines, into storage vesicles in sympathetic nerves. If the hypothesis were correct, then treatment with reserpine would prevent uptake of the radioactive dopamine into the vesicles and therefore prevent visualization of the sympathetic nerves.

After the testing, the dog was returned to its kennel. Later I received a phone call from a very concerned veterinarian. The dog lay in a corner, listless, almost motionless. Its tail was tucked underneath it, and the dog would not wag its tail when a caretaker approached. It seemed poorly responsive, it would not eat, and its blood pressure was low. The dog turned out not to be ill, in the sense of, say, being in septic shock from an infection. Instead it had a form of acute depression and dysautonomia, both of which could be ascribed to reserpine. Blocking uptake into vesicles prevented conservative recycling of the norepinephrine stored in those vesicles. Normally, norepinephrine leaks from them into the cytoplasm ("cell juice"), but what leaks gets taken back up. Because of the inability to recycle the norepinephrine, the sympathetic nerves rapidly became depleted of the neurotransmitter. This was the basis for the low blood pressure. Indeed, the leaf of the plant from which reserpine was isolated, *Rauwolfia serpentina*, was the first successful drug treatment for hypertension. The same blockade of amine recycling took hold in the animal's brain, causing depletion of norepinephrine, dopamine, and serotonin. As you will learn later, depletion of these amines in the brain produces several important effects on behavior and mood. Depletion of dopamine causes decreased spontaneous movement, decreased oral intake, and possibly a tendency to depression. Depletion of norepinephrine probably decreases vigilance behavior and may also tend to depression. Depletion of serotonin probably also tends to depression. Depletion of all three chemicals in the brain probably produced depressed affect in the dog.

Kinky Hair Disease

Dopamine-beta-hydroxylase (DBH) is an enzyme that speeds up the conversion of dopamine to norepinephrine. This particular enzyme contains copper, and the activity of the enzyme depends on copper. Several years ago, a colleague asked whether the fact that DBH is a copper enzyme might prove useful in the diagnosis of a disease called Menkes disease or "kinky hair disease." Menkes disease is a genetic disease. A baby with this disease can seem normal at birth, except for peculiar hair that is a light tan-orange and kinky and exhibits twisted hair shafts. The baby soon fails to meet milestones of development, deteriorates neurologically, and dies in childhood.

Menkes disease occurs only in boys. The mutation that causes the disease is on the X chromosome. A mutation is like a typo in the genetic encyclopedia. The encyclopedia consists of two sets of 23 volumes each. The last two volumes are the same size in girls (each volume is X), whereas the last two differ in size in boys (the larger volume X, the smaller Y). In boys with the mutation on their single X chromosome, the disease is expressed, but in girls with the mutation on one of their two X chromosomes, the disease is not expressed, because the other X chromosome is normal. If a mother who carried the mutation on one of her X chromosomes were pregnant with a boy, the chances would be 50-50 that the boy would have the disease (if the X chromosome from the mother had the mutation) or would not have the disease (if his X chromosome from the mother lacked the mutation). Unfortunately, kinky hair disease cannot be diagnosed by the usual prenatal testing. Meanwhile, in at-risk pregnancies, it is important to diagnose the disease soon after birth, because if the baby had the disease, and if the disease were caused by a particular mutation, then the baby could respond to injections of copper, but the treatment must begin within a few weeks of birth.

Consistent with the requirement of copper for normal DBH activity, the plasma of at-risk babies who actually have Menkes disease contains more dopamine than normal for a given amount of norepinephrine. As shown in the diagram (fig. 27), patients with Menkes disease all have a neurochemical pattern indicating low DBH activity. Detecting this pattern has so far

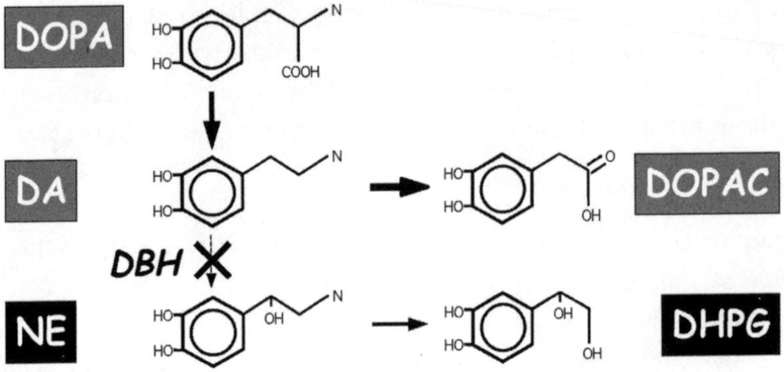

Fig. 27. Any disorder or disease associated with decreased dopamine-beta-hydroxylase (DBH) activity causes a buildup of DOPA and dopamine compared with norepinephrine and DHPG.

proven perfectly sensitive and specific in diagnosing the disease in at-risk newborns.

Menkes disease is not the only disease that involves decreased DBH activity. Rarely, adults with orthostatic hypotension (a fall in blood pressure when the patient stands up) lack DBH activity because of a problem with the gene for this enzyme. As discussed later, patients with DBH deficiency are unable to produce norepinephrine in sympathetic nerves. Other than orthostatic hypotension, surprisingly little else seems wrong in these patients, despite the fact that mice with genetic deficiency of the same enzyme do not survive even to birth. No one has resolved this paradox so far.

Production of adrenaline and other catecholamines requires some vitamins and minerals. Dopamine in the body comes from DOPA. To make DOPA requires the mineral iron. Production of dopamine from DOPA, and therefore production of all the catecholamines, depends on the availability of pyridoxal phosphate, which is vitamin B_6. The conversion of dopamine to norepinephrine in the body requires ascorbic acid, which is vitamin C, as well as the minerals, magnesium and copper. "Stress formulas" vary in their contents of these minerals, but they all contain vitamins B_6 and C.

The Search for the Omega Sign

Once produced in the vesicles in sympathetic nerves, norepinephrine is released from the nerve terminals by a process called exocytosis. Exocytosis is the key element in the theory of chemical neurotransmission, first proposed by T. R. Elliott in 1904 (*J. Physiol.* 31:xx–xxi). Elliott was a student of

Langley, the same Langley who coined the phrase, "autonomic nervous system."

Elliott had noted that stimulation of sympathetic nerves and injection of adrenal gland extract produced similar effects in the body. In a stroke of genius, he hypothesized that the similarity resulted from a chemical like adrenaline actually being released from the nerves and acting on nearby cells. In a brief note published in the *Journal of Physiology*, he wrote: "a mechanism developed out of the muscle cell, in response to its union with the synapsing sympathetic fibre, the function of which is to receive and transform the nervous impulse. Adrenalin(e) might then be a chemical stimulant liberated on each occasion when the impulse arrives at the periphery."

It took until the early 1920s for experimental proof of this concept to emerge, and the scientist who provided that proof, Otto Loewi, received a Nobel Prize in 1936 for his discovery of the first neurotransmitter, acetylcholine. It was not until much later that scientists considered how neurotransmitters actually are released from nerves.

The theory of exocytosis is fairly simple to state but has proven devilishly difficult to test. According to the theory chemical neurotransmission results from physical movement of the bubblelike vesicles containing the neurotransmitter toward the cell membrane, fusion of the vesicle membrane with the cell membrane, poration at the site of fusion of the two membranes, and entry of the contents of the vesicles into the fluid outside the cell. Among those contents is the neurotransmitter, which diffuses a short way to reach receptors on the membrane of the target cells.

One of the ways to test the theory of exocytosis would be by direct visualization. If the vesicle membrane actually fused with the cell membrane, and a hole formed at their junction, then if one looked under an electron microscope at the nerve terminal, one should see little "omega signs" or see the vesicle contents coming through the cell membrane (fig. 28). Only relatively recently has this type of direct visualization come about by highly sophisticated techniques. One of the mysteries so far has been the very small percentage of vesicles in which the contents are actually found poking their way through the membrane surface.

A Better Inner World through Recycling

Several types of nerve cells recycle their chemical messengers. Sympathetic nerves possess an ingenious processing mechanism that simultaneously inactivates the released chemical messenger norepinephrine, recycles the norep-

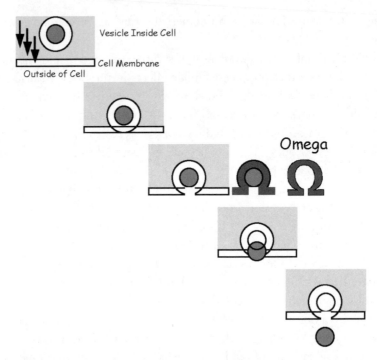

Fig. 28. The theory of exocytosis predicts that if you looked at a nerve releasing its chemical messenger, you would see objects that looked like the Greek letter omega.

inephrine, limits its actions spatially to a small volume, and modulates the amount of delivery of the message to the target cells for a given rate of release. The processing mechanism is reuptake of the neurotransmitter from the fluid outside the cells (extracellular fluid). For discovering the role of reuptake, rather than simple metabolic breakdown by an enzyme, in inactivation of neurotransmitters, Julius Axelrod shared the Nobel Prize for Physiology or Medicine in 1970. He carried out this work at the NIH in the same Building 10 where I sit.

The reuptake process by nerves is relatively specific for the particular neurotransmitter. One might even define the type of nerve cell by the neurotransmitter it takes up. For the catecholamines, norepinephrine, adrenaline, and dopamine, reuptake takes place by a process originally called "uptake-1," in contrast with "uptake-2" by cells other than nerve cells. Now we know that uptake-1 involves at least two different transporters, which physically transport the neurotransmitter molecules into the cells. The transporter for norepinephrine is called the cell membrane norepinephrine transporter, or NET. The transporter for dopamine is called the dopamine transporter, or DAT. One of the peculiarities of the functioning of these transporters is that, although dopamine is more avidly taken up by the DAT than norepinephrine is, dopamine is also more avidly taken up by the NET than norepinephrine is. From the point of view of nerves that release norepinephrine, dopamine acts mainly or only as an intermediary in the production of norepinephrine, so maybe there would be an advantage to the nerves sopping up any dopamine that happens to escape into the fluid around the cells, to maximize availability for norepinephrine production; or maybe dopamine uptake via the NET provides an alternative method for production of norepinephrine besides synthesis from scratch within the nerves, because, as noted above, dopamine can be made in and enter the bloodstream from a variety of nonneuronal cell types. We exploited this neurochemical quirk in developing a form of dopamine tagged with radioactivity to visualize sympathetic nerves in people by PET scanning, as you will read about later. The sympathetic nerves take up the radioactive dopamine via the NET.

The recycling process is completed by reuptake of catecholamines from the cytoplasm into storage vesicles, by a different and less selective transporter, called the vesicular monoamine transporter, or VMAT. Because of the NET, the concentration of norepinephrine in the cytoplasm normally exceeds that in the fluid around noradrenergic cells by manyfold, and because of the VMAT, the concentration of norepinephrine in the vesicles normally exceeds that in the cytoplasm also by manyfold. As a result of these processes acting in series, the concentration of norepinephrine in the storage vesicles normally is several thousand times the concentration in the extracellular fluid. Now that's recycling!

At least five types of perturbation interfere with catecholamine recycling. Every one exerts profound effects both inside the brain and out (fig. 29). The first is cocaine, which is a classic inhibitor of uptake-1. The heart depends heavily on uptake-1 to inactivate norepinephrine released from local sympathetic nerves, and cocaine administration can evoke severe heart problems, such as heart failure and even sudden cardiac death in apparently healthy people. A notorious example was Len Bias, the University of Maryland basketball star who died of the cardiac toxic effects of cocaine. The second is the class of drugs for depression called tricyclic antidepressants. Some tricyclics are desipramine, imipramine, nortriptyline, and amitriptyline (brand names Norpramin, Tofranil, Pamelor, and Mylan). Another

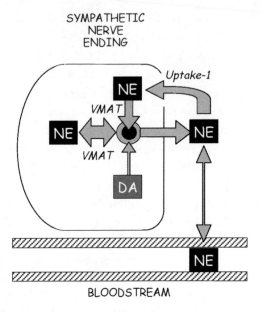

Fig. 29. Sympathetic nerves recycle norepinephrine.

antidepressant that is not a tricyclic but is thought to work at least partly by inhibiting the NET is venlafaxine (Effexor). In general, tricyclic antidepressants inhibit uptake-1 and also decrease sympathetic nervous system outflows from the brain. As a result, they do not produce nearly as great an increase in the delivery of norepinephrine to its receptors in the heart as cocaine does. The third is a type of drug that blocks the VMAT. Reserpine is the classic example of this type of drug. By depleting the stored chemical messengers outside the brain, reserpine usually drops blood pressure, and by depleting messengers inside the brain, it can produce depressed mood, as illustrated in the case of the depressed dog discussed previously. The fourth is a genetic mutation of the NET. This has been described so far in only one family. Because of decreased ability to recycle norepinephrine, people with this mutation have excessive delivery of norepinephrine to its receptors in the heart in situations that activate sympathetic nervous system outflows. One of these situations is simply standing up, and so NET deficiency constitutes a rare cause of postural tachycardia syndrome (POTS), in which an inability to tolerate prolonged standing (orthostatic intolerance) is coupled with an excessive heart rate response to standing (postural tachycardia). Among other findings in POTS with NET deficiency is a predisposition to panic, possibly associated with excessive delivery of norepinephrine to receptors in the brain. The fifth is excessive "leakiness" of the storage vesicles. Normally, because of the enormous concentration of norepineph-rine in storage vesicles, norepinephrine leaks passively out of the vesicles at a high rate into the cytoplasm. Correspondingly, however, by way of the efficient VMAT, the norepinephrine is taken back up into the vesicles. For the VMAT to function requires a concentration gradient for hydrogen ion between the cytoplasm and the inside of the vesicles, with the vesicle con-tents acidic. In any situation in which the cytoplasm becomes acidic, such as anoxia (lack of oxygen), there is an increased net leakage from the vesi-cles, which taken to an extreme can deplete sympathetic nerves of their neu-rotransmitter and thereby disable them. This may help explain why patients in shock can rather suddenly have a vicious cycle of fall in blood pressure, buildup of acid in the bloodstream, and loss of sympathetic cardiovascular tone, leading to worsening of the fall in blood pressure and death within minutes.

Of Mice and Men and Wine and Cheese

Although catecholamines are recycled efficiently in sympathetic nerves, a small percent of norepinephrine and dopamine present in the cytoplasm of sympathetic nerves undergoes metabolic breakdown by a process that is sped up by the enzyme, monoamine oxidase (MAO) (fig. 30).

In the brain, MAO plays key roles in mood. Drugs that inhibit MAO and that get into the brain are effective antidepressants. Conversely, genetic deficiency of MAO activity causes extraordinary hyperactivity and aggres-

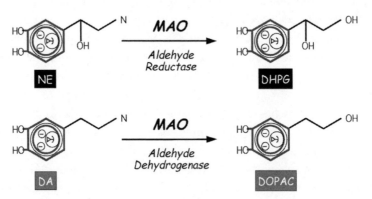

Fig. 30. The enzyme, MAO, plays a key role in the metabolic breakdown of norepinephrine and dopamine.

siveness in mice and men. A Dutch family with this deficiency attained notoriety for antisocial behavior, murder, and violent rape.

I use the phrase "mice and men" because both murine and human MAO deficiency produces severe aggressive behavioral disorders, but only in the males. The gene for MAO is present on the X chromosome. You may recall from the section on kinky hair disease that in boys with a mutation on their single X chromosome, the disease is expressed, but in girls with the same mutation on one of their two X chromosomes, the disease is not expressed and the girls are asymptomatic carriers. This means that in the family with "bad seed" from mutation of the MAO gene, none of the girls would have the disorder, but half of the at-risk boys would.

No discussion of MAO would be complete without wine and cheese. Red wine and hard cheeses contain abundant tyramine. Tyramine is an indirectly acting sympathomimetic amine. That is, it doesn't exert effects by itself, but it increases release of norepinephrine from sympathetic nerves. The released norepinephrine increases the blood pressure and the force of the heartbeat. Ordinarily, relatively little of ingested tyramine makes its way to the bloodstream because of an effective gut-blood barrier made up of a variety of enzymes, one of which is MAO. Patients taking an MAO inhibitor have a relatively permissive gut-blood barrier for substances that normally would be broken down by MAO in the gut, one of which is tyramine. Sympathetic nerves take up tyramine, by way of the cell membrane norepinephrine transporter, the NET, discussed in the preceding section. This means that the tyramine that has penetrated the gut-blood barrier can get into the sympathetic nerves. Once inside the nerves, tyramine in the cytoplasm gets taken up into the vesicles, by way of the vesicular monoamine transporter (VMAT), and once inside the vesicles, tyramine accelerates leakage of norepinephrine from the vesicles, possibly by alkalinizing them and decreasing the hydrogen ion gradient required for concentration of norepinephrine in the vesicles. Norepinephrine then builds up in the cytoplasm and can go backward through the NET to reach the fluid surrounding the cells or leave the vesicles that have fused with the membrane surface and have the "omega sign" opening to the extracellular fluid. By these mechanisms, norepinephrine is delivered to its receptors on cardiovascular cells, and the blood pressure and force of the heartbeat increase. In people taking an MAO inhibitor, such as for depression, ingestion of tyramine therefore can produce a paroxysmal increase in blood pressure or evoke an abnormal heart rhythm. If you were taking an MAO inhibitor for depression, you wouldn't want to attend a wine-and-cheese party.

There are two genes for MAO near one another on the X chromosome, and there are two corresponding forms of MAO, called MAO-A and MAO-B. Sympathetic nerves express only MAO-A, whereas many other cell types express both forms. It is thought that the enzymatic gut-blood barrier for tyramine depends mainly on MAO-A. Theoretically, the "cheese effect" would apply only to drugs that inhibit MAO-A or inhibit both forms of MAO. In particular, selegiline (also called l-deprenyl, with brand name Eldepryl), which is used to treat Parkinson disease is a relatively selective MAO-B inhibitor, and so it is much less likely to cause a cheese reaction than drugs that inhibit MAO-A.

The Getaway Car Analogy

Suppose you were a bank robber and you parked your getaway car at the curb outside the bank. Would you keep the car idling? Of course you would. If you shut the car down, then it would take longer for you to get away just when you had to, and if the ignition happened to fail at the crucial time, that would be the end of the whole operation and your career as a bank robber. Suppose you decided not to rob the bank on that particular day. Would it have been worth it to keep the getaway car in idle? Of course. You would certainly have needed it, had you decided to rob the bank. What if you decided to "case the joint" for a whole week, and you had to put gas into the car's tank. It still would be worthwhile to keep the car idling. Now what if you decided that, after several months of reconnaissance and many fuel refills, you aren't gong to rob the bank after all. Just from the wear and tear of having had the car in idle all that time, the engine's life span probably would be shortened because of a buildup of harmful deposits inside. If the added fuel contained a contaminant, this could have accelerated the buildup of gunk. If the car had been manufactured with a defective catalytic converter, or a slightly misaligned piston, this also could have accelerated the accumulation of gunk. If the engine oil, even if formulated according to the original manufacturer's specifications, tended to break down with prolonged heat and pressure, this would promote gunk buildup too. If you waited long enough, and there were enough built-in and added-on harmful factors at work, so much grunge might build up that the engine would

REAL LIFE

ANALOGY

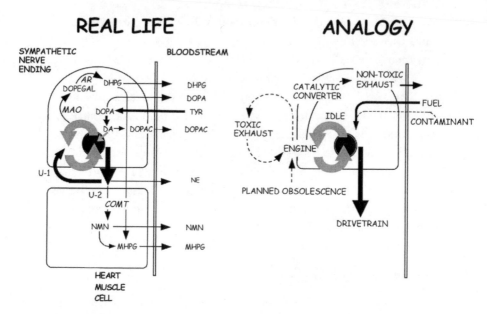

Fig. 31. Catecholamine systems of the body are like a getaway car.

fail entirely. Even if none of these factors alone would have ever caused a problem in the normal life span of the car, together they could have built up sufficient gunk to kill the engine. Despite the extraordinarily complex design and manufacture of the car, and its obvious importance for you, you might well decide to tow it to the junkyard and sell it for scrap. Nevertheless, you could still decide in the end that it had been worthwhile to keep that car idling at the curb.

The getaway car analogy applies to several topics in this book, including Darwinian medicine and mechanisms of development of chronic diseases of the elderly. For now, the analogy applies to the "vesicular engines" in the sympathetic nerves (fig. 31). The brain keeps those engines in idle all the time, ready to get you away when an emergency such as a fight-or-flight situation requires you to floor the accelerator and escape. Having that engine idling ensures that you can release norepinephrine in abundance on short notice.

There is no way you can recycle norepinephrine perfectly. Some of what leaks from the vesicles into the cytoplasm undergoes metabolic breakdown by enzymes, including monoamine oxidase. These enzymes literally are catalytic converters. One prediction from the getaway car analogy is that if a person had a genetic change resulting in decreased activity of one of those enzymes, then toxic by-products of the incomplete breakdown of catecholamines could lead to sufficient buildup of "gunk" inside cells so that they wouldn't work right any more, or even die. The high rate of leakage of norepinephrine from vesicles into the cytoplasm, and the high rate of re-uptake back into the vesicles by way of the VMAT, would at first seem like a waste of energy. What good could this possibly do, as opposed to having a stable pool of norepinephrine that doesn't leak? My colleague at the NIH, Graeme Eisenhofer, came up with an insightful explanation, which he calls "gearing down." If there were a stable pool of vesicles, then it can be shown mathematically that an emergency requiring sustained norepinephrine release would rapidly dissipate that pool. It would be impossible for synthesis of norepinephrine from scratch (the rate of which can only about double) to keep up with the irreversible loss of norepinephrine from the tissue (the rate of which can go up manyfold). But if there were continuous leakage of norepinephrine from the vesicles, and continuous replacement of the norepinephrine by ongoing synthesis, then the organism could maintain a high rate of release of norepinephrine for a much longer time.

The Atavistic Catecholamine

So far, this chapter has dealt mainly with adrenaline, the hormone released by the adrenal gland, and with norepinephrine, the neurotransmitter released by sympathetic nerves. What of dopamine, the third member of the catecholamine family? Until relatively recently, dopamine was thought to function merely as an intermediary in the production of norepinephrine and adrenaline. Beginning in the 1950s and 1960s, researchers began to obtain evidence that dopamine does exert effects in its own right, both inside and outside the brain. For the discovery that dopamine is a neurotransmitter in the brain and that loss of dopamine in a particular neurochemical pathway in the brain causes the movement disorder in Parkinson disease, Arvid Carlsson of Sweden shared the 2000 Nobel Prize for Physiology or Medicine.

While Carlsson was doing this work, Leon Goldberg, an American, proposed the existence of specific receptors for dopamine. These receptors are especially prominent in kidney tubule cells. Goldberg found that stimulation of dopamine receptors in the kidney increases excretion of sodium and

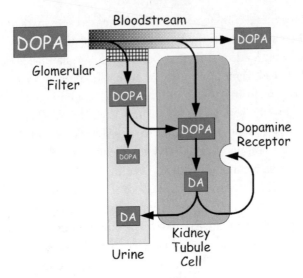

Fig. 32. In the kidneys, dopamine comes from DOPA taken up from the bloodstream.

water in the urine. Dopamine given by intravenous infusion is used widely today to treat severe disorders, such as decompensated heart failure, that produce sodium and water retention.

Where does the endogenous dopamine come from that normally occupies these receptors? At first it was thought that dopamine in the kidney was derived from specialized sympathetic nerves. Since the 1970s, however, evidence has accrued for a different mechanism that probably antedated hormones and the sympathetic nervous system in evolution, because such a system does not require a bloodstream or a brain. This is why I call dopamine the "atavistic catecholamine."

There is no good single word to describe the operation of this type of system. Researchers have used the term *autocrine/paracrine*. This means that the effector chemical, in this case dopamine, is produced in, released by, and acts on the same or nearby cells (fig. 32).

How can dopamine be produced in ordinary kidney cells, which don't possess enzymes like tyrosine hydroxylase and the various required cofactors? The answer seems to come from the uptake of DOPA from the circulation. Therefore, although the dopamine system is an autocrine/paracrine system, it does require a bloodstream. But where does DOPA in the bloodstream come from? Unfortunately, although we know fairly well how the story of the atavistic catecholamine ends, we don't know for sure how it begins. At least some of DOPA in the bloodstream comes from sympathetic nerves. We know this, because destruction of sympathetic nerves supplying a given organ decreases or eliminates local entry of DOPA into the veins draining that organ. In humans this has been shown in the limbs of patients who have had a surgical sympathectomy and in the hearts of patients with a heart transplant or with a loss of cardiac sympathetic nerves as part of a disease process. Sympathetic nerves supplying the kidneys themselves do not contribute significantly to DOPA in the bloodstream, because patients with a kidney transplant have a normal ability to make dopamine in the transplanted kidney. We also know that a substantial amount of DOPA in the bloodstream comes from the diet. Healthy people who have no caloric intake for 72 hours have clearly decreased but nevertheless readily detectable DOPA in their plasma. The amount of DOPA itself is much too small in a normal diet to account for the concentration of DOPA in the plasma; however, the diet does contain abundant phenylalanine and tyrosine and proteins that can be broken down to these amino acids, which in turn can be converted to DOPA in cells that express the appropriate enzymes. In particular, we now know that a variety of cells in the gastrointestinal tract that are not nerve cells nevertheless have the ability to produce DOPA from tyrosine. It is even possible that dietary tyrosine might be converted to DOPA without requiring an enzyme at all.

You may ask, if the body has a third catecholamine system, in which dopamine plays the key role, then do patients with Parkinson disease have abnormal functioning of the DOPA-dopamine autocrine/paracrine system? No one knows.

"First I Secreted a Hell of a Lot of Adrenaline"

About the same time that von Euler identified norepinephrine as the neurotransmitter of the sympathetic nervous system, disproving Cannon's notions about sympathin E and sympathin I, Ahlquist proposed a different explanation for the impressively large variety of effects of the two rather simple chemicals. Ahlquist's idea was that catecholamines differentially stimulate specific receptors—adrenergic receptors, or adrenoceptors. In 1948, he suggested that there were two types of adrenoceptors, alpha and beta. Norepinephrine would stimulate alpha adrenoceptors, the synthetic catecholamine, isoproterenol, would stimulate beta adrenoceptors, and adrenaline would stimulate both types of adrenoceptors. Numerous studies, using drugs and more recently molecular genetic tools, have by now not only

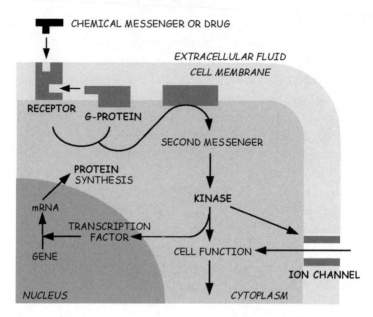

Fig. 33. Receptors in the cell membrane mediate the effects of adrenaline and similar chemicals.

confirmed this suggestion but actually provided the molecular structures of adrenoceptors and the mechanisms that link occupation of the receptors at the surface of the target cells to processes inside those cells.

The discovery of adrenoceptors led to the development of novel, highly successful drugs to treat many common and important disorders, such as hypertension, abnormal heart rhythms, coronary artery disease, and heart failure. For the development of beta-adrenoceptor blockers, which remain key agents in the treatment of hypertension, angina pectoris, and abnormal heart rhythms, Sir James Black shared the Nobel Prize for Physiology or Medicine in 1988.

Adrenoceptors such as beta adrenoceptors in the cell membrane transmit information via specific "G proteins" (the "G" standing for guanine-nucleotide-regulatory proteins). The G proteins are located near the receptors on the inner portion of the cell membrane (fig. 33). For the discovery of G proteins and their significance in cellular activation by adrenaline, Alfred G. Gilman and Martin Rodbell shared the Nobel Prize in Medicine in 1994.

Describing to an audience of colleagues his reaction to the news that he had won a Nobel Prize, as reported in the *Washington Post*, Gilman quipped,

"First, I secreted a hell of a lot of adrenaline and then that reached my adrenergic receptors and they responded via the G proteins."

In the liver, adrenaline liberates the vital metabolic fuel, glucose. This is a major way that adrenaline increases blood glucose levels. The release of glucose by adrenaline takes place partly by stimulating the breakdown of glycogen to form glucose in the liver. The breakdown of glycogen, in turn, involves a rather complex cascade of biochemical events. For this cascade to begin requires formation of a messenger substance inside the cells, cyclic adenosine monophosphate (cAMP). The discovery of cAMP, the first identified intracellular messenger ("second messenger," the first being the hormone itself, in this case adrenaline), depended on studies of the fractions of cell homogenates that were required for the hormonal effects of adrenaline and another hormone, glucagon, in the liver. For the discovery of cAMP, E. W. Sutherland received the 1971 Nobel Prize for Physiology or Medicine.

Medical textbooks often include imposing-looking charts that list the numerous types and subtypes of adrenoceptors and dopamine receptors (table 2). The remarkable array of receptors contrasts starkly with the small family of chemicals that reach those receptors. The multiplicity of receptors for catecholamines probably follows the principle of natural selection favoring the evolution of multiple effectors, for the reasons outlined earlier.

IM 21/2 N 1025

On an unusually hot day in Philadelphia in late March 1990, an elderly, diabetic, hypertensive, black woman, who had worked as a laundry folder for 27 years, complained to her coworkers of feeling dizzy, wobbly, and weak while at her usual job of folding laundry. She felt worse as the day wore on. By a few days later, her doctors agreed that the patient had suffered a stroke. She never returned to work again and applied for worker's compensation, claiming that the physical stress (high environmental temperature) and mental stress (routine overtime work) of her job had combined to precipitate the stroke.

The medical records sent to me for analysis weighed several pounds, yet I found that something was missing. On the morning of her stroke, the patient had had an appointment with her eye doctor. When she left for the appointment, she felt well. When she returned before lunch, she felt bad. What did the eye doctor observe? The note was missing from the records sent for review.

Table 2. Catecholamine receptor types, subtypes, G proteins, and second messengers

Subtype	G protein	Second messenger	Agonist	Antagonist
α_1	G_q/G_{11}	Phospholipase C-β	Phenylephrine	Prazosin
α_{1A}	G_q/G_{11}	Phospholipase C-β		
α_{1B}	G_q/G_{11}	Phospholipase C-β		
α_{1D}	G_q/G_{11}	Phospholipase C-β		
α_2	G_i, G_o	Inh. adenyl cyclase[a]		Yohimbine
α_{2A}	G_i, G_o	Inh. adenyl cyclase	Oxymetazoline	
α_{2B}	G_i, G_o	Inh. adenyl cyclase		Prazosin[b]
α_{2C}	G_i, G_o	Inh. adenyl cyclase		Prazosin[b]
β	G_S	Adenyl cyclase	Isoproterenol	Propranolol
β_1	G_S	Adenyl cyclase	Dobutamine	Metoprolol
β_2	G_S	Adenyl cyclase	Terbutaline	
β_3	G_S	Adenyl cyclase		
D1-like		Adenyl cyclase	Fenoldopam	
D1 (D1A)		Adenyl cyclase		
D5 (D1B)		Adenyl cyclase		
D2-like	G_i, G_o	Inh. adenyl cyclase	Bromocriptine	Raclopride
D2	G_i, G_o	Inh. adenyl cyclase		Haloperidol
D3		Inh. adenyl cyclase		
D4		Inh. adenyl cyclase		Clozapine

[a]inh., inhibited
[b]Prazosin also blocks α_1-adrenoceptors nonselectively.

Eventually I received it. The note was in the usual physician's scrawl. It contained the cryptic notation, "1M 21/2 N 1025." After looking over other eye clinic notes written by other doctors, I interpreted the notation as: "1% Mydriacil, $2\frac{1}{2}$% NeoSynephrine at 10:25 AM." This meant that, at 10:25 AM, eye drops to dilate her pupils had been instilled. NeoSynephrine is a brand name for phenylephrine. Phenylephrine not only dilates the pupils but, when injected systemically, constricts blood vessels by binding to receptors for norepinephrine. Could the phenylephrine in the eye drops have entered the bloodstream and increased her blood pressure acutely, precipitating the stroke? I did a computerized bibliographic search of MEDLINE and culled several research articles about systemic effects of NeoSynephrine eye drops. One that I found in the medical library reported that not only can phenylephrine in eye drops enter the bloodstream and increase blood pressure but also that this effect was most pronounced in hypertensive diabetics. From this I inferred that an iatrogenic explanation—that the doctor caused the problem—could account for the patient's stroke better than could the stress of her job. At the time the patient reported beginning to feel bad, she actually wasn't at the job at all. The note also showed that she had received a drug that could have precipitated a stroke by increasing blood pressure acutely. When apprised of the possibility that the hypertensive effects of the eye drops could have precipitated the patient's stroke, the expert for the claimant had to agree.

Frau Schwandt's Cold

In the early 1960s, chemists of a German drug company came up with what they thought would be an effective treatment for nasal congestion. The drug, clonidine, which has an imidazoline chemical structure, constricted blood vessels in a manner similar to phenylephrine, the alpha-1 adrenoceptor agonist sold as NeoSynephrine, but with a longer duration of vasoconstrictor action. In 1962, the secretary to the medical director, a Frau Schwandt, came down with a bad cold, and the medical director applied a dilute solution of clonidine to the mucus membranes of her nose. Soon after, Frau Schwandt fell asleep. She didn't wake up until the next day, and her blood pressure fell substantially. Soon afterward it was found that clonidine enters the central nervous system, producing sedation and dropping sympathetic nervous system outflows to the cardiovascular system. The company creatively redirected its marketing strategy, and the drug was developed and is still indicated for treating hypertension. The drug has also been used successfully to treat conditions as diverse as alcohol and opiate withdrawal, baroreflex failure, and attention deficit hyperactivity disorder. Researchers have not settled yet on whether clonidine works in humans by stimulating alpha-2 adrenoceptors, imidazoline receptors, or both. Ironically, the active ingredient in NeoSynephrine 12-hour nose spray is not phenylephrine but oxymetazoline, another imidazoline that does not enter the central nervous system as does clonidine.

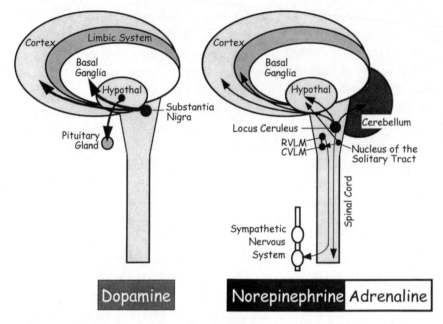

Fig. 34. Catecholamine pathways in the central nervous system. RVLM, rostral ventrolateral medulla; CVLM, caudal ventrolateral medulla.

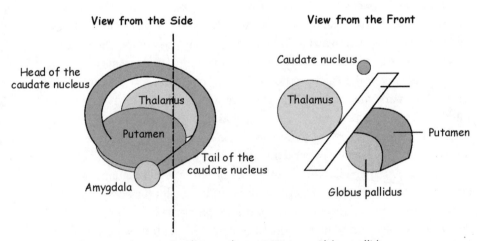

Corpus striatum = Caudate nucleus + Putamen + Globus pallidus

Lentiform nucleus = Putamen + Globus pallidus

Fig. 35. The "basal ganglia," where loss of dopamine terminals causes the movement disorder in Parkinson disease.

A Play-Doh Model of the Brain

The concepts introduced by Carlsson about dopamine in the brain led to an avalanche of research about catecholamines in psychiatry and neurology. A tremendous amount of attention has by now been paid to catecholamine systems in the brain.

Catecholamine cells in the brain occur in two norepinephrine and three dopamine pathways (fig. 34). Several different functions of dopamine have been proposed, in the three chemical pathways. The nigrostriatal system is the main source of dopamine in the brain and the main determinant of dopamine effects on movement. Patients with Parkinson disease experience particular difficulty with "pill-roll" tremor at rest and with initiating and terminating movements, presumably because of nigrostriatal dopamine deficiency. The nigrostriatal system courses from a tiny cluster of pigmented cells in the substantia nigra ("black substance") in the midbrain portion of the brainstem to much larger structures toward the middle front of the brain. These structures have collectively been called the "basal ganglia." The nomenclature for the components of the basal ganglia is notoriously complex (fig. 35). The basal ganglia include the caudate (tail-like) nucleus and lenticular (lenslike) nucleus. The lenticular nucleus, in turn, consists of the putamen and globus pallidus. The corpus striatum, often simply called the striatum, consists of the caudate, putamen, and globus pallidus. One would think the striatum and basal ganglia would be synonymous, but some authorities include other components in the basal ganglia.

The mesolimbic (or mesocortical, or mesolimbocortical) system sends dopamine fibers from the substantia nigra to parts of the limbic system, such as the amygdala, and several associated structures, such as the anterior cingulate cortex, septal nuclei, and nucleus accumbens. It is thought that this system is dysfunctional in schizophrenia, because many effective drugs for schizophrenia appear to work by blocking the effects of dopamine released in this system. In the mesolimbic system, dopamine seems to increase locomotion and positive reinforcement, not so much due to pleasurable reward sensations as due to an enabling action that decreases the threshold for initiating responses.

Finally, the tuberoinfundibular (or tuberohyophyseal) system delivers dopamine from cells in the hypothalamus to the pituitary gland. Dopamine in the pituitary gland inhibits production of prolactin. In postpartum women who don't want to breast-feed, a single injection of bromocriptine, which stimulates dopamine receptors, causes cessation of lactation.

Complete destruction of all dopamine systems in the brain produces a syndrome of decreased movement, inattention, decreased food intake, and decreased fluid intake; it gives the appearance of generalized behavioral unresponsiveness. This "dopamine deficiency syndrome" applies to all voluntary acts requiring motivation, sustained alertness, and receptiveness to sensory input. Animals deficient in dopamine fail to initiate coordinated movements and fail to orient to sensory stimuli. Motivated behaviors are not eliminated, but the arousal threshold appears to be increased before the behaviors are elicited. Most of the research in this area has depended on administration of a neurotoxin to produce chemical destruction of dopamine cells and terminals; however, the same neurotoxin also destroys norepinephrine cells and terminals, and researchers have paid surprisingly little attention to the interactions between norepinephrine and dopamine systems in the brain.

Conversely, increased occupation of dopamine receptors in the brain, such as produced by DOPA, amphetamines, or drugs that stimulate dopamine receptors directly, produces hyperactivity, stereotyped involuntary movements, agitation, psychosis, and risk taking. Patients with Parkinson disease who take dopamine receptor stimulants therefore can have a surprisingly high frequency of an unusual side effect, gambling.

Norepinephrine also is an established neurotransmitter in the brain, but very little is known about what it does in humans. Based on studies in animals, norepinephrine, rather than acting as a direct inhibitor or stimulator of neuronal function, seems mainly to modify responsiveness to other inputs. Activation of the locus ceruleus, the brainstem source of most of the norepinephrine in the brain, biases attention toward novel, rapidly changing signals from sense organs monitoring both the outside and inner worlds. Norepinephrine in the locus ceruleus system may therefore play a role in vigilance behavior and in registration of distressing events into long-term memory. A pathway from norepinephrine-producing cells of the locus ceruleus down the spinal cord seems to contribute to "stress-induced analgesia." Lower in the brainstem, norepinephrine-producing cells participate in neurocirculatory reflexes. Most of the evidence for such a role has come from studies of the baroreflex in laboratory animals. For instance, norepinephrine-producing cells exist at high concentration in the nucleus of the solitary tract (NTS). The NTS is the main site of termination of input from the baroreceptors to the brain. From the NTS, nerve fibers branch widely as they ascend to higher levels of the central nervous system, such as the hypothalamus and amygdala. Conversely, as part of coordinated behavioral, emotional, and autonomic nervous system responses, descending pathway traffic in fibers from higher centers to the NTS can reset the barostat and redefine "normal" blood pressure. A loss of norepinephrine-producing cells in the NTS can help explain why some neurodegenerative diseases feature extreme swings of blood pressure.

Despite the fact that both dopamine and norepinephrine are established neurotransmitters in the brain, and despite the apparent involvement of dopamine systems and norepinephrine systems in determining responses to environmental and internal inputs, interactions between dopamine systems and norepinephrine systems have received remarkably little research attention, especially in humans, and no concepts have emerged to explain whether and how these two types of catecholamine systems work together in health or disease.

The Nobel Chemicals

Discoveries about norepinephrine, adrenaline, and dopamine have led to many Nobel Prizes. These discoveries relate directly to regulation and dysregulation of the inner world by the autonomic nervous system and development of several novel, successful, rational treatments for major diseases. This section presents some of these discoveries together, to discuss, in brief, ideas that receive more attention elsewhere in this book, to provide a kind of summary for this long chapter, and to affirm the continuing importance of catecholamine systems in science and medicine.

After Ahlquist's 1948 suggestion that there were two types of adrenoceptors, alpha and beta, researchers worldwide directed their attention to the molecular structures of adrenoceptors, the mechanisms that link occupation of the receptors at the surface of the target cells to processes inside those cells, and development of novel treatments for diseases, based on drugs that blocked or stimulated adrenoceptors. As noted above, for the development of beta-adrenoceptor blockers, Sir James Black shared (with Gertrude B. Elion and George H. Hitchings) the Nobel Prize for Physiology or Medicine in 1988.

Discoveries related to the mechanisms determining cellular activation after adrenoceptor occupation led to at least three other Nobel Prizes. As noted above, for the discovery of G proteins, Alfred G. Gilman and Martin Rodbell shared the Nobel Prize for Physiology or Medicine in 1994; for the discovery of cAMP, the first identified intracellular messenger E. W. Sutherland received the 1971 Nobel Prize; and for the discovery of phosphorylation as a key step in the activation or inactivation of cellular processes, Edmond H. Fischer and Edwin G. Krebs shared the 1992 Nobel Prize.

After release of norepinephrine from sympathetic nerves, the norepinephrine undergoes inactivation mainly by a conservative recycling process, in which sympathetic nerves take up norepinephrine from the fluid bathing the cells—a process called uptake-1. Once back inside the nerve cells, most of the norepinephrine undergoes uptake back into storage vesicles. Julius Axelrod's studies about the disposition of catecholamines introduced the idea that termination of the actions of some neurotransmitters depends on neuronal reuptake. Axelrod shared with U. S. von Euler the 1970 Nobel Prize for Physiology or Medicine. As noted above, von Euler received the Nobel Prize for identifying norepinephrine as the neurotransmitter of the sympathetic nervous system.

Release of norepinephrine in response to traffic in sympathetic nerves of course depends on the existence of functional sympathetic nerve terminals. The development and continued existence of sympathetic nerves in an organ depend on a continuous supply of a nerve growth factor. The discovery of nerve growth factor arose importantly from studies of sprouting of nerve filaments from sympathetic ganglia cells. For discovering the first known neurotrophic factor, Stanley Cohen and Rita Levi-Montalcini shared the 1986 Nobel Prize for Physiology or Medicine.

Arvid Carlsson and Paul Greengard shared the most recent Nobel Prize for Physiology or Medicine that depended on catecholamine research, in 2000. Both these scientists focused on the "third catecholamine," dopamine. Until about the 1950s, dopamine had been assumed not to have any specific function in the body beyond serving as a chemical intermediary in the production of adrenaline and norepinephrine. Carlsson discovered that dopamine in the brain acts as a neurotransmitter in its own right and is of great importance in regulation of movement. Loss of dopamine in a particular pathway in the brain produces the movement disorder defining Parkinson disease, and replenishment of dopamine by administration of its precursor, L-DOPA, results in rapid improvement in movement. Carlsson also demonstrated that effective drugs to treat schizophrenia work by blocking dopamine receptors in the brain. Greengard discovered that communication between nerve cells mediated by catecholamines takes place by a relatively slow, diffuse process, called slow synaptic transmission, which probably underlies phenomena such as mood and vigilance and also modulates fast synaptic transmission, as in speech, movement, and sensation.

We need to know much more about the roles of catecholamines in the transmission of information to and within the brain. If the overall goal of physiological research is to identify the "algorithms" the body uses to maintain the internal environment, the means to achieve this goal may be the elucidation of mechanisms by which homeostats operate during stress, reset during distress, and malfunction in disease. Medical history predicts that catecholamine research will spearhead this quest.

The brain has at its disposal many effectors to control the inner world, in addition to the components of the autonomic nervous system described classically by Langley and Cannon. These other effectors operate according to the same principles as those that apply to the traditional components of the autonomic nervous system.

First, they all work by way of chemical messengers. Many of these messengers are hormones, released into the bloodstream and acting at sites remote from the site of release. Some are neurotransmitters, released from nerves and acting on target cells that are also nerve cells or nonneuronal cells. Recent studies have also increasingly described autocrine/paracrine substances produced in, released from, and acting on the same or nearby cells. Second, each of the chemical messengers produces effects on target cells by way of multiple types and subtypes of receptors, specialized proteins on or in the target cells that determine how the cells respond to a specific messenger. Using a relatively small ensemble of chemical instruments, the brain can play a huge number of cellular works. Third, occupation of receptors typically incites complex, parallel cascades of intracellular events. Fourth, the same chemical messengers exert actions in body organs outside the brain, such as the kidneys and heart, and also on centers in the brain itself. In most cases we remain ignorant about how or even whether the functions of the same chemicals outside and inside the brain relate to each other. Fifth, homeostats regulate other effectors as they do the components of the traditional autonomic nervous system, according to the principles of the operation of homeostatic systems such as negative feedback, multiple effectors, and effector sharing. Finally, effectors participating in regulation of the inner world of the body interact with members of the adrenaline family as the chemical messengers, often in multiple ways and at multiple sites. This chapter conveys some of the richness of these interactions.

The Axis Powers

The shell of the adrenal gland, the adrenal cortex, is derived from an embryological origin entirely different from that of the core of the gland, the adrenal medulla. Cells in both layers, however, release important hormones into the bloodstream. The adrenal medulla releases adrenaline and other catecholamines. The adrenal cortex releases cortisol, aldosterone, and other steroids. The hormones of the adrenal cortex are called adrenocortical steroids.

A key chemical difference between steroids and catecholamines is that steroids are fatty. All steroids of the body are made from cholesterol. Unlike catecholamines, steroids can readily enter the brain from the bloodstream to produce effects directly on cells that determine release of the steroids into the bloodstream in the first place. This allows the systems involving steroids as chemical messengers to be regulated by negative feedback, not indirectly via information carried by nerves to the brain but directly by the chemical messengers themselves. Steroids also cross cell membranes readily and exert effects on receptors on the nucleus inside.

The system regulating secretion of cortisol by the adrenal cortex is the hypothalamic-pituitary-adrenocortical system, called the HPA system. The system consists of the innermost portion of the hypothalamus, a complex cluster of nerve cells at the top of the brainstem; the front portion of the pituitary gland, located at the tip of a stalk hanging from the base of the middle of the brain; and the outer portion of the adrenal gland, the adrenal cortex. Researchers refer to the HPA system as the "HPA axis."

In humans the most prominent hormone regulated by the HPA axis is cortisol. Cortisol is a "glucocorticoid," because it comes from the adrenal cortex and increases blood glucose levels. Patients with excessive release of cortisol by the adrenal cortex, such as in Cushing disease, tend to have high blood glucose levels (diabetes mellitus), and patients with failure of the adrenal cortex, such as in Addison disease, tend to have low blood glucose levels (hypoglycemia).

Cortisol also inhibits inflammation. The anti-inflammatory effects of hormones of the adrenal cortex figured prominently in the stress theory of Selye, about which you will read in the next chapter. At high doses, glucocorticoids given as drugs can improve the condition of patients with inflammatory diseases, but they also increase susceptibility to certain types of infection. In failure of the adrenal cortex, the patient has a tendency to go into shock during exposure to a variety of stressors. No one knows for sure why people require normal adrenocortical function to weather acute stress. Deficiency of circulating glucocorticoids increases the leakiness of microscopic blood vessels, tends to decrease the responses of the heart and blood vessels to catecholamines, increases the likelihood of hypoglycemia, and reduces blood volume. These effects may combine to increase the tendency for circulatory collapse.

As with adrenaline, cortisol influences virtually all body organs, although the effects develop much more slowly than do those of adrenaline. Ordinarily, even a massive single dose of a glucocorticoid produces remarkably few harmful or persistent side effects, whereas a massive single dose of adrenaline evokes acute heart failure, backup of blood into the lungs, abnormal heart rhythms, and death.

Persistently elevated glucocorticoid levels can produce a form of diabetes mellitus. Body fat redistributes, resulting in central or truncal obesity and a moon-faced appearance. Increased metabolic breakdown of proteins leads to muscle wasting. Increased fragility of the skin causes easy bruising. Because of retention of sodium by the kidneys, there is a tendency to high blood pressure and to swelling from fluid accumulation. Psychiatric disturbances such as depression develop frequently, and gastrointestinal bleeding can occur. Inhibition of inflammation increases susceptibility to some infections, such as by viruses, fungi, and tuberculosis.

Selye's stress syndrome included enlargement of the adrenal gland, inhibition of inflammation, and gastrointestinal bleeding. Although he never realized it, activation of the HPA axis can explain all three defining components of the stress syndrome.

Corticotropin, or ACTH (an abbreviation for adrenocorticotropic hormone), a small protein, enters the bloodstream from the pea-sized pituitary gland. ACTH stimulates cortisol production and secretion by the adrenal glands. Within the brain, in the hypothalamus, which sits at the top of the brainstem and from which the stalk extends to the pituitary gland, another small protein is released, which acts locally on the ACTH-secreting cells. This small protein is corticotropin-releasing hormone (CRH), or corticotropin-releasing factor (CRF). It is thought that, in response to a variety of stressors, CRH release from the hypothalamus causes or contributes to the release of ACTH by the pituitary gland. Some have even dubbed CRH the "master stress hormone."

The HPA axis interacts in several ways with catecholamine systems.

The study of these interactions and identification of their roles in chronic diseases are important parts of research in scientific integrative medicine. Here are a few of these interactions:

—The HPA axis and sympathetic nervous system are alternative effectors for multiple homeostatic systems. As one would predict from the principle of compensatory activation, stimulating one system tends to inhibit activity of the other, and destruction of one system tends to increase activity of the other. Therefore, administration of glucocorticoids decreases sympathetic nervous system outflows, whereas surgical removal of the adrenal glands or pituitary gland increases sympathetic nervous system outflows.

—Administration of CRH in the brain increases not only levels of ACTH in the bloodstream but also levels of adrenaline and norepinephrine, consistent with stimulation of both the sympathetic nervous system and adrenomedullary hormonal system. CRH also stimulates cells of the locus ceruleus, the main source of norepinephrine in the brain. This stimulation might play a role in the decreased pain sensitivity, increased vigilance, and augmented memory retention in situations associated with distress.

—Glucocorticoids facilitate adrenaline synthesis in the adrenal medulla by promoting activity of the enzyme that converts norepinephrine to adrenaline. This explains why decreased adrenaline production occurs in pathological states involving decreased pituitary release of ACTH, failure of the adrenal cortex, or decreased cortisol production.

The Adrenal Bonbon

The adrenal gland is like a bonbon. It has an outer layer, the adrenal cortex, and a filling, the adrenal medulla. The outer layer and filling have completely different embryological origins in fetal development. In mammals, including humans, the cells arrange themselves with the steroid-producing cells on the outside and the catecholamine-producing cells on the inside.

This is not a quirk of evolution. Because of this arrangement, and the flow of blood from cortex to medulla, the medulla is bathed in very high local levels of the steroids, much higher levels than are ever attained in the blood reaching other organs. One of the main steroids of the adrenal cortex is cortisol. In addition to its many effects on metabolism in the body,

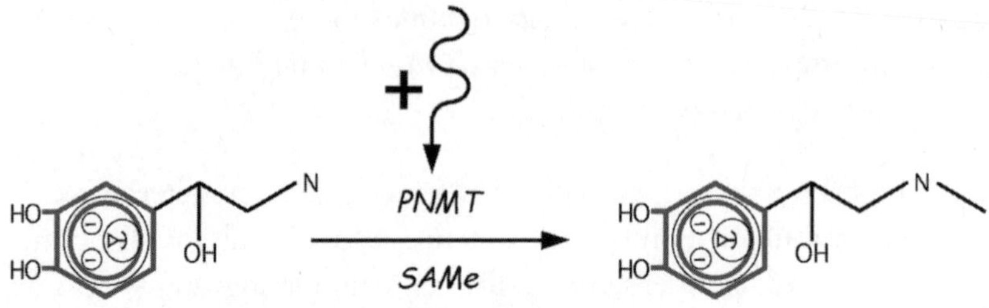

Fig. 36. Cortisol made in the adrenal cortex helps regulate production of adrenaline in the adrenal medulla. SAMe, S-adenosyl-L-methionine.

cortisol in the adrenal medulla contributes importantly to the production of adrenaline. It does so by increasing the production of phenylethanolamine N-methyltransferase (PNMT) (fig. 36). Therefore, diseases associated with decreased secretion of cortisol, such as Addison disease (a disease that President John F. Kennedy had), pituitary gland failure, and genetic diseases involving decreased production of cortisol, are associated with decreased production of adrenaline. Adrenaline increases blood sugar levels, and decreased adrenaline production may contribute to the tendency of patients with Addison disease to suffer from low blood sugar. People who take high doses of glucocorticoids as medication decrease production of glucocorticoids by their own adrenal glands because of a form of negative feedback regulation. The end result in these cases is also decreased PNMT activity, decreased adrenaline production, and probably blunted adrenaline responses to stressors.

The Water Works and Kosher Pickle Treatment

Ever since our ancestors emerged from water to live on dry land, water deprivation has threatened survival. The aquaporin-vasopressin system is a major effector for maintaining total body water content. Vasopressin acts in the kidneys to increase the efficiency of recycling of water. The urine becomes concentrated and scanty. This is why vasopressin also has been called the antidiuretic hormone, or ADH.

Vasopressin is produced in specific cells of the hypothalamus, transported in fibers to nerve terminals in the rear portion of the pituitary gland, and released from the posterior pituitary gland directly into the bloodstream. Vasopressin therefore is a classical neuroendocrine substance.

Aquaporins were discovered by my medical school classmate, Peter Agre, who received the 2003 Nobel Prize in Chemistry for this discovery. Aquaporins are a class of proteins that act as channels for transporting water across cell membranes. Aquaporin 2 (AQP2) is a vasopressin-sensitive water channel that migrates from the cytoplasm to the cell membrane in response to occupation of vasopressin receptors on the cell surface. Other aquaporins are expressed in the kidneys, and genetic deficiency of AQP1 is required for mice to concentrate the urine in response to water deprivation, even if vasopressin receptors are occupied. Clinically, AQP2 deficiency manifests as an unusual cause of diabetes insipidus where the kidneys are insensitive to vasopressin.

Increased serum osmolality, reflecting a decrease in the amount of water diluting solutes in the serum, potently stimulates vasopressin secretion. Decreased cardiac filling, such as occurs during shock from blood loss, also stimulates vasopressin release. Together, the two homeostatic systems that use vasopressin as a shared effector work together to compensate for water deprivation.

What if you were to drink a half-gallon of salt water? Both your blood volume and serum osmolality would increase. The increased blood volume would tend to decrease vasopressin release, because of stimulation of the volustat, whereas the increased osmolality would tend to increase vasopressin release, because of stimulation of the osmostat. These two opposite effects can cancel out each other, so that vasopressin levels may not change at all.

By promoting excretion of concentrated urine, vasopressin increases retention of water when water is available to drink. Water retention, in concert with decreased filtration of the blood in the kidneys, can explain low serum sodium concentrations (hyponatremia) in disorders that feature edema, such as heart failure. Conversely, alcohol inhibits secretion of vasopressin. This is why people have an urge to urinate after drinking alcohol.

When I was a medical student, we had a patient with severe high blood pressure, heart failure, and voracious thirst. Her serum sodium concentration was low. A common treatment for low serum sodium is to withhold water, because people can't stop urinating or stop losing water in sweat, so withholding water forces the sodium concentration upward. But for this patient, not drinking was a torment, and she just couldn't do it. The intern thought of infusing a concentrated saline solution by vein to raise the serum sodium concentration, but she was already in heart failure, and this would have increased the work of her heart and filled her lungs with fluid, making matters worse. So he decided on a compromise and prescribed that she eat a large kosher pickle. By the kosher pickle treatment, he thought the serum sodium concentration might increase, without worsening the heart failure; but he was wrong, her condition worsened, and the serum sodium concentration remained low.

The mistake here might have been avoided by considering a principle of scientific integrative medicine, which is to treat the patient, not the number. The patient had severe hypertension, heart failure, and voracious thirst. All these proved to be due to a drastic increase in production of renin by one of her kidneys, which in turn was due to a narrowing of the artery delivering blood to that kidney. Because of activation of the renin-angiotensin-aldosterone system, levels of angiotensin II probably were very high, and angiotensin II constricts blood vessels, increasing the blood pressure, and also potently stimulates water drinking by effects in the brain. Angiotensin II also stimulates release of the potent salt-retaining steroid, aldosterone, by the adrenal glands, forcing the kidneys to retain sodium. The appropriate treatment here would be to alleviate the underlying problem, the constriction of the artery to the patient's kidney. The low serum sodium concentration was the result of high vasopressin levels, which were evoked by her heart failure, which was caused by severe high blood pressure and excessive sodium retention, which was caused by the activation of the renin-angiotensin-aldosterone system, which was caused by the low perfusion pressure of the kidney, which was caused by the narrowing of the artery. Treating the low serum sodium concentration itself by the kosher pickle treatment would not remove the stimulus to vasopressin release and if anything would exacerbate it. When the constriction was relieved surgically, however, the patient's heart failure resolved, the blood pressure came down, and the serum sodium concentration normalized.

As its name "vasopressin" implies, exogenously administered vasopressin increases blood pressure via constriction of blood vessels. Vasopressin produced in the body probably does not participate importantly in blood pressure regulation in healthy humans; however, when the other major effectors for blood pressure regulation are destroyed, then blood pressure can come to depend on vasopressin.

Vasopressin also augments inhibition by baroreflexes of sympathetic nervous system outflows but does not appear to interact directly with members of the adrenaline family.

Salt Sense

According to evolutionary biologists, our ancestors' ancestors' ancestors emerged from a saline environment. Ever afterward they have had to deal with surroundings lacking readily available salt. Terrestrial organisms developed impressively efficient means to conserve sodium (table salt is sodium chloride) by recycling this key element. The renin-angiotensin-aldosterone system (RAS) plays a dominant role in the maintenance of sodium balance in the body. Dietary sodium restriction stimulates RAS activity; sodium loading virtually shuts it down.

The kidneys filter the blood by millions of leaky blood vessels coiled into tiny ball-like tufts called glomeruli (singular, glomerulus). Blood cells themselves normally cannot pass through the holes in the glomeruli, but the watery part of the blood, containing sodium, does pass through. The filtered fluid (filtrate) then enters tiny tubes, tubules. Cells lining the tubules take up the filtered sodium and put it back in the bloodstream. The sodium that escapes this recycling stays in the filtrate and eventually leaves the body in the excreted urine.

Specialized tubule cells in the macula densa ("dense spot") monitor the concentration of sodium in the filtrate that has passed through the glomeruli (fig. 37). When the amount of sodium falls below a certain level, the macula densa cells send a message to other nearby cells, called juxtaglomerular cells, located in the walls of the blood vessels heading toward the glomeruli. The juxtaglomerular cells release into the bloodstream the first effector chemical of the RAS, renin.

The same juxtaglomerular cells also act as sensors themselves. They detect stretch, and therefore the distending pressure, in the blood vessels. A fall in the distending pressure leads to release of renin. Therefore, not just one but two homeostats regulating the RAS exist in the kidneys. The main monitored variables for regulation of the RAS are the pressure in the blood vessels approaching the glomeruli and the concentration of sodium in the glomerular filtrate.

Stretch receptors in two other places outside the kidneys also contribute to regulation of release of renin. These are the "low-pressure" baroreceptors located especially in walls of the chambers at the entry to the heart and the "high-pressure" baroreceptors located especially in the walls of the carotid arteries, the arteries that deliver blood to the brain. When the amount of blood filling the heart falls, such as by a fall in blood volume, or when the

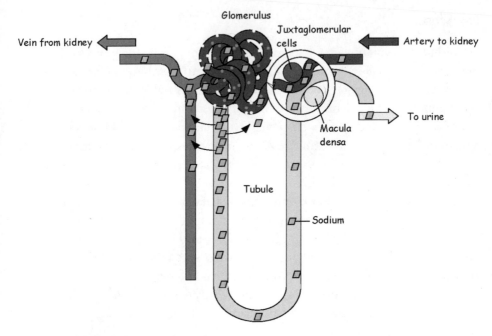

Fig. 37. The kidney recycles sodium.

blood pressure in the carotid arteries falls, such as from relaxation of blood vessels, the brain acts on this information to direct an increase in renin release.

Conceptually, the homeostat that regulates renin release to maintain blood volume as monitored by the low-pressure baroreceptors can be called the "volustat," and the homeostat that regulates renin release to maintain blood pressure as monitored by the high-pressure baroreceptors can be called the "barostat."

Renin has no known activity of its own, but it does act as an enzyme to speed up the conversion of a protein, angiotensinogen, to a peptide (a short chain of amino acids) called angiotensin I. Angiotensin I also has no known physiological action, but another enzyme, angiotensin-converting enzyme (ACE), speeds up the conversion of angiotensin I to angiotensin II. Angiotensin II is one of the most potent known chemicals in the body that constrict blood vessels. Angiotensin II therefore increases blood pressure. On a weight basis, angiotensin is four to eight times as potent a vasoconstrictor as norepinephrine is in healthy individuals. Predictably, both ACE inhibitors and angiotensin II inhibitors are effective and widely used to treat hypertension.

Another key effect of angiotensin II, which helps establish the RAS as the body's main system regulating sodium balance, is to stimulate the adrenal cortex to release aldosterone. Aldosterone potently stimulates reabsorption of sodium from the tubules in the kidneys by increasing exchange of sodium for potassium. Because of this indirect effect, activation of the RAS increases blood pressure not only by constricting blood vessels, via the direct constrictor effect of angiotensin II, but also by increasing blood volume, via the sodium retention produced by aldosterone.

In the brain, angiotensin II elicits thirst. In fact, angiotensin II is the most potent known stimulant of water intake. It also evokes salt hunger and increases secretion of vasopressin and ACTH from the pituitary gland. These effects link the RAS, the body's main system regulating sodium balance, with the vasopressin system, a major system regulating water balance, and with the HPA axis, one of the body's main systems regulating metabolism, inflammation, and the experience of distress.

Components of the RAS system interact in several ways with systems that use the three members of the adrenaline family as chemical messengers. In the adrenal gland, angiotensin II evokes release of adrenaline. Conversely, adrenaline, by way of stimulating beta-2 adrenoceptors, activates the RAS system. In the brain, angiotensin II increases sympathetic nervous system outflows, thereby augmenting the release of norepinephrine from sympathetic nerves. In the adrenal cortex, dopamine inhibits aldosterone release in response to angiotensin II. The renin-angiotensin-aldosterone system and sympathetic nervous system are alternative effectors that the brain has available for maintaining appropriate levels of blood pressure, blood volume, cardiac filling, and the amounts of sodium and potassium in the body.

Your Own Brand of Morphine

In the brain and in other organs, you produce morphinelike opiates, in what is called the endogenous opioid system. Collectively, these chemicals are called endorphins. This system contributes to the extent of pain you feel in response to a noxious stimulus and also to the remarkable lack of pain during some forms of stress, sometimes called stress-related analgesia.

One class of endogenous opioids, enkephalins, is packaged together with members of the adrenaline family and released with them during stimulation of the adrenal gland. Another endogenous opioid, beta-endorphin, is a portion of a precursor peptide that is also the precursor of ACTH, which directs the release of cortisol from the adrenal glands. CRH, the putative "master stress hormone of the brain," increases plasma levels of both ACTH and beta-endorphin.

Many types of stress increase circulating levels of beta-endorphin, and increases in beta-endorphin levels correlate tightly with those of adrenaline during real-life stress in humans. The role or roles of endogenous opioids in the regulation of the sympathetic nervous system and adrenomedullary hormonal system remain incompletely understood. Most reports have suggested indirect inhibitory effects.

Studies about physiological roles of endogenous opioids have relied heavily on the use of naloxone, a drug that blocks effects of all endogenous opioids. Naloxone is short-acting but very effective in the treatment of opiate overdose. Opioid antagonism by naloxone can reverse septic, hemorrhagic, or endotoxic shock, consistent with the view that endogenous opioids participate in the apparently paradoxical inhibition of the sympathetic nervous system that occurs in these conditions.

High enkephalin concentrations in the spinal cord suggest involvement of enkephalins in the transmission of pain information to the brain. Injection of beta-endorphin or the opioid receptor stimulator fentanyl into the cerebrospinal fluid space produces analgesia, and both have been used to treat pain in patients with terminal cancer. Release of beta-endorphin in the brain might be the basis for analgesia produced by acupuncture and placebos.

Novel, painful stimulation evokes distress and struggling. In terms of the homeostat theory, these are associated with the resetting of multiple homeostats, resulting in changes in values for many neuroendocrine parameters. In rats, subcutaneous injection of a drug that produces painful tissue trauma elicits large increases in arterial plasma levels of ACTH, adrenaline, and norepinephrine. Levels of adrenocortical steroids also increase substantially, whereas levels of sex steroids decline.

Concentrations of the endogenous opioid, beta-endorphin, in the bloodstream increase during pain. Exaggeration of experienced pain and of neuroendocrine activation in humans treated with the opiate antagonist naloxone demonstrates compensatory activation. Strenuous exercise typically increases pain thresholds, probably because of the release of endogenous opiates. This can explain why foot blisters produced by friction during running or skating hurt noticeably more after than during the exercise. High circulating levels of adrenaline may also ameliorate pain, because third molar extraction elicits increases in levels of both adrenaline and beta-endorphin, and injection of adrenaline attenuates the beta-endorphin response. In other words, endogenous opiates and adrenaline might be alternative effectors in modulating pain. Activation of descending pathways from the brain inhibits transmission of pain signals, probably by occupation of alpha-2 adrenoceptors on cells in the dorsal horn of the spinal cord. Drugs that act as central alpha-2 adrenoceptor agonists are therefore being developed for the treatment of chronic pain.

Growth and maintenance of sympathetic nerves and of cells transmitting sensory impulses require the same nerve growth factor. Patients with mutation of the gene for the trk A nerve growth factor receptor have congenital insensitivity to pain. Overexpression of nerve growth factor in nerve helper cells enhances pain after a nerve constriction injury. Whether patients with reflex sympathetic dystrophy (complex regional pain syndrome, type I) have abnormal sympathetic innervation or function remains a subject matter for research.

Thinking teleologically, in situations involving physical trauma, you would want to release not only adrenaline, to decrease bleeding and preserve blood flow to vital organs, but also chemicals to deaden pain. In "fight or flight" situations, adrenaline enhances delivery of blood to vigorously exercising skeletal muscle and might also interfere with transmission of painful sensations such as from blisters or wounds. In situations evoking distress, but in which you could neither fight nor flee, your brain might opt instead for a "playing dead" reaction, like that of a cornered opossum, the skin cold, heart pulsations undetectable, and pain dulled to ensure unresponsiveness to a probing predator. Sympathetic nervous shutdown and high adrenaline and beta-endorphin levels attend the human equivalent of playing dead— fainting.

Cytokines

Over the past two decades, more than 200 different proteins and their receptors have been identified that come under the broad heading of "cytokines." The exact functions of most of these proteins in the body economy are unknown. Many play roles in different steps of cascades of immunity or allergic responses. Some are growth factors for particular types of cells, such as white blood cells, red blood cells, scar cells, and nerve cells. In general, cytokines are autocrine/paracrine factors, because they act on the same or nearby cells. In contrast with other autocrine/paracrine factors, such as dopamine, however, the source or target cells for cytokines are in the bloodstream or lymphatics. That is, the source or target cells are themselves delivered to several organs and tissues.

The classification and nomenclature of cytokines are very difficult. Researchers have grouped them not only by chemical structure and putative role but also by the type of receptor. Different cytokine types can share the same receptor, and single cytokine types can bind to more than one receptor. For instance, for the interleukins, a subgroup of cytokines produced in white blood cells, at least eighteen different interleukins bind to at least sixteen different receptors. Cytokines can also act in synergy or in antagonism of others. Different cytokines work in concert with each other in networks or cascades, with diverse effects on different body systems.

Given this enormous variety, understanding the roles of cytokines in regulation of the inner world and in allergic, autoimmune, inflammatory, degenerative, and other types of diseases remains in its infancy.

A substantial but indirect literature has accumulated in the general area of interactions between interleukins—cytokines produced by white blood cells—and catecholamines. Interleukins produced by monocytes and promoting inflammation include interleukin-6 (IL-6), interleukin-8 (IL-8), and tumor necrosis factor (TNF-alpha). In general, infusion of catecholamines promotes secretion of IL-6, apparently via stimulation of beta-adrenoceptors, consistent with a generally pro-inflammatory effect.

Sex

As with digestive processes, sexual activity declines during periods of sustained exertion or distress. Decreased circulating levels of sex steroids such as testosterone in men reflect this phenomenon. Indeed, in at least some situations, a direct negative relationship exists between the change in the testosterone level and the change in the adrenaline level. Infusion of adrenaline decreases testosterone levels, and testosterone administration decreases adrenaline levels.

Sympathetic nervous system activity, as indicated by plasma norepinephrine levels, tends to be higher in the luteal, premenstrual phase of a woman's cycle than in the follicular phase, which precedes ovulation. One might speculate that women with premenstrual tension syndrome have high plasma norepinephrine or adrenaline levels during the luteal phase, but studies to date do not appear to have addressed this issue directly.

It is well known that women experiencing distress can have irregular periods, dysfunctional uterine bleeding, or failure to ovulate. This may have been part of the basis of establishing guilt in the biblical trial of the adulterous woman, as discussed in the section on "biblical lie detection" in the chapter about distress.

Exactly how distress inhibits brain mechanisms determining fertility in women remains unknown. Most research attention has focused on the hypothalamic-pituitary-adrenocortical system, not catecholamine systems. Corticotropin-releasing hormone interferes with release of gonadotropin-releasing hormone (GnRH), the main factor regulating release of sex-related hormones by the pituitary gland and therefore reproductive and sexual behavior. Cortisol inhibits release of both GnRH and luteinizing hormone, which prompts ovulation and sperm release. Cortisol also acts directly in the testes and ovaries, attenuating production of the male and female sex hormones testosterone, estrogen, and progesterone.

Leptin

The discovery in the mid-1990s that fatty tissue releases a peptide hormone—leptin—led to an avalanche of research about fat as an endocrine organ. Obese people were found to have high plasma levels of leptin. At first it was thought that leptin inhibition would treat obesity. Instead, researchers found that the brain possesses leptin receptors and that stimulation of leptin receptors causes weight loss, not weight gain. People with inherited leptin deficiency are overweight, and treatment with leptin reverses the obesity, mainly by effects on satiety and satiation.

Since leptin's discovery researchers have described other peptides (short chains of amino acids) released from fat, including tumor necrosis factor-alpha and adiponectin. Moreover, ghrelin, which stimulates appetite, and cholecystokinin, glucagon-like peptide-1, and peptide YY3-36, which promote satiety, are released from the gastrointestinal tract. Neuronal information from the gastrointestinal tract travels to and from the brain via the vagus nerve. In the brain, neuropeptide Y, agouti gene-related peptide, and orexin stimulate appetite, and melanocortins and alpha-melanocortin-stimulating hormone promote satiety. Corticotropin-releasing hormone suppresses appetite. Some of these peptides not only act on but also are produced within the brain.

No integrated concept about calorie intake, body metabolism, and obesity has emerged yet from this complexity. The sympathetic nervous and adrenomedullary hormonal systems must interact with these many peptides and with the hypothalamic-pituitary-thyroid axis, but researchers have only begun to understand how. A few facts have emerged, however. First, the hypothalamic-pituitary-thyroid axis and sympathetic nervous system act as alternative effectors, because hypothyroid humans and thyroidectomized animals have high plasma norepinephrine levels via compensatory activation of the sympathetic nervous system effector. Second, patients with pure autonomic failure, who lack a functioning sympathetic nervous system, have normal leptin levels, whereas patients with pheochromocytoma and high norepinephrine levels do not have leptin suppression, meaning that leptin and the sympathetic nervous system do not appear to be alternative effectors, even though obese people generally have both increased leptin levels and increased sympathetic nervous system outflows. Third, adrenaline injection decreases leptin levels, whereas patients with congenital adrenal hyperplasia, which entails decreased adrenaline biosynthesis, have elevated leptin levels, meaning that the adrenomedullary hormonal system and leptin may act as alternative effectors.

The scientific integrative medicine approach can help understand how genetic changes already present at birth lead to degenerative diseases decades later, at the other side of life. This chapter develops a theory about this linkage; the starting point is stress as a scientific idea.

A Brief History of Stress

Bernard and the Milieu Intérieur

About 150 years ago, Claude Bernard concentrated on the fundamental physiological issue of the time: Do living beings share a vital essence beyond understanding by physical or chemical laws? Or can principles based on observation and experimentation explain bodily processes? These were the opposing views of the vitalist and determinist schools. Bernard was the foremost proponent of the determinist view. His creed was that by scientific observation, one could grasp the laws governing and so predict the activities of body systems. The foundation of what he called "scientific determinism" was the criterion of deduction from experiment. If the experimental conditions were identical, then the experimental results would be the same, that is, the results would be determined.

For most of medical history, the opposing vitalist doctrine dominated medical thought. You have already read about Galen's teachings concerning the "spirits" and their relationships to the functions of body organs. In the independent Chinese tradition, the *Yellow Emperor's Canon of Medicine* contains remarkably similar associations between the "vital essence" and internal organs.

> The kidney . . . receives the vital essence from the other organs: heart, spleen, liver, and lungs. So when other organs are full, the kidney gives a vital essence. When a person is getting on in age, her internal organs deteriorate and her vital essence is drained.

Jing qi, the same as *zheng qi,* refers to the matter considered the essence of life and its functions. It usually refers to the essence acquired after birth and the essence contained in internal organs. . . .

Evil *qi,* the opposite of vital *qi,* refers to all factors that cause one to fall ill. . . .

Deficiency of *qi,* in traditional Chinese medicine, refers to the pathological phenomenon resulting from the deficiency of vital *qi* or exhaustion of primordial *qi.*

Fright disturbs the heart *qi.*

The heart is the seat of Mind. Mind can be hurt by fear, panic, and worrying beyond measure.

When a person is born, all the organs of his body keep functioning under the direction of the [sic] autonomic nervous system.

In constructing a stress theory that would fit with scientific integrative medicine, the ability to test derivative ideas—hypotheses—by observation and experiment would strongly favor the theory of Bernard over vitalist theories. Bernard's theory answered the question about why body systems function as they do by proposing the purpose of maintaining a stable internal environment. Scientific integrative medicine answers the question about why disorders develop and worsen over time by proposing that they constitute long-term consequences of regulation of the inner world.

Cannon and Homeostasis

Regarding the issue of purposiveness, Cannon wrote, in his *The Way of an Investigator,*

> Since a response in the organism has certain definite consequences, however, we should frankly regard them as being integrated with what has immediately preceded them. The various stages in the response that lead to the consequences may then be looked upon as *purposive.* If a crumb lodges in the larynx, for example, nerve impulses pass to the lower brain stem and, reflexly, impulses are discharged to abdominal muscles so that a cough results and the crumb is expelled. The sensory and neuromuscular sequences of the reflex action are all meaningless unless the aim is considered, unless attention is paid to the end effect toward which the complicated act is directed. (Cannon, 1945)

One can extend Cannon's example to note that stroking the tracheal lining evokes a coordinated, effective cough reflex, even in unconscious individuals; indeed, doctors depend on this reflex for pulmonary toilette in intubated, comatose patients. The apparent goal directedness and coordination of this reflex does not imply either that the patient senses the suctioning catheter consciously or coughs voluntarily, just as the apparent purposiveness of a thermostat does not imply that the thermostat is either conscious of or "wants" to maintain the temperature of a room.

Probably Cannon's most important overall scientific contribution was in affirming Bernard's concept of the *milieu intérieur* by demonstrating repeatedly, in a brilliant series of experiments in the early 1900s, that stability of the internal environment depends on the adrenaline family.

Maintaining the numerous monitored variables of the inner world requires continuous monitoring and coordination. The monitoring depends on perceptions of the outside world and sensations from the inside, and the coordination depends on the existence and functioning of a large but limited number of effectors, including effectors that use members of the adrenaline family as the chemical messengers. Adjustments in activities of the sympathetic nervous system and adrenomedullary hormonal system accompany virtually every human action and reaction and, in particular, are the main means for acute regulation of cardiovascular function—from the subtle, unconscious shifts of the distribution of blood volume that occur each time a person stands to the desperate distress syndrome of shock.

According to Cannon, the most important process determining the evolution of physiological and even psychological patterns of response has been essentially the same process determining the development of anatomic patterns—natural selection. As he wrote in *The Wisdom of the Body*, "The perfection of the process of holding a stable state in spite of extensive shifts of outer circumstance is not a special gift bestowed upon the highest organisms but is the consequence of a gradual evolution" (Cannon, 1939).

Specifically, Cannon taught that the "sympathicoadrenal system" evolved to help maintain homeostasis in emergencies, such as traumatic hemorrhage, exercise to exhaustion, and fight-or-flight encounters. In general, the effects of activation of the system would increase the chances of survival.

One would predict from this view that, in many disorders, alterations in sympathetic nervous system activity reflect an attempt at compensation to maintain homeostasis, rather than reflect a primary abnormality of the system itself. This is the essence of the problem in elucidating the role of the sympathetic nervous system in several common diseases and in distinguishing primary from secondary forms of dysautonomia (discussed in chap. 8).

During emergency situations such as fight-or-flight encounters, values for many monitored variables attain new levels but are regulated at those levels, redefining homeostasis temporarily. Cannon did not recognize this. The newer concept of allostasis incorporates this redefinition.

Selye and the General Adaptation Syndrome

The theories of Bernard and Cannon did not include stress itself as a scientific construct nor the relationship between stress and disease. Hans Selye concentrated on these issues. Selye popularized stress as a scientific and medical idea. Having observed as a medical student that sick patients seemed to share a "syndrome of just being sick," he eventually elaborated a theory in which stress would be a stereotyped syndrome shared by all organisms in their interaction with the environment.

According to Selye's theory, stress is the sum of all the wear and tear on the body at a given time. This definition seems quite straightforward and convincing; however, for a theory to have value it must not only explain but also predict. It must not only account for phenomena but also lead to hypotheses that observation or experiment can test. A key problem with Selye's definition is its circularity. How do you know if you are stressed? You have more wear and tear. How does this wear and tear come about? From stress. How can you reduce wear and tear? By reducing stress. How can you reduce stress? By taking "stress pills." How do you know the pills work? They reduce wear and tear. But what if they don't work? Then they haven't reduced your stress. One researcher put it this way: "Stress, in addition to being itself, and the result of itself, is also the cause of itself."

I am not implying here that there is no such thing as wear and tear on the body. There is. There even may be ways to measure it and even to minimize or prevent it. In chapter 12 I offer a theory to explain it, in terms of acute and long-term effects of stress. The issue I am raising here is the circularity inherent in defining stress only in terms of wear and tear. One can gauge the scientific value of a theory by its ability, potentially, to disprove itself, by generating an hypothesis that fails to predict the experimental observations. Unbreakable circularity is a sure sign of a weak theory.

Note that I am not referring to theories such as Selye's as being the truth or not. It is a rule of scientific thinking that one can prove a theory to be false, but one can never prove a theory to be true. The measure of a theory is value, or usefulness, or richness, or even fertility, but not truthfulness. We humans filter and color our internal and external perceptions, our memories, and our simulations in anticipation of future events. We confuse consensus with truth, which we approach best by obtaining evidence independent of us. The "ur-scientist" relishes searching for truth and always has doubts about having attained it.

From the beginning, in a letter to the scientific journal, *Nature*, in 1936, Selye emphasized that the stress response was nonspecific. The same stress response would be brought on regardless of the stimulus. After specific responses were removed from consideration, a nonspecific syndrome would remain. Although nonspecific with respect to the inciting agents, the stress response itself would consist of a specific pathological pattern, with three components: enlargement of the adrenal glands, shrinkage of the thymus gland (associated with atrophy of the lymph nodes and inhibition of inflammatory or immune responses), and ulcers or bleeding in the stomach or gastrointestinal tract. A decrease in the circulating number of eosinophils, a particular type of white blood cell, was added later to this triad.

The stress response was also thought to have characteristic stages, in a triphasic "general adaptation syndrome." The first phase would be a rapid "alarm" reaction. After an undefined length of time, a longer-lasting stage of "resistance" would ensue, with increased resistance to the particular stressor but decreased resistance to other stimuli. A balance of "syntoxic" and "catatoxic" hormones of the adrenal cortex would characterize the stage of resistance. The adrenal corticosteroids (cortisol in humans) were thought to be syntoxic, in that they would help the body to put up with aggressors by acting as "tissue tranquilizers," inhibiting defensive reactions such as immune and inflammatory responses. Catatoxic agents were thought to be pro-inflammatory, destroying aggressors by destructive attack by enzymes. The stage of resistance would end with depletion of "adaptation energy," ushering in the final stage, "exhaustion," characterized by resurgence of activity of the adrenal gland, gastrointestinal ulcers, immunological failure, and death.

According to Selye's theory, stress is not necessarily harmful. Relatively late in his career, he coined the term "eustress," for stress that is not harmful and possibly even helpful to the body, and "distress," for damaging or unpleasant stress. Excessive, repeated, or inappropriate stress responses were viewed as maladaptive, and Selye coined the phrase "diseases of adaptation" to refer to situations in which the general adaptation syndrome would become derailed. If abnormal (hyper-, hypo-, or dysadaptive) stress responses did not directly cause these diseases, then they were thought to predispose the individual to develop them, based on tendencies Selye called "conditioning factors." Selye proposed an immense list of diseases of adaptation. Hyperfunctional and dysfunctional conditions included Cushing disease, adrenal gland tumors, pheochromocytomas, hypertension, inflammation of blood vessels, kidney failure, rheumatic and inflammatory diseases, gouty arthritis, peptic ulceration, diabetes, allergic and hypersensitivity disorders, and psychosomatic disorders. Hypofunctional conditions included Addison disease, cancer, and diseases of resistance in general. The most severely affected targets were thought to be the cardiovascular system, the joints, and metabolism.

Selye's stress theory became and remains popular. Among other things, the theory provided a ready explanation for how any distressing experience could lead to or worsen virtually any disease state. The theory also aroused intense controversy. Bombastic publicity amplified the theory's controversiality.

Although Selye's stress theory has certainly provoked much thought and research, the theory has proven deficient in several crucial respects. You read before that circularity decreases the testability and therefore the value of a theory. Four circularities vitiated Selye's theory. (1) Stress was the condition producing the general adaptation syndrome; however, the occurrence of the syndrome was the only means by which the existence of the condition could be deduced. (2) Conditioning factors could explain any deviation from the predicted pattern of stress-induced lesions; however, the presence of conditioning could be detected only by this deviation. (3) The only means to determine whether a particular stress was a distress or eustress was the occurrence of observable tissue damage or shortened survival. (4) If there were no pathological consequences to a stress response, then the active and passive defenses were viewed as in balance, but if there were pathological consequences, then this was viewed as due to an imbalance and maladaptation. The only way to determine whether such an imbalance had occurred was by its presumed pathological effects.

Cannon, to whom Selye referred as the "Great Old Man," was one of the first critics of Selye's theory. Cannon's critique centered on the doctrine of nonspecificity and the implicit assumption that a stereotyped response pattern would be adaptive, regardless of the stressor. Because a nonspecific stress response would not have provided an advantage in natural selection, a stereotyped stress response should not have evolved. This criticism was ironic, because it could have been used against Cannon's own view of the survival value of activation of the sympathoadrenal system in all emergencies threatening homeostasis.

One can also argue that the basis for similarities in responses to different stressors in Selye's research was not the nonspecificity of responses of the body to any demand but that all the stressors used in Selye's experiments produced fear or anxiety, resulting in similar effects across the experiments. This was the basis for the critique by John Mason, and it still stands.

Selye also overemphasized analogies to inflammation and the role of the adrenal cortex in the stress response. Finally, by dwelling on only one effector, he could detect the presence or absence of stress only by the presence or absence of adrenal gland activation; however, many other effector systems participate in different stress responses, as discussed later in the section on primitive specificity. Because Selye never incorporated these other systems adequately in his theory, he did not consider possible adaptive patterning of responses of these systems.

Homeostat resetting redefines homeostasis. In his classic book for lay people, *The Stress of Life*, Selye suggested resetting of the hypothalamic-pituitary-adrenocortical system during stress:

> It had been claimed a few years ago that . . . a real increase of corticoids in the blood could never develop during stress. . . . But as I found to my surprise in 1940, during stress this moderator system is largely by-passed. It turned out that the alarm signals (discharged from the various cells of our tissues during stress) can stimulate ACTH-secretion, even when the concentration of corticoids in the blood reaches the highest attainable levels. . . . If the feedback mechanism were perfect we could never survive a seriously stressful experience. (Selye, 1956)

A Homeostatic Definition of Stress

The "homeostat theory" defines stress as a condition, in which expectations, whether genetically programmed, established by prior learning, or deduced from circumstances, do not match the current or anticipated perceptions of the internal or external environment, and this discrepancy between what is observed or sensed and what is expected or programmed elicits patterned, compensatory responses.

This sensation requires a comparative process, in which the brain compares available information with set points for responding (fig. 38). This

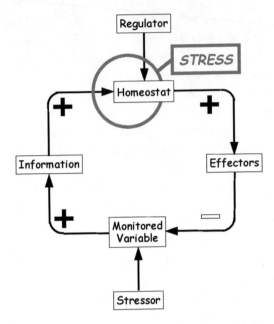

Fig. 38. In stress the organism senses a disruption or a threat of disruption of homeo-stasis.

brings us back to the HVAC analogy (see chap. 1). Feedback about temper-ature reaches a thermostat set for a certain temperature. When the thermo-stat senses a sufficiently large discrepancy between the measured tempera-ture and the set temperature, the thermostat directs changes in the operation of effectors, reducing the discrepancy. As discussed previously, the body has many such homeostatic comparators, which have been called "homeostats." Each homeostat compares information with a set point for responding, de-termined by a regulator. The homeostat uses effectors to regulate values of the monitored variable. It is the state of sensed discrepancy that defines stress. The organism responds not to the external or internal perturbation itself but to changes in values of the variable that the sensor actually monitors.

Several treatments used in modern medicine entail artificial homeostats to replace deranged stress systems. In patients with diabetes mellitus, the glu-costat fails to regulate blood glucose levels adequately. An implanted glucose sensor can measure levels of the monitored variable and regulate the rate of an insulin injection. To treat patients with orthostatic hypotension due to pure autonomic failure, in the 1980s my colleague at the NIH, Dr. Ronald Polinsky, developed a "sympathetic neural prosthesis," consisting of a transducer to monitor blood pressure and an injector to infuse norepinephrine, so that when the patient would stand, the monitor would sense the fall in blood pressure, and the pump would infuse norepinephrine to maintain blood pressure within a set range. The implantable electrical defibrillator (automated implanted defibrillator, AID) constitutes perhaps the most extreme example of an artificial homeostat. No natural compensatory mechanism has ever evolved against ventricular fibrillation, an invariably and rapidly lethal loss of cardiac rhythm. Ventricular fibrillation is tantamount to sudden death. Electrical countershock can reverse ventricular fibrillation; however, the survivors are highly susceptible to develop ventricular fibrillation again. The implanted defibrillator senses the loss of cardiac rhythm, diagnoses ventricular fibrillation, and delivers a defibrillatory shock.

According to the current definition, even a simple homeostatic reflex, such as the baroreflex, can reflect stress, when a perceived discrepancy between a set point for a monitored variable and information about the actual level of that variable elicits compensatory responses that decrease the discrepancy. Is stress defined in this way too general to be meaningful, since stress responses would encompass virtually all physiological and psychological adjustments? As discussed at the beginning of this chapter, the value of the definition will depend on the ability to generate hypotheses that testable observations or experimentation can measure. Homeostatic systems seem to operate according to several principles, presented below; and from them one can derive testable hypotheses.

Given the multiplicity of homeostatic systems, predictions about patterns of responses to stressors that potentially affect many homeostats, each of which may have particular gains and time constants for several effectors, would seem to require sophisticated computer modeling. Nowadays this is quite doable. One would prefer this complexity over the alternative—regressing to Selye's doctrine of nonspecificity.

Stress Response Patterns

The body's responses to different forms of stress occur in relatively specific patterns that help maintain appropriate levels of monitored variables such as temperature, blood pressure, blood glucose, and blood oxygen tension. A general theme of these patterns is that they are automatic, involuntary, and unconscious, but once the organism senses that the compensatory adjustments are not maintaining or will not maintain levels of the monitored variables, then the situation typically reaches consciousness, the brain directs the adrenal gland to release adrenaline into the bloodstream, and the individual experiences distress.

The "Cephalic" Phase

The "cephalic" phase of digestion takes place after, during, and even in anticipation of a meal. "Cephalic" refers to the head. The idea is that digestive processes begin even before the stomach fills with food, because of the actions of the brain. The brain directs an increase in parasympathetic nervous system outflow to the gut via the vagus nerve. The parasympathetic nervous system stimulation in turn augments release of digestive hormones, such as insulin and gastrin, evoking acid secretion in the stomach. Surgical cutting of the vagus nerve (vagotomy) has for many years been used to decrease gastric acid release.

Increased vagus nerve traffic to the gut also evokes peristalsis, the gut motions that move the food through the digestive tube like squeezing a tube of toothpaste at the bottom moves the contents toward the top. By way of a "gastrocolic reflex," an urge to have a bowel movement often follows. You may have had this uncomfortable sensation while driving after eating a large meal at a restaurant.

Sympathetic nervous system outflows to several organs also increase after a meal. This finding belies the notion that the parasympathetic and sympathetic nervous systems always antagonize each other. The mechanisms of sympathetic nervous system stimulation after a meal are complex. By way of increased vagal outflow and elevated glucose levels after a meal, insulin secretion by the pancreas goes up, and insulin increases sympathetic nervous system outflows, both by actions of insulin in the brain and by reflexive responses to insulin-induced relaxation of blood vessels. Pooling of blood in the gut decreases cardiac filling and stimulates sympathetic nervous system outflows reflexively.

In response to elevated levels of glucose in the bloodstream, plasma adrenaline levels tend to decrease. After eating a meal, then, vagal parasympathetic and sympathetic nervous system outflows increase, whereas adrenomedullary hormonal system outflow if anything decreases.

Crurifragium

Standing up, like eating and digesting a meal, seems simple because the body's responses to this challenge are rapid, unconscious, involuntary, and automatic; however, these responses actually reflect complex changes and interactions among a variety of effector systems. When you stand up, the blood pools in the legs and pelvis because of gravity. This rapidly decreases the return of blood to the heart. In the heart, "low-pressure" baroreceptors virtually immediately sense the perturbation, eliciting powerful reflexive adjustments in activities of a variety of effectors that maintain delivery of blood to the brain, lungs, and heart. The brain also receives information about the altered orientation of the body in space, the altered point of view seen by the eyes, and the altered state of contraction of antigravity muscles.

The main effector for the rapid, reflexive adjustments in blood flow to body organs when you stand up is the sympathetic nervous system. Within seconds the rate of traffic in sympathetic nerves to skeletal muscle of the legs approximately doubles, and the plasma norepinephrine level also doubles within minutes. Other effectors, such as the renin-angiotensin-aldosterone and vasopressin systems, play minor and more delayed roles. Therefore, patients with failure of the sympathetic nervous system always have a fall in blood pressure when they stand up (orthostatic hypotension) and usually have an inability to tolerate prolonged standing (orthostatic intolerance) because of dizziness or lightheadedness. Neither vasopressin nor the renin-angiotensin-aldosterone system can compensate for failure of the sympathetic nervous system to maintain blood pressure during orthostasis. Adrenaline levels in the bloodstream increase, but generally not to such an extent as to produce effects as a hormone.

Standing up also elicits automatic adjustments in behavior, in the sense of altered contraction of skeletal muscle, mediated by the somatic nervous system. The main behavioral response is leg muscle pumping. Leg muscle pumping enhances venous return to the heart and therefore helps to maintain blood pressure and blood flow to vital organs.

Chances are you are no more aware of muscle pumping when you stand up than you are of the automatic changes mediated by the autonomic nervous system. In this situation responses of the two main components of the peripheral nervous system, the somatic and autonomic, occur together in a built-in pattern. You can exploit this association to improve toleration of standing. Voluntarily contracting foot, calf, thigh, and buttocks muscles enhances venous return to the heart and at the same time increases sympathetic nervous system outflows to the skeletal muscle, constricting local blood vessels.

People condemned to death by crucifixion by the ancient Romans could last several days while nailed upright to a wooden cross. *Crurifragium* refers to smashing the shinbones. By eliminating leg muscle pumping as a means to return blood to the heart against gravity *crurifragium* would almost immediately bring on loss of consciousness and death of the victim—"mercy killing."

As discussed previously (see chap. 1), muscle pumping probably also prevents orthostatic hypotension in climbing snakes, whereas water snakes, which appear to lack this capacity, develop orthostatic hypotension when tilted in a tube.

Don't Swim after a Big Meal

An impressive array of homeostatic systems interact complexly and dynamically during exercise to maintain appropriate delivery of metabolic fuels, remove metabolic waste products, and maintain levels of key monitored variables such as core temperature and blood flow to the brain. Multiple homeostats monitor and regulate levels of oxygen, carbon dioxide, and acidity of the blood; filling of the heart via information from low-pressure baroreceptors; blood pressure via high-pressure baroreceptors; levels of metabolic waste products via input from "metaboceptors" in the exercising muscle; glucose; the osmolality of the serum; and temperature via sensors in the skin and brain.

Blood pressure normally increases during exercise, especially because of increased sympathetic nervous system outflows to the cardiovascular system. It is thought that there are three determinants of the increase in blood pressure attending exercise. First is "central command" by the conscious brain. Second is input to the brain from baroreceptors, which sense average blood pressure, the pulse pressure (the systolic minus the diastolic blood pressure), the heart rate, and cardiac filling. Third is input from other types of internal sensors, including mechanical, chemical, and pain sensors in the exercising muscle. These determinants interact dynamically, depending on the type (isometric versus isotonic), duration, intensity, and time of onset of the exercise, as well as on the individual's perceptions and even thoughts.

As exercise continues, production of heat increases. Body temperature would increase correspondingly, except for the reflexes aroused by temperature-sensitive cells in the hypothalamus at the top of the brainstem. These reflexes activate sympathetic cholinergic nerves to sweat glands, while inhibiting sympathetic noradrenergic nerves to blood vessels in the skin. This pattern results in sweating and flushing, augmenting heat loss and prevent-

ing dangerous increases in blood temperature. At the same time, sympathetic nervous system outflow to the heart increases markedly. The amount
of blood pumped by the heart per minute increases, and the blood is distributed especially to the exercising skeletal muscle and to the skin. During
prolonged exercise, by-products of the high rate of metabolism accumulate,
and the oxygen debt increases. Beyond an "anaerobic threshold," secretion
of adrenaline augments further the rate and force of the heartbeat and also
constricts veins and kidney blood vessels. Meanwhile, the renin-angiotensin-
aldosterone, vasopressin, and hypothalamic-pituitary-adrenocortical systems are recruited. The requirement for supplying glucose to exercising
muscle appears to determine the adrenaline response, because infusion of
glucose during exercise attenuates that response, without greatly affecting
the sympathetic nervous system response, as indicated by plasma norepinephrine levels.

Short-term changes in homeostatic settings during stress generally enhance the long-term well-being and survival of the organism. Responses
during exercise provide an obvious example. During exercise, homeostatic
resetting caused by altered "central command" releases sympathetic nervous system outflows from baroreceptor restraint, enabling vasoconstrictor
tone to counter the effects of vasodilator substances that if unopposed would
decrease blood pressure and flow to the brain.

Your mother probably warned you not to go swimming after eating a
large meal. After a large meal, by a variety of mechanisms blood flow redistributes to the gut, to aid in digestion. This redistribution occurs at the ex-
pense of blood flow to the skeletal muscle. If you were to exercise heavily
after a meal, you might have less ability to deliver glucose and oxygen to the
exercising muscle; at the same time, waste products of metabolism in the
skeletal muscle could build up beyond the capacity of the circulation to remove them. The net effect could be painful muscle cramping. If the cramping occurred while you were over your head in water, you might not be able
to swim to safety.

If You Can't Stand the Heat...

The sympathetic nervous system endows mammals with a most remarkable
ability to maintain internal temperature. Without an intact sympathetic
nervous system, mammals cannot survive prolonged exposure to either hot
or cold environments. Failure of the sympathetic nervous system therefore
can manifest clinically as heat or cold intolerance. As people age, they have

less ability to activate or inhibit the sympathetic nervous system appropriately in response to altered environmental temperature. This loss of plasticity explains why old people are more susceptible to death from heat stroke in the summer and hypothermia in the winter; and probably why many U.S. retirees migrate south in winter. The locals refer to them as "snowbirds."

Two key responses of the sympathetic nervous system explain the ability of people to withstand extremes of heat. The first is thermoregulatory sweating. Heat exposure reflexively releases acetylcholine from sympathetic nerves supplying the skin. Acetylcholine is especially potent at evoking sweating, which can exceed a liter per hour. The loss of the watery sweat from the skin surface cools the skin by evaporation.

Thermoregulatory sweating involves diffuse sweat secretion, including onto the skin of the upper trunk and face. Emotional sweating involves more selective activation of sweat glands in the palms and soles. Gustatory sweating after eating spicy foods is prominent on the forehead. Norepinephrine probably plays only a small role in thermoregulatory sweating, and acetylcholine seems to be the main chemical messenger released from sympathetic nerves for this purpose. Patients with an inborn inability to produce norepinephrine but with retained ability to produce acetylcholine have normal thermoregulatory sweating.

A different type of sweat comes from glands in the underarm, in the pigmented region surrounding the nipples, and in the genital skin. The secretion is thick, from its contents of proteins. The functions of this form of sweat remain obscure; they might be part of sexual signaling. Release of norepinephrine from sympathetic nerves supplying these sweat glands appears to contribute to emotional sweating of the underarms.

The second response of the sympathetic nervous system that enables people to withstand heat is a fall in the constrictor tone of blood vessels in the skin. The relaxation of the blood vessels in the skin increases the delivery of the blood to the skin surface, where the blood is cooled by loss of heat to the outside world.

Injected adrenaline can also elicit sweating; however, a high level of adrenaline in the bloodstream also reduces delivery of blood to the skin because of constriction of skin blood vessels; the type and location of sweating may also be inefficient for evaporative heat loss. Instead, the skin becomes moist but cold—"clammy." This is the "cold sweat" of emotional distress. Adrenaline release can explain the progressively increasing pulse rate and the feeling of impending doom in people unable to cope longer with heat exposure. In the amazing cooking experiment described in chapter 1 regarding Dr. Charles Blagden and colleagues, who exposed themselves and survived in a chamber heated to above the boiling temperature of water, effects of adrenaline seem eventually to have induced Blagden to end the experiment.

When people suffer heat stroke and shock, they usually look pale rather than flushed. This could reflect adrenaline release and consequent adrenaline-induced constriction of skin blood vessels. Meanwhile, adrenaline increases the body's overall rate of metabolism and heat production. A vicious cycle may develop, with adrenaline producing ever-greater heat production while interfering more and more with heat loss, a positive feedback loop that can end rapidly in death.

Through Thin Ice

Exposure to cold to also elicits unconscious, automatic responses of the sympathetic nervous system. Under ordinary circumstances these responses suffice to maintain the core temperature, without the experience of distress. The sympathetic nervous system activation constricts blood vessels in the skin, produces goose bumps, and causes the hair to bristle (piloerection). These changes have the net effect of decreasing evaporative heat loss. Instinctive behavioral responses, such as shivering and moving about, increase total body metabolic activity and help keep up the core temperature. Activity of the adrenomedullary hormonal system also tends to increase during cold exposure, but to a lesser extent than does the activity of the sympathetic nervous system.

When the core temperature actually falls after cold exposure, despite the activation of the sympathetic nervous system and the adrenomedullary hormonal system, the ability of the brain to direct behaviors such as shivering and repetitive body movements declines, and the core temperature spirals downward as lethargy followed by unconsciousness and death ensue.

Exposure of the face to cold water stimulates nerve endings and evokes the "diving reflex." In the diving reflex, both sympathetic nervous system and parasympathetic nervous system outflows increase. The pulse rate falls precipitously, and blood vessels in the skin, gut, skeletal muscle, and kidneys constrict. If the individual has fallen through ice and breathing has ceased, blood oxygen levels fall, carbon dioxide levels increase, and the blood becomes more acidic as waste products of metabolism accumulate. Chemoreceptors in the walls of the carotid arteries and in the brainstem sense these changes, augmenting the reflexive increases in sympathetic nervous system outflows. Humans sometimes survive prolonged immersion in ice-cold water, such as in near drowning in partially frozen lakes, because of decreased total body, brain, and heart metabolism and probably because of catecholamine-mediated redistribution of blood flow toward the heart and brain. The record for the longest survival of out-of-hospital cardiac arrest—four hours—belongs to a 41-year-old man who fell overboard into icy water near Bergen, Norway.

Altered Dietary Salt Intake

The renin-angiotensin-aldosterone system dominates the complex pattern of responses to alterations in dietary salt intake. Several homeostats monitoring the amount of filling of the heart, blood pressure, blood flow to the kidneys, and sodium filtered by the kidney all use the renin-angiotensin-aldosterone effector. The prominence of this system fits beautifully with aldosterone functioning as the main salt-retaining hormone of the body.

Salt deprivation also leads to salt-seeking behavior and a preference for salty food, and aldosterone can act in the brain to increase salt appetite. Deprivation of salt, without concurrent deprivation of water, would not be expected to increase the osmolality of the serum. Accordingly, vasopressin levels change relatively little in this situation. Conversely, dietary salt loading can virtually shut down the renin-angiotensin-aldosterone system, with little change in vasopressin levels.

Sympathetic nervous system outflow to the kidneys increases during dietary salt restriction, but adrenaline levels do not change. Dietary salt loading substantially increases urinary excretion of dopamine and L-DOPA, suggesting compensatory activation of the DOPA-dopamine system in ridding the body of excess salt.

Weightlessness

Weightlessness during space flight constitutes a novel and unique stressor in evolution. The human body does not possess mechanisms to counter effects of rapid reexposure to the earth's gravity during reentry after prolonged space flight. Instead, the body's responses to the weightlessness of space flight appear to reflect reflexive adjustments that evolved to adjust to recumbency or water immersion. In zero-gravity conditions, astronauts have a redistribution of blood volume away from the legs and pelvic organs and toward the heart. The absence of gravity also increases blood volume in the head, producing fullness of the face, nasal congestion, and distended neck veins. Probably from the increased venous return to the heart and stimulation of "low-pressure" baroreceptors, sympathetic nervous system outflow to the kidneys decreases, promoting excretion of sodium and water, and blood volume falls.

Upon reexposure to the earth's gravity, the blood pools in the legs and pelvic organs, and cardiac-filling pressures and stroke volume decrease. The sudden decrease in venous return to the heart, coupled with the low blood volume, can help explain the poor tolerance of standing up that returning astronauts experience.

Hemorrhage to the Point of Shock

In response to most local or mild stressors, patterned alterations in glandular activity or distribution of blood flow mediated by the sympathetic nervous system might suffice, without distracting the organism. One may view the sympathetic nervous system effector as a "housekeeping" system and the adrenomedullary hormonal system effector as a "distress" system. In general, stressors that pose perceived immediate threats to life or that compromise distribution or utilization of essential nutrients evoke marked increases in adrenaline secretion, whereas sympathetic nerve traffic may increase markedly, change little, or even decrease.

Throughout mammalian evolution, traumatic hemorrhage has posed a threat to survival. Numerous systems have evolved to counter this threat. The blood volume depletion during hemorrhage decreases venous return to the heart and reflexively stimulates effector systems that tend to restore cardiac filling. The pattern of responses to blood loss depends on whether activation of the sympathetic nervous system alone suffices to redistribute blood flow and maintain blood pressure and blood flow to the brain. If so, then the individual notices nothing special. This is why chronic, slow bleeding from a cancer of the gastrointestinal tract can go on unnoticed for so long.

In humans, blood donation provides a useful model for studying responses to small decreases in blood volume and thereby in cardiac filling. After donation of about one unit of whole blood (480 mL, 7 mL/kg), increments in plasma levels of norepinephrine exceed those of epinephrine, and levels of vasopressin, atrial natriuretic peptide, and renin activity remain unchanged. Heart rate stays about the same, and blood pressure, if anything, increases. Blood loss sufficient to decrease blood pressure recruits activities of several neuroendocrine systems, including the adrenomedullary hormonal system and hypothalamic-pituitary-adrenocortical system. After a rapid fall in blood volume beyond a critical amount—about 30% of blood volume—the individual notices something "wrong" and experiences distress. In this phase, activity of the sympathetic nervous system can actually fall, whereas levels of adrenaline and vasopressin increase markedly, accompanied by activation of the renin-angiotensin-aldosterone system.

High levels of adrenaline in the bloodstream in the setting of severe hemorrhage can explain concurrently elevated blood glucose levels, because the adrenomedullary hormonal system is a shared effector for both the barostat and glucostat.

Sugar-free

Glucose is so important in the body economy and so many situations alter glucose utilization that a large number of effectors contribute to regulation of levels of this vital fuel and react rapidly to deprivation of glucose (glucoprivation). Hypoglycemia, a low blood glucose level, poses a metabolic threat to all cells. In contrast with mild hemorrhage, where regionally selective increases in sympathetic nervous system activity redistribute blood volume and effectively counter mild challenges to cardiovascular homeostasis, even mild hypoglycemia necessitates global—i.e., hormone—responses to counter the challenge to metabolic homeostasis. Adrenomedullary hormonal system activation, insulin dissipation, and glucagon secretion dominate bodily responses to hypoglycemia. Glucagon deficiency increases dependence on adrenaline for glucose counterregulation, illustrating the principle of compensatory activation, and glucagon itself rapidly increases plasma adrenaline levels, illustrating direct interactions among effectors. Other hormones, such as growth hormone, cortisol, beta-endorphin, vasopressin, renin, and prolactin, play minor or as yet unknown roles in glucose counterregulation.

Hypoglycemia elicits hunger. The central mechanisms are unknown. Parasympathetic nervous system stimulation to the gut seems to constitute the final pathway for this response; vagal activation in turn stimulates gastric production of acid and pepsin and increases gut motility.

Decreases in blood glucose levels too small for the individual to notice increase circulating adrenaline levels, with little if any concurrent sympathetic nervous system activation as indicated by circulating norepinephrine levels. Selective adrenomedullary hormonal system activation during hypoglycemia constitutes key evidence for differential regulation of the sympathetic nervous and adrenomedullary hormonal systems during exposure to different stressors, in contrast with Cannon's concept of the unitary sympathicoadrenal system. Ironically, it was Cannon who first demonstrated that hypoglycemia evokes release of adrenaline into the bloodstream.

Throttled

Blockage of the airway produces asphyxiation, or suffocation, manifested by the biochemical triad of decreased arterial oxygen and increased carbon dioxide concentrations and a buildup of acid in the blood. Each of these probably serves as a monitored variable in regulation of ventilation. Chemical sensors, called chemoreceptors, located especially in the carotid bodies adjacent to the carotid sinuses, respond to decreased arterial oxygen, increased carbon dioxide, and increased blood acidity. Chemosensitive cells in the brainstem respond to the same stimuli. Asphyxiation always increases adrenaline levels drastically. A low blood oxygen level alone produces only small increases in plasma levels of catecholamines. Reflexive ventilatory stimulation, by decreasing carbon dioxide and increasing the pH of the blood, restrains the sympathetic nervous system response. The word *asphyxiation* comes from the Greek for lack of pulse, not lack of breathing.

Pain

Cannon probably was the first to describe adrenaline release into the bloodstream in response to pain. According to Cannon, activation of the sympathicoadrenal system during pain would facilitate fight-or-flight behaviors that throughout evolution have been associated with the experience of pain. Catecholamine systems probably participate indirectly in several ways in coordinated responses to pain.

Novel, painful stimulation evokes distress and struggling. Blood levels of ACTH and adrenaline increase, whereas levels of sex steroids fall. Circulating levels of the endogenous opioid, beta-endorphin, also increase during pain. Exaggeration of experienced pain and of neuroendocrine activation in humans treated with the opiate antagonist, naloxone, demonstrates compensatory activation.

Strenuous exercise typically increases pain thresholds, probably because of release of endogenous opiates. This explains why, for instance, foot blisters produced by friction during running or skating hurt noticeably more after than during the exercise.

High levels of adrenaline in the bloodstream may also ameliorate pain. In people undergoing wisdom tooth extractions, plasma levels of both adrenaline and beta-endorphin increase, and injection of adrenaline attenuates the beta-endorphin response.

Activation of descending norepinephrine pathways inhibits transmission of pain signals, probably by occupation of alpha-2 adrenoceptors in the spinal cord.

Nerve growth factor promotes sprouting of sympathetic nerves and pain sensor cells. Thus, patients with an inherited abnormality of the nerve growth factor receptor have congenital insensitivity to pain. (Whether they have arrested development of the sympathetic nervous system remains unknown.) Overexpression of nerve growth factor may help to explain neuropathic pain following trauma.

Sex Again

Components of the autonomic nervous system must work together for normal sexual function. Classically, parasympathetic nervous system activation plays a major role in initiating and maintaining penile erection, whereas sympathetic nervous system activation plays a role in ejaculation. Penile erection results from engorgement of veins. This engorgement seems to depend on release of the gaseous chemical messenger nitric oxide, either from nerves or as a messenger inside cells after the binding of acetylcholine to its receptors on the cell surface.

Dopamine delivered from the hypothalamus to the pituitary gland inhibits production of the hormone prolactin. This effect explains why injection of bromocriptine, which stimulates a type of dopamine receptor, prevents lactation in women postpartum who do not want to breast-feed.

In men, masturbation to orgasm is associated with increased plasma levels of norepinephrine but not of adrenaline. The process involves motion but not distress!

6 | Distress

Distress is a form of stress with additional characteristics: consciousness, aversiveness, observable signs, and adrenal gland activation.

Characteristics of Distress

Consciousness

The occurrence of stress does not require consciousness. Selye would have agreed with this assertion, because he claimed that stress reactions can occur in anesthetized animals, in lower animals without nervous systems or undergoing mechanical damage to denervated limbs, and even in cells cultured outside the body. In contrast, distress does require consciousness, because distress involves not only a challenge to homeostasis but also a perception by the organism that homeostatic mechanisms may not suffice—that is, conscious interpretation of sensory information and simulation of future events.

This is a more generalized statement of the concept of psychological stress as a consequence of a perceived inability to cope. The sense of an inability to cope or of a lack of controllability is basic to psychological theories about feelings associated with distress. An organism experiences distress when it perceives the inadequacy of compensatory adjustments to either a psychological or physiological stressor.

Aversiveness

Distressed organisms avoid situations that may produce the same experience. Distress therefore is negatively reinforcing, motivating escape and avoidance learning. The experience of distress would be expected to enhance vigilance behavior and long-term memory of the distressing event. These adaptive neurological adjustments seem to involve catecholamines in the brain.

Most animals can react instinctively not only to a stressor but also to symbolic substitutes that resemble the natural stimulus. Monkeys become visibly upset upon exposure to a snake, without ever having seen one before; rabbits freeze when a hawk-shaped shadow glides by; male stickleback fish attack any red object in their territory; and mallards scurry to the water in response to a foxlike piece of red-brown skin dragged along the edge of the pond.

The plasticity afforded by learning decreases the likelihood of inappropriate instinctive responses to symbolic cues. One definition of learning is modification of behavior based on experience. According to this definition, learning requires memory. Even "primitive" animals have the capacity to learn to withdraw or escape from noxious stimuli or to habituate after prolonged or repeated exposure to a stimulus. These forms of learning mirror each other, the former a sensitization and the latter a desensitization. The fact that primitive animals have these capabilities indicates the remarkably ancient and durable survival advantage of learning.

Classical (or Pavlovian) conditioning represents an important refinement of these responses (fig. 39). Habituation and sensitization exemplify nonassociative learning, where the organism learns about single stimuli. In contrast, classical conditioning (and operant conditioning, to be discussed shortly) involves learning associations among stimuli.

In classical conditioning, repeated pairing of a neutral stimulus (e.g., a bell ringing) with an unconditioned stimulus (UCS) that elicits an instinctive unconditioned response (UCR—e.g., salivation at the presentation of meat powder to a hungry dog; limb withdrawal after a local shock) results eventually in the elicitation of the UCR (or components of it) by the previously neutral conditioned stimulus (CS). The CS elicits a conditioned response (CR). For instance, depending on the UCS with which the ringing is paired, a dog may salivate or withdraw its leg when the bell rings. Pavlov taught that the acquisition of conditioned reflexes requires cerebral cortices; however, even invertebrates such as the sea snail, *Aplysia*, have the capacity to learn by classical conditioning.

Although most classical conditioning experiments involve an external UCS, such as an electric shock to the skin, this does not imply that the UCS must be external. For instance, rats can acquire hyperglycemia as a CR after repeated pairing of a previously neutral cue with injections of insulin. Pavlov himself demonstrated classically conditioned nausea and vomiting after repeated pairing of a CS (approach of the experimenter) with an internal UCS (evoked by injected morphine).

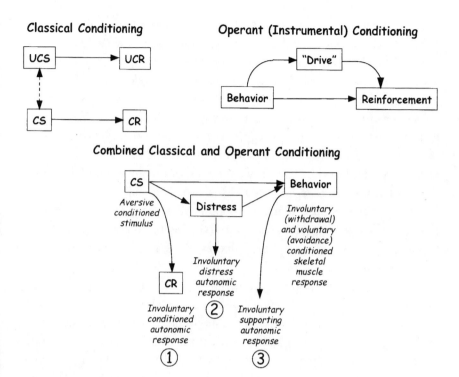

Fig. 39. Three ways autonomic responses can be learned by conditioning.

Instrumental, or operant, conditioning, represents a more advanced form of learning that requires a cerebral cortex. In instrumental conditioning, the likelihood of a behavior increases when the behavior leads to positive reinforcement (reward) and decreases when the behavior leads to negative reinforcement (punishment). Conversely—but circularly—reinforcement can be defined as an event that strengthens the response it follows. The conditioning is "operant" in that the individual's behavior operates on the environment, determining the occurrence of reinforcement; and the conditioning is "instrumental" in that the learning is a means to an end, with the occurrence of reinforcement contingent on the behavior. Operant conditioning therefore differs from Pavlovian conditioning, in which the delivery of the reinforcement occurs independently of the individual's behavior.

Both forms of conditioning require remembering an association between reinforcement and behavior. In Pavlovian conditioning, behavior (the UCR and CR) depends on the reinforcement (the UCS), whereas in operant conditioning, reinforcement depends on the behavior.

In avoidance learning, a form of operant conditioning, the individual learns to avoid negative reinforcement by producing behaviors that decrease the likelihood of that reinforcement. According to one psychology theory, the punishment increases the experience of fear or anxiety, and learning the avoidance behavior reduces the drive. This is where the present view of distress enters the picture. If an organism experienced distress consistently in a given situation, subsequent perception of reexposure to the situation would elicit distress as a classically conditioned response. Thus, in the morphine experiment described by Pavlov, when the experimenter entered the room, the dog became "restless," not as a CR to morphine injection but as a CR to the experimenter himself. In anthropomorphic terms, the dog recognized that every time the experimenter entered the room, suffering followed, and this realization elicited a feeling of anxiety as a CR in response to the CS of the experimenter.

Situations evoking distress typically involve a complex interplay of classically conditioned and operantly conditioned behaviors, as well as a complex interplay of skeletal muscle and autonomic responses. A concrete example may help here: What happens when a speeder notices a red flashing light in the rear-view mirror? From prior experience, being caught speeding causes delay, confrontation, and humiliation, all delivered by a UCS in uniform. The light therefore is a CS, signifying an approaching car containing an aversive UCS.

Aversive CRs entail at least two types of behavioral response. One is a rapid, involuntary, conditioned withdrawal response. The response may be so rapid, the individual may not have time to consider the significance of the CS. The sheer rapidity of withdrawal (or escape) responses helps explain their endurance in evolution. Virtually instantaneously, the speeder's right foot lifts from the accelerator—a skeletal muscle withdrawal CR. A second response is avoidance. The basis for learning avoidance behavior is the reinforcement provided by reducing the distress. The speeder may flip down the rear-view mirror, rendering the red light less glaring, or turn on the cruise control, rapidly adjusting the car speed to a rate within the legal limit, or even search for a raffle ticket from a recent fund-raising campaign of the police benevolent association! These avoidance behaviors would decrease the distress.

The same aversive CR would elicit three types of autonomic response. The speeder's heart rate might increase—a visceral CR, because the red light has been paired in the past with confrontation and humiliation, and these constitute a UCS, increasing sympathetic nervous system outflow to the heart. The speeder experiences distress, and this also increases cardiac sympathetic outflow. Third, sympathetic nervous system outflows change to support the circulation during the conditioned skeletal muscle contractions.

Here is a novel prescription to treat drowsiness while driving—voluntarily putting oneself into a situation evoking anger. Try this sometime when you feel drowsy driving: intentionally slow down, to the point that the driver behind honks, flashes lights, speeds past, yells and gesticulates going by, and reenters your lane close in front of you. I bet this would wake you up! You would be voluntarily exposing yourself to a UCS to elicit a vigilance UCR.

Communication

A third characteristic of distress, in addition to consciousness and aversiveness, is evocation of signs that others can interpret as indicating the emotional state and intent of the organism. Darwin emphasized that the various outward manifestations of emotion provide important means of communication that have survival value.

Darwin also proposed that physiological arousal, by intensifying emotions, amplifies further the physiological stress responses that accompany those emotions. This constitutes a psychophysiological positive feedback loop. From the previous discussion, such a loop is unstable. Flight can degenerate to self-destructive panic, anger to frenzy, fright to collapse, and defeat to suicide.

Perceptions of signs of distress by other members of the species elicit involuntary, instinctive responses. Here is how the Nobel Prize–winning ethologist Konrad Lorenz described the behavior of two fighting wolves after one submitted and extended its neck to the victor:

> A dog or wolf that offers its neck to its adversary . . . will never be bitten seriously. . . . Since the fight is stopped so suddenly by this action, the victor frequently finds himself straddling his vanquished foe in anything but a comfortable position. So to remain, with his muzzle applied to the neck of the "under-dog" soon becomes tedious for the champion and, seeing that he cannot bite anyway, he soon withdraws. . . .
>
> Why has the dog the inhibition against biting his fellow's neck? Why has the raven an inhibition against pecking the eye of his friend? . . . Should the raven peck, without compunction, at the eye of his nest-mate, his wife or his young, in the same way as he pecks at any other moving and glitter-

ing object, there would, by now, be no more ravens in the world. Should a dog or wolf unrestrainedly and unaccountably bite the neck of his pack-mates and actually execute the movement of shaking them to death, then his species also would certainly be exterminated within a short space of time. (Lorenz, *King Solomon's Ring*, 1952, 188–191)

This principle applies analogously in humans: the fiercest combat usually ends abruptly when one side shows universally understood signs of surrender and submission.

The communication value of external signs of distress helps to explain the continued elaboration of observable components of distress responses in modern society, despite the relative rarity of true fight-or-flight reactions in humans. Even in the wild, all social animals continually elicit and instinctively comprehend psychosocial cues.

Alterations in sympathetic nervous and adrenomedullary hormonal system activity often produce these external signs. For instance, sympathetic nerves to skin blood vessels mediate facial blushing, indicating embarrassment or humiliation. In a confrontation between two people, if one turns pale, quivers, averts his eyes, mumbles, and exposes his palms, and the other flushes, stands erect, glowers, shouts, and clenches his fists, the former evinces signs of submission and capitulation, and the latter signs of dominance and triumph. In evolution, these signs may have been by-products of genetically determined neurocirculatory adjustments supporting fleeing and fighting. In modern society, they serve signal functions of their own.

Emotional-behavioral states such as anger, panic, defeat, boredom, elation, and depression, seem contagious. Epidemics of coughing disturb concerts, people yawn together, crowds stampede in panic, soldiers rampage, teenage girls at rock concerts swoon and faint. In 1994, several members of an emergency room team fainted after taking care of a woman with terminal cancer of the ovaries. Perhaps the uriniferous odor of her breath from kidney failure triggered this response.

Instinctive communication of distress can operate even across species. Reading about the instinctively communicated distress of a dog convinced me that O. J. Simpson killed his wife. You probably remember the case. O. J. Simpson, the football star turned movie star, stood accused of having slashed his wife, Nicole Brown Simpson, to death in a fit of jealous rage. He did, however, have a potential alibi. Witnesses had seen him later that night at the airport, and he made it there in time for an 11:45 PM flight. If the murder had occurred late enough in the evening, then too little time would have elapsed for Simpson to have committed the crime and then been driven to the airport. The case hinged on the timing of the murder. The forensic evidence could not pinpoint the timing accurately enough to reject the alibi.

Neighbors testified that they remembered a dog wailing outside that night. Eva Stein and Louis Karpf, Nicole Simpson's next door neighbors, heard and saw a dog barking strangely between about 10:15 and 10:47 PM. Another neighbor, Steven Schwab, was walking his own dog when, at about 10:55 PM, he saw an Akita barking at the corner near the murder site. The dog had blood on its legs. Another neighbor reported hearing a dog's "plaintive wail" at about 10:15 PM. Nicole Simpson Brown's pet Akita emitted that wail.

You might ask how these people, months later, could remember the exact time at which they heard a dog bark. Dogs bark all the time; no one remembers a bark. But this wasn't a bark. This was a wail, a "plaintive wail." Wailing instinctively conveys the misery of grief. It is almost as if the individual is sharing the agony that a loved one suffered while dying. This communication is generated instinctively, and it can be understood instinctively, even by members of an entirely different species. It is a sign of distress in both humans and dogs. Throughout evolution, communication of this experience has offered important information relevant to survival. The incident, the circumstances, the timing, and one's sensations, emotions, and actions become etched in memory. The assault, struggle, and death of its master, which evoked the wail by Nicole Brown Simpson's pet dog, must have occurred beforehand. If so, then there would have been enough time for O. J. Simpson to have committed the crime, leave the scene, and ride to the airport.

Adrenal Activation

A fourth characteristic of distress is adrenal gland activation, with enhanced release of catecholamines from the adrenal medulla and steroids from the adrenal cortex. Increased release of adrenaline constitutes perhaps the most sensitive chemical index of this activation.

Several studies have supported a closer link between adrenomedullary hormonal system and hypothalamic-pituitary-adrenocortical responses than between adrenomedullary hormonal system and sympathetic nervous system responses during distress. Public speaking markedly increases plasma levels and urinary excretion of adrenaline and cortisol, with only small changes in norepinephrine excretion. In humans playing a video game, responses of ACTH levels correlate positively with responses of adrenaline levels but not with norepinephrine levels. In rats, passive avoidance elicits large plasma adrenaline and corticosterone responses but small plasma norepinephrine responses. Concurrent adrenocortical and adrenomedullary activation in distress provides an explanation for the adrenal "bonbon" arrangement, with the cortex surrounding the medulla, despite their very different embryological origins.

Cannon viewed the neuronal and hormonal components of the sympathoadrenal system to act as a unit—the "sympathicoadrenal" system—in preserving homeostasis. According to the present conception, specifically the adrenomedullary hormonal component characterizes distress; sympathetic nervous system outflows can increase, decrease, or stay the same.

Biblical Lie Detection

The Bible contains a unique and remarkable instance of trial by ordeal, of a woman accused by her husband of adultery. Visible signs of emotional distress (trembling, pallor, abdominal swelling, and failure to ovulate or menstruate) signified guilt. Several of these signs result from automatic, involuntary, unconscious activation of systems in which members of the adrenaline family serve as the chemical messengers. The ancients must have recognized that these signs, by revealing emotional distress, could constitute evidence of guilt—about the same rationale as in modern "lie detection."

The priest would conduct the trial according to a specific ritual. He would loosen the woman's hair, place a meal offering of barley meal in the woman's hands, take "holy water" in an earthen vessel, adding to the water dust from the floor of the tabernacle, and then incant: "If thou has gone aside, being under thy husband, and if thou be defiled . . . this water that causeth the curse shall go into thy bowels, and make thy belly to swell, and thy thigh to fall away" (Numbers 5:19–21). The accused woman would reply, "Amen, amen" (the first use of the term in the Bible). The woman would then drink the test potion. If she had been unfaithful, her belly would swell and her thigh would "fall away."

Emotional distress, via members of the adrenaline family, causes the hair to stand out. We all have heard "hair-raising" stories that make us "bristle" with horror. Loosening the hair enabled the community to see if this reaction would occur. By the priest placing the meal in her hands, attention would focus on them. All could witness whether her hands trembled or appeared pale. Both signs can be elicited by the hormonal actions of adrenaline and norepinephrine. The woman had to say publicly, "Amen, amen." Perhaps the community would detect distress in her voice. (Nowadays one can buy an "Emotion Reader," a computerized voice analyzer that measures "stress levels.") If the woman were guilty, then drinking the test potion would cause her belly to swell. Apparently, she would not be able to digest. Adrenaline potently relaxes involuntary muscle of the gut. Indeed, this relaxation provided the basis for the first successful method, by Walter Cannon, for detecting adrenaline release during emotional distress. Finally, the woman's "thigh" would "fall away." We can guess the meaning of *fall away* from the prediction that, if the woman were innocent, she would conceive. Today we know that women experiencing emotional distress often have irregular periods or fail to ovulate.

Adrenal gland activation alone does not itself produce distress. The experience of distress requires both physiological arousal and appropriate cognition by the organism, as proposed by Schachter and Singer in their classic 1962 study. Although several emotions include distressing elements (e.g., fear, anxiety, panic, guilt), other emotions do not (e.g., libido, joy), yet adrenomedullary hormonal system activation accompanies even positive emotional experiences. This activation of itself does not imply the experience of distress, because such an experience requires appropriate cognitions and because adrenomedullary hormonal system activation can accompany even nondistressing emotions; however, in organisms with a functional adrenomedullary hormonal system, the absence of adrenomedullary activation excludes the experience of distress.

With repetition of exposure to a situation evoking distress, the organism habituates, in the sense that effector components whose expression depends on novelty or unpredictability recede; concurrently, however, the organism becomes hyperreactive to other potential stressors. Habituation to a stressor recalls the stage of resistance, the second phase of Selye's general adaptation syndrome; however, in the stage of resistance, all the components of the unitary stress response would diminish, not only those components dependent on novelty or unpredictability. The occurrence of "stressor switch hyperresponsiveness," or dishabituation, would violate Selye's doctrine of nonspecificity, because the stress response in this setting would depend on the type of stressor.

Homeostat resetting accompanies distress and implies an allostatic change. Whether repeated distress causes or contributes to development of chronic diseases might then depend on whether the associated allostatic changes increase allostatic load. Chapter 12 fleshes out this concept.

Distress versus the General Adaptation Syndrome

How does the present view of distress differ from Selye's general adaptation syndrome? First, as noted above, Selye's theory emphasized the nonspecificity of the general adaptation syndrome. According to the present conception, the elicitation of distress responses depends on the character, intensity, and meaning of the stressor as perceived by the organism and on the organism's perceived ability to cope with it.

Second, distress responses—as all stress responses—are viewed here as compensatory in origin and purpose, attempting in some way to mitigate the effects of a stressor. This applies not only to nervous system or hormonal aspects of those responses but also to psychological aspects, such as conditioned and instrumental avoidance learning.

Third, according to Selye, the general adaptation syndrome consisted of a series of well-defined stages: alarm, resistance, and exhaustion; however, experimental results have not consistently confirmed either the habituation or exhaustion of adrenomedullary hormonal system responses after chronically repeated episodes of distress. The present theory does not depend on these stages.

Fourth, the present theory views distress as a consciously experienced condition. Neither adrenomedullary nor hypothalamic-pituitary-adrenocortical activation per se implies the experience of distress. Because Selye never developed a clear distinction between stress (which could be conscious or unconscious) and distress, his theory did not state whether an experiential requirement would distinguish them.

Fifth, the present theory does not assume that distress causes disease. Distress, though unpleasant, is not by definition pathological. Selye characterized distress as unpleasant or harmful, without separating these two very different characteristics. He never incorporated the relationship between distress and disease explicitly in his theory; he appears to have added distress as a concept long after he proposed maladaptation from excessive or inappropriate stress responses or the operation of "conditioning factors." For instance, the index to his treatise about stress and diseases of adaptation, published in 1950, does not include an entry under "distress"; and in his book for laypeople, *Stress without Distress*, he did not elaborate on the relationship between distress and disease.

Perhaps Selye recognized the paradox of stress as simultaneously homeostatic and pathological. Rather than concluding that the relationship between stress and disease was a matter for research, he simply defined a new term, distress, to denote stress that causes disease. As suggested above, he seems to have developed this idea rather late in his career. Writers about stress, in general, have also not recognized this paradox of Selye's theory and have either assumed the linkage between stress and psychiatric and physical disease or else have adopted the term, distress, without explaining its meaning specifically.

It has been suggested that chronic, frequent repetition of even mild "defense reactions" can produce high blood pressure. This notion is a largely unproven tenet of psychosomatic medicine. The present conception implies no necessary link between stress or distress and the long-term development of physical disease. This does not mean that acute stress, by evoking increases in levels of hormones such as adrenaline, cannot evoke severe and even fatal cardiovascular events. For instance, a large plasma adrenaline response during exercise in a patient with coronary heart disease can augment myocardial oxygen consumption, promote platelet aggregation, and destabilize heart electrical activity, resulting in heart attack or sudden death. Nor does this suggest a lack of reasonableness for the assertion that chronic emotional distress has pathological consequences. Rather, the present conception views the pathological effects of stress and distress as a matter for experimental testing, especially using longitudinal, controlled studies.

Fight Isn't Flight

The following discussion develops the theme that the body's automatic responses, mediated by smooth muscle, during "fight" differ from those during "flight," as well as during "fright" and "defeat," just as the patterns of movement and posture, mediated by skeletal muscle, differ, even though all four types of response contain an element of distress.

Walter Cannon introduced the phrase, "fight or flight," about a century ago. He thought that these emotionally charged situations would elicit essentially the same activation of the "sympathicoadrenal" system. Observations dating back at least to the time of Charles Darwin disagree with this notion. Terror does share several features with rage—trembling, hyperventilation, fast pulse rate, sweating, and bristling. Movements and postures obviously distinguish fear and anger, however, and one would expect that the different behavioral responses would require different supportive changes in regulation of the inner world.

In his classic book, *The Expression of the Emotions in Man and Animals*, Darwin described the main signs that distinguish extreme fear (terror) from extreme anger (rage). The following discussion considers four such differences—the state of effective tone of skeletal muscle, the tone of smooth muscle in blood vessels of the skin, the tone of smooth muscle in the wall of the gut, and the tone of smooth muscle regulating secretion by glands.

The trembling associated with fear represents a form of ineffective skeletal muscle contraction, contrasting with the more obviously purposeful, concerted, yet largely involuntary skeletal muscle contraction that produces clenched fists, grimacing, and upright or advancing posture that are associated with anger. One may speculate that trembling provided an evolutionary advantage as a form of skeletal muscle "idling" prior to escape.

Trembling also communicates extreme emotional intensity. Humans shake during both terror and rage. The words, "agitate," "quiver," and "quake" imply both shaking and a state of emotional upset, without necessarily indicating fear or anger; however, in the absence of signs of purposeful skeletal muscle contraction, and in the presence of other signs discussed below, trembling usually indicates intense fear. Classical writers most commonly have used trembling for this purpose.

I shudder at the word (Virgil, *The Aeneid* II, 204).

Less than a drop of blood remains in me that does not tremble; I recognize the signals of the ancient flame (Dante, *Purgatorio*, XXX, Line 46).

Right as an aspes leef she gan to quake (Chaucer, *Troilus and Criseyde* III, 656).

What man dare, I dare:
Approach thou like the rugged Russian bear,
The arm'd rhinoceros, or the Hyrcan tiger,
Take any shape but that, and my firm nerves
Shall never tremble (Shakespeare, *Macbeth* III, 4, 99).

Darwin also associated terror with muscular weakness, in contrast with the association between rage and contraction of skeletal muscle:

We may . . . infer that fear was expressed from an extremely remote period, in almost the same manner as it now is by man; namely, by trembling, the erection of the hair, cold perspiration, pallor, widely opened eyes, the relaxation of most of the muscles, and by the whole body cowering downwards or held motionless. . . .

The excited brain gives strength to the muscles, and at the same time energy to the will. The body is commonly held erect ready for instant action, but sometimes it is bent forward towards the offending person, with the limbs more or less rigid. The mouth is generally closed with firmness, showing fixed determination, and the teeth are clenched or ground together. Such gestures as the raising of the arms, with the fists clenched, as if to strike the offender, are common. Few men in a great passion, and telling some one to begone, can resist acting as if they intended to strike or push the man violently away.

The trembling associated with extreme fear may result from high circulating adrenaline levels, because adrenaline given intravenously elicits trembling in humans. Patients who have panic reactions evoked by particular drugs have both marked trembling and large increases in plasma adrenaline concentrations.

The state of contraction of smooth muscle cells in the walls of the blood vessels in the skin determines whether the skin looks pale or flushed. Constriction of skin blood vessels causes pallor, and dilation of skin blood vessels causes flushing. These colors also differentiate terror from rage. In many animal species, including humans, the color red signifies aggressive feeling and intent. When enraged, we "see red," and our "blood boils." When we surrender, we wave a white flag. The English adjectives, "pale," "wan," and "pallid," denote not only whiteness but also feebleness or weakness. "Sanguine" denotes not only bloodiness but also confidence. "Ruddy" denotes not only redness but also vigor. We "seethe" with anger but "freeze," turn "pale as a ghost," and turn white with fright. Among Olympic athletes competing in combat sports, those wearing red uniforms are more likely to win.

These skin color changes are automatic, involuntary, and unconscious. Predictably, they result from patterned changes in activities of components of the autonomic nervous system. During rage, release of the chemical messenger, acetylcholine, and possibly nitric oxide, contributes to the flushing, whereas during fear, release of adrenaline from the adrenal gland probably produces the pallor.

The lizard species, *Anolis carolinensis*, is also called the American lizard.

Anoles are popular pets. They change color according to their temperature, humidity, mood, and health. Fighting between male anoles increases plasma levels of both norepinephrine and adrenaline within 30 seconds, accompanied by a darkening of a spot behind their eyes. Remarkably, the more aggressive the combatant, and the more likely it will win, the quicker the spot darkens; the winners have higher plasma norepinephrine levels than the losers do. Castration increases the time to darkening of the eyespot. This finding suggests that testosterone contributes to the eyespot darkening. At least in anoles, testosterone and the sympathetic nervous system appear to work together to increase social dominance.

The state of contraction of gastrointestinal smooth muscle constitutes a third general distinction between terror and rage. You already read about the Old Testament "trial by ordeal" to test a woman accused by her husband of adultery. Failure to digest a type of potion, the "water of bitterness," would produce swelling of the abdomen and indicate guilt. This swelling would have reflected expansion of the stomach due to relaxation of the smooth muscle in the stomach wall and therefore failure to move the potion through. You also already read that Cannon first demonstrated release of adrenaline during emotional distress from the relaxation a strip of gastrointestinal muscle produced by the blood of a cat exposed to a barking dog. Cannon's demonstration gives a rationale for biblical "lie detection."

Possibly from parasympathetic activation and intestinal peristalsis, coupled with loss of voluntary sphincter control and adrenaline effects, individuals in distress defecate. In rats, the rate of feces production has been used as a quantitative index of anxiety. In the film, *Shoah*, Franz Suchomel, former SS Unterscharfuhrer at the Treblinka death camp, recalls with sardonic detachedness the "death panic" of Jews in the tunnel to the gas chambers:

> In the "funnel" the women had to wait. They heard the motors of the gas chambers. Maybe they also heard people screaming and imploring. As they waited, "death panic" overwhelmed them. "Death panic" makes people let go. They empty themselves, from the front or the rear. So often, where the women stood, there were five or six rows of excrement. . . . When this "death panic" sets in, one lets go. It's well known that when someone's terrified, and knows he's about to die. . . .

The state of tone of smooth muscle in glands provides a fourth physiological difference between terror and rage. Darwin wrote that during terror,

The salivary glands act imperfectly; the mouth becomes dry, and is often opened. . . . One of the best-marked symptoms is the trembling of all the muscles of the body; and this is often first seen in the lips. From this cause, and from the dryness of the mouth, the voice becomes husky or indistinct, or may altogether fail.

Anxiety-provoking situations generally inhibit production of saliva. The inability to produce saliva is a well-known component of stage fright in musicians. A teacher of the French horn is reported to have admonished a student with performance anxiety, "You can't play the French horn if you can't make spit." In contrast, during rage, production of saliva increases, perhaps as an evolutionary remnant before predatory attack. As noted previously, in the Bible spitting in another's face signaled aggressive contempt.

The relative amount of adrenomedullary hormonal system and sympathetic nervous system activation provides a fifth distinction between rage and terror—between "fight" and "fright." In general, situations producing panic or anxiety increase adrenaline levels proportionately more than they increase norepinephrine levels. For instance, in people with acute flight phobia, actual flying increases heart rate, blood pressure, perceived anxiety, and plasma adrenaline levels, whereas plasma norepinephrine levels remain unchanged. In professional hockey players, selective increases in norepinephrine excretion accompany aggressive, active emotional display, whereas selective increases in urinary adrenaline excretion accompany tense and anxious but passive emotional behaviors.

Adrenomedullary hormonal system activation during fright intensifies but probably does not cause the emotional experience. Patients with pheochromocytomas have high circulating catecholamine levels due to catecholamine release by the tumor, but the patients do not have excessive anxiety. Adrenaline when administered exogenously amplifies emotional experiences but does not elicit any specific emotion. Moreover, plasma adrenaline levels required for healthy people to discriminate between infusions of adrenaline or saline exceed those typically noted in situations eliciting distress.

As the intensity of an emotion increases, the tendency to evince locomotor activity increases. The continuum of fear ranges from boredom to unexpressed but experienced anxiety to visible, trembling terror to uncontrollable panic and headlong flight. The continuum of anger ranges from boredom to visible annoyance to rage to uncontrollable frenzy. The autonomic patterns accompanying fear or anger probably depend importantly on the extent of expression of the locomotor behaviors—that is, on the amount of activity or passivity.

Any of several reaction patterns can occur as fear intensifies. The organism may tremble but otherwise remain attentive and motionless (the "freezing" or "fright" reaction); it may attack defensively (the "defense reaction"); it may suddenly attempt to flee; or it may suddenly lose consciousness in a "playing dead" or "defeat" reaction. Species vary in their tendencies for these instinctive behaviors. The triggers and mechanisms causing abrupt shifts among these reaction patterns remain mysterious.

Darwin recognized that extreme fear can evoke sudden loss of consciousness in lower animals and in humans: "A terrified canary-bird has been seen not only to tremble and to turn white about the base of the bill, but to faint; and I once caught a robin in a room, which fainted so completely, that for a time I thought it dead" (Darwin, 1965, 77). Psychological theorists have viewed fainting as an expression of helpless defeat, when the individual perceives the futility of either fighting or fleeing in an emotionally distressing situation, and the central nervous system directs a physiological response pattern resembling primitive "playing dead" reactions. Many situations in modern-day life, such as undergoing blood sampling at the doctor's office, receiving an injection of dental anesthetic, witnessing a traumatic automobile accident, or receiving tragic news in public, can cause distress without the possibility of coping by fighting or fleeing.

In fainting, activity of the sympathetic nervous system decreases or even disappears completely, while activity of the adrenomedullary hormonal system increases drastically. Concurrently, the parasympathetic nervous system usually is activated, and levels of endogenous opioids and vasopressin increase. This pattern sets the stage for multiple positive feedback loops, discussed in more detail in chapter 8. Standing for a long period, warm external temperature, and delayed ingestion of a meal increase the likelihood of developing a fainting reaction, possibly because these stimuli require sympathoneural activation to maintain venous return to the heart.

One may ask what survival advantage a "giving up" or defeat reaction provided in evolution. Predators may instinctively avoid eating an animal they have not killed, because eating any discovered carcasses would pose an infectious or toxic threat to health. Thus, when attacked opossums enter a deathlike trance, the predator may shake the animal but may eventually lose interest in the prey that looks and feels already dead. Years ago a young woman camping in the Pacific Northwest was approached by a grizzly bear and fainted. The bear scratched and threw her, but she lived to tell the tale. Within a species, including humans, combat usually ends abruptly when one of the combatants displays a defeat reaction, so that the "underdog" survives. A defeat reaction may also arouse altruistic behavior in others. Finally, "giving up" may sacrifice consciousness to allay pain and suffering.

Hypothalamic-pituitary-adrenocortical (HPA) activation seems especially prominent in distressing situations perceived as novel. When no coping behavior is possible, novel or threatening conditions are associated with both HPA and adrenomedullary hormonal system activation. Most evidence supports the view that repeated exposure to distressing stimuli attenuates responses of ACTH and corticosterone levels in rats, with generally maintained responses of plasma levels of catecholamines. Early clinical studies about HPA activation in stressful situations did not take into account separately the factors of novelty, predictability, and controllability. During repetition of exhausting bicycle exercise, physiological and performance measures are reproducible, whereas responses of ACTH, cortisol, and vasopressin levels diminish with increasing experience.

Chronic, repeated exposure to a distressing stimulus augments plasma catecholamine responses to a novel distressing stimulus—"dishabituation." The response to either a physiological or psychological stimulus evoking distress therefore depends importantly on the previous experiences of the organism, refuting Selye's doctrine of nonspecificity.

In 1942, Cannon described "voodoo death," based on reports that aboriginal natives in Australia, South America, Africa, and New Zealand had weakened and died within days of being tabooed by a shaman. Cannon proposed that activation of the sympathicoadrenal system would elicit a form of positive feedback loop: "A vicious circle is then established; the low blood pressure damages the very organs which are necessary for the maintenance of an adequate circulation, and as they are damaged they are less and less able to keep the blood circulating to an effective degree." To explain the low blood pressure, Cannon suggested that adrenaline would reduce blood volume; a more modern explanation might impute direct heart muscle damage from high adrenaline levels in the bloodstream. As a medical student I attended an extraordinary clinicopathological conference about a patient who had died of voodoo death. As I recall, the patient felt doomed to die on a certain day. As that day approached, the patient refused food or drink and died on the appointed day, not with a rapid pulse rate, as one might expect adrenaline to produce, but with a progressive fall in pulse rate and eventual cessation of the heartbeat, perhaps by excessive outflow of the parasympathetic nervous system to the heart.

The Nose of God

The Hebrew word for nose is used in at least 275 different verses of the Old Testament. For almost the entire Old Testament, the nose is used symbolically, and English translations do not refer to the nose when used in this manner. Whereas the heart of the Bible symbolizes inner thought, a person's "self-talk," invisible to the outside observer, *ahf*, the nose, reveals a particular behavioral-emotional state: rage.

In Jacob's deathbed farewell to his sons, near the end of Genesis, he recalls how Simeon and Levi had led an expedition to kill Shechem, Shechem's father Hamor, and their entire town after Shechem had raped Dinah, Jacob's daughter. In Genesis 49:6–7 Jacob berates Simeon and Levi for their acts of deceit and murder:

> Let not my person be included in their council,
> Let not my being be counted in their assembly.
> For when angry they slay men,
> and when pleased they maim oxen.
> Cursed be their anger so fierce,
> and their wrath so relentless.
> I will divide them in Jacob,
> Scatter them in Israel.

Literally, Jacob is cursing their noses.

The nose as the organ of rage is also used in the description of the attributes of God, in Exodus 34:6–7: "The Lord passed before him and proclaimed: 'The Lord! The Lord! A God compassionate and gracious, *slow to anger*, abounding in kindness and faithfulness, extending kindness to the thousandth generation, forgiving iniquity, transgression, and sin.'" Literally, God has slow nostrils.

The word for nose is commonly associated with another word, the Hebrew root for which is *charah*. The exact meaning of *charah* is not clear, but the word always refers to externally observable, extreme emotional upset. The best English translation for *charah* would be "flare," which refers to widening, as in flared nostrils, as well as to sudden, bright burning, or signaling by means of a hot light. Flared nostrils would provide a visible sign of distress. *Charah* appears for the first time in Genesis 4:5–6, when God pays heed to Abel's offering but not to Cain's.

> Cain was much *distressed* and his face fell.
> and the Lord said to Cain, "Why are you *distressed*,
> and why is your face fallen?
> Surely, if you do right,
> There is uplift.
> But if you do not do right,
> Sin couches at the door;
> Its urge is toward you,
> Yet you can be its master."

The verses quoted here presage a theme in modern jurisprudence about attempts to invoke stress-induced temporary insanity as a legal defense for murder. The attempts virtually always fail.

The muscles that control the size of the nostrils are called the alae nasi, from the Latin for "wings of the nose." When a person becomes enraged, the alae nasi contract and widen the nostrils involuntarily and unconsciously. Given this automaticity, one would predict that the autonomic nervous system would contribute to the flaring of the nostrils in rage, and this seems to be the case. Administration of the drug, alpha-methylDOPA, which inhibits sympathetic nervous system outflows, decreases the muscular tone of the alae nasi. In other words, inhibition of the sympathetic nervous system limits the ability of the nostrils to flare. Conversely, exercise potently stimulates the sympathetic nervous system and decreases the resistance of the nose to the flow of air, partly because of nostril flaring. Asphyxia and nicotine share the characteristic of evoking release of adrenaline into the bloodstream, and in anesthetized dogs, brief periods of asphyxia or injection of nicotine stimulate the alae nasi and widen the nostrils. Flaring of the nostrils in enraged people therefore provides an externally visible, instinctively communicated sign of the behavioral-emotional state of rage, and members of the adrenaline family cause or contribute to this sign.

Stimulation of the sympathetic nervous system acts in two ways to increase the exchange of air via the nose. Not only do the nostrils widen but also the blood vessels in the mucus membranes constrict. Since the air in the lungs is about at body temperature, which is usually warmer than the temperature in the outside world, these effects would be expected to increase the temperature of the exhaled air, especially in the setting of an increased rate or depth of breathing, which adrenaline also produces. It is therefore no coincidence that flared nostrils and hot exhalation go together. A hot blast from flared nostrils, due to effects of members of adrenaline's chemical family, would fit perfectly with the frequent biblical usage of God destroying by a hot blast from the nose. Independently of the biblical tradition, many different cultures include a legendary fire-breathing dragon. We humans when enraged instinctively "breathe fire."

Stress Toons

Cartoonists often exploit the autonomic nervous system in their work, because changes in autonomic nervous system functions produce observable effects that communicate the emotions and intentions of the characters. Cartoonists convey these emotions and intentions immediately using a few strokes.

Students of Pupils

Cartoonists are great students of the pupils of the eyes. Constriction of the pupils conveys startle, unequal pupils show disorientation, and large pupils indicate cuteness, as shown in the illustration in the preface.

Pinpoint pupils during startle result from a sudden increase in the parasympathetic nervous system outflow to the muscles of the eye that regulate pupil diameter. The nerves release the neurotransmitter, acetylcholine, which binds to specific receptors in the sphincter muscle of the pupils, causing them to constrict. Simultaneously, stimulation of parasympathetic nervous system outflow to the heart causes a sudden fall in the heart rate and decrease in the efficiency of conduction of electricity within the heart. This is why when you are startled, your heart "skips a beat." Destruction of sympathetic nerves supplying the iris muscle also constricts the pupil. In 1852, Claude Bernard demonstrated constriction of the pupil, drooping of the eyelid, and loss of sweating on the side of destruction of the sympathetic nerves supplying the head. A physician named Horner described a patient with the same triad, which in English-speaking countries came to be called Horner syndrome. In France the same condition is called Bernard-Horner syndrome or simply Bernard syndrome.

Cartoonists often use the sudden appearance of unequal pupils to convey a state of severe confusion or disorientation. Trauma to the head can produce enough accumulation or blood or swelling of the brain to increase pressure on the third cranial nerve, the optic nerve, which carries autonomic nerve fibers from the brainstem to the muscle controlling the size of the pupil. The pupil on the affected side dilates. In medical slang this is called a "blown pupil." Clinicians worry when they see unequal pupils in a patient, especially when the inequality develops rapidly, because this could be a sign of a catastrophe inside the head.

Enlargement of both pupils has an entirely different significance. Cartoonists enlarge the pupils to convey cuteness or romantic allure. According to legend, large pupils are thought to increase attractiveness. Italian women would instill into their eyes "belladonna," meaning "beautiful woman." Belladonna, an extract of the plant *Atropa belladonna*, blocks receptors for acetylcholine.

In a cover article by Eckhard H. Hess in *Scientific American* in April 1965, Hess hypothesized that interesting or pleasing stimuli produce pupil dilation, whereas unpleasant or distasteful stimuli produce pupil constriction.

> It is said that magicians doing card tricks can identify the card a person is thinking about by watching his pupils enlarge when the card is turned up, and that Chinese jade dealers watch a buyer's pupils to know when he is impressed by a specimen and is likely to pay a high price.

Hess reported that when men viewed a picture of a woman's face that had been retouched to show enlarged pupils, the men's own pupils dilated, compared with their response to the same picture but with the woman having constricted pupils. Most of the men thought the two pictures were identical, but some did report that one was "more feminine" or "prettier," or "softer." Why would enlarged pupils in a woman increase her allure to a man? By nonverbally demonstrating her own interest in him!

Scared to Death

Cartoonists recognize, and readers instinctively appreciate, that fear in response to a sudden, unexpected threat develops along a continuum of intensity. Here are some tricks of the trade about how cartoonists depict these stages, based on responses of components of the autonomic nervous system.

The first stage of fear is startle, or the shock of alarm. The hair is lifted slightly off the head. The person "flips his wig." Erection of the hair reflects increased sympathetic nervous system outflow to the hair follicles. The pupils are constricted, from parasympathetic nervous system activation, and the eyes are transfixed on the source of the fear. Both eyebrows are lifted.

The second stage is fright. The eyes bulge out, the person sweats and trembles, from the effects of adrenaline, the hair rises further, the mouth slackens open, indicating a loss of voluntary control of skeletal muscle, and there is no saliva. The third stage is extreme fright. The hair not only stands out but also is frayed. The cheeks puff with vomit, because parasympathetic nervous system activation has caused the guts to churn, while adrenaline prevents forward propulsion of ingested food. The person becomes dissociated and no longer fixes his gaze on the source of fear. In the last stage, the person loses consciousness and turns blue. The pupils are fixed and dilated, or the eyes are replaced by Xs, and the face swells from edema fluid.

Breathing Fire

Cartoonists draw anger also along a continuum of intensity. The first stage is annoyance. An eyebrow is lifted, the person looks straight at the object of anger, and the nostrils flare slightly. The hair is raised slightly off the head, the mouth downturned, the pupils constricted—hence the statement, "His eyes were pinpoints of hate." The second stage is anger. The head is red and enlarged, the teeth are bared, the nostrils enlarged further, and the eyes are squinty and positioned higher on the face. There is increased salivation because of parasympathetic and sympathetic nervous system activation. The third stage is rage. Now the face is beet red, the skin so hot that smoke rises from the scalp or comes out of the flared nostrils. The teeth are very prominent and the mouth is open as if to bite. The fourth stage is frenzy. The person is now dissociated and no longer focuses on the victim. The eyes bulge out, and the tongue falls out of the mouth, signaling delirium. Slurpy drool descends from the mouth, consistent with the protein-rich saliva released from catecholamine effects.

The Best Defense

A few decades ago, researchers began to study the "defense response." This is a particular pattern that stimulation of certain brain centers evokes, which has components of Cannon's emergency fight-or-flight pattern. If you visualized a threatened cat, you would have the defense response in mind. The eyebrows are raised, the pupils are dilated, the hair stands out, the back is arched, the teeth are bared as the lips pull back, and the individual emits a characteristic saliva-laden screech or hiss. This is a display that warns of impending attack.

The individual's appearance in the defense response is not exactly the same as that before attack from rage or predation, and cartoonists appreciate these distinctions. In rage or predatory attack, the eyes are squinted, as if the muscles of the eyelids are protecting them, and the pupils are if anything constricted; the skin is flushed rather than pale. In terror or passive fear, the mouth contains decreased saliva (Gulp!) and the skeletal muscle tone is slackened. You stand up to defend yourself, but you cringe, crumble, or collapse with fright.

7 | Stress in Evolutionary Perspective

Science depends on measurement. Measurement is the key link in the circular chain of the scientific method. The chain consists of observation, induction of an explanatory concept, derivation of a testable hypothesis, prediction, experimental design, measurement, data analysis, and inference, which enlighten further observation. Hopefully, accumulating experimental information leads us not in circles but up spirals, serpentine helices of increased understanding.

History teaches that medical scientific discovery and improving technology go hand in hand. The same measurement that renders science powerful, however, also renders it difficult and restrictive. Certainly it is easier to hold on to beliefs or to pass on legends without measuring anything. In particular, for many centuries doctors misdiagnosed and maltreated patients based on the "spirits," as taught by the second-century Greek physician Galen. The history of medicine is replete with examples of sickness and death caused by doctors acting on their philosophies.

Why Evolution Is a Worthwhile Theory and Creationism Isn't

Scientists and theologians share the quest to comprehend existence by trying to understand how things came to be the way they are. Theologians do this by derivation from the assumption that phenomena do not just happen. Everything has a purpose, a design, and so there must be a Creator. This lends a sense of meaning to existence. That meaning may remain forever obscure, but although we may never fathom the design, we can appreciate the effects of that design in observable reality and live out our lives in humble thanks.

As a corollary, discrepancies, paradoxes, and inconsistencies in our lives as actually lived must be apparent and not real. Perhaps they teach, by spurring attempts to resolve them through insights into deeper meanings.

STRESS IN EVOLUTIONARY PERSPECTIVE   165

Regardless, they do not and cannot lead to rejection of the core belief, because ultimately the religious person accepts the limited comprehension of the human mind.

Creationism depends essentially on this assumption of the inability of the human mind to understand the origin and meaning of existence. One cannot comprehend the Creator, at the creation, in history, now, or ever. Creationism assigns more importance to revelation than to prediction. All creationist explanations derive from the assumption of purpose. Purposes exist, and they are ultimately divine, even if the human mind cannot "divine" them. Epiphany is a feeling of the revelation of the meaning and purpose of existence.

Scientists spend their time formulating, testing, applying, revising, and rejecting theories. Theories, like articles of religious faith, reflect attempts to comprehend existence by derivation from one or a few elementary principles. But there are crucial differences. For one thing, theories, despite their logical derivation, are not assumed to be either true or false. Indeed, theories cannot reveal the Truth. One judges a theory not by the ability to account for phenomena, nor by the pleasant sense of insight or revelation, but by the ability to generate hypotheses that observation or experiment can test. The distinguishing characteristic of a worthwhile theory is not explanation but prediction. Theories have tenuous existences, because they ultimately survive only by the correspondence of observed phenomena with predictions. Once a theory makes a prediction that observation or experimentation fails to verify, the theory must undergo modification or rejection. One may of course attempt to rationalize contrary results—inappropriate or erroneous experimental methods or design, illogical derivation or inferences, biases, complicating factors, statistical variation, and so forth—but eventually, after failed attempts at replication or negative results of valid alternative experiments, the scientist must let go of even the most closely held theory.

The strong scientist questions everything, assumes the least, and thinks continuously about how to go about testing theories. The main articles of scientific faith are in the method itself; in the assumption of logic of the universe and of life, where everything potentially is comprehensible by the human mind; in observations and experimental evidence that transcend the observer and experimenter; and in conformance of replicated results with fact. This is why, in science, fabrication of results is a cardinal sin.

Vitalism and Mechanism

Vitalism holds that life processes are uniquely different from physicochemical phenomena and so are beyond understanding by physicochemical laws. Vitalist explanations always have offered a pleasing sense of order and purpose. You already read that according to the influential ancient Greek physician Galen, the veins distributed the "natural spirit" formed in the liver, the arteries distributed the "vital spirit" formed in the heart, and the nerves distributed the "animal spirit," associated with sensation and emotion, formed in the brain. For 1,400 years, the heart was viewed not as a pump but as a furnace, imbuing the blood with the "vital spirit" and igniting a biological flame that would literally heat the body. Traces of vitalism remain in modern "holistic" and "new age" medicine.

The opposite of the vitalist view, the purely mechanist view, holds that physical and chemical laws can explain all physiological processes, with no need to posit intervening influences such as "goals" or "purposes" for those processes. Mechanistic theories have also received criticism, for two reasons. First, mechanism, considered cursorily, does not seem to account for organized complexity, which of course is a characteristic of all higher organisms. Isn't the whole greater than the sum of the parts? Mechanistic theories, however, do not have to ignore the fact of organization. In particular, Charles Darwin proposed his theory of evolution, a type of mechanistic theory, exactly to explain the complexity of the structure and the apparent purposefulness of the emotional behavior of organisms. Modern-day Darwinians emphasize that genetic variation and natural selection can explain organized complexity, even without an overall design. Second, how can one apply a mechanistic theory to explain goal-directed behaviors, which precede their effects? A mechanistic theory need not require responses only to past events. Organisms have a variety of mechanisms of proactivity that are built-in (instinctive), readily acquired early in life (imprinted), learned by association (conditioned), or even invented (simulated). For instance, a chess computer can simulate consequences of alternative actions and, according to programmed algorithms, choose the move most likely to produce checkmate, even if the computer has never experienced the situation before or made that move. The ability to simulate provides a ready mechanistic explanation for anticipatory stress responses in higher organisms.

The theory of evolution contains two, and only two, elements. The first is that the offspring of an individual can differ from that individual itself.

The second is that such differences matter. Offspring of sexually reproducing organisms differ from the parents mainly because of genetic recombination and mutation. Genetic recombination refers to mixing of segments of chromosomes. All our cells except germ cells (sperm and eggs) contain 23 pairs of chromosomes, long chains of deoxyribonucleic acid (DNA). To form a germ cell, the DNA in the precursor cell replicates, and then the cell divides twice, reducing the complement of chromosomes to 23 individual strands. Before the first division, segments of the paired chromosomes can exchange places, or cross over. This means that the germ cells contain chromosomes that, considered as entire units, did not exist previously. Mutation refers to changes in the structure of the chromosomes themselves, with a portion deleted or replicated or with a specific link in the DNA chain, called a nucleotide, changed to a different one.

A classical creationist argument against evolution is the randomness alternative: if there were no design to the universe, then creation would have had to occur by random events, and how could so much complexity, so apparently purposive, have arisen by chance alone? Variation of itself, even across a very large number of generations, cannot account for life's organized complexity; but variation constitutes only half of evolutionary theory.

Evolutionary theory claims that the organized complexity of living things arose from the operation of natural selection on intergenerational variation. Natural selection can reduce drastically the number of generations leading to a particular genetic arrangement. The English ethologist Richard Dawkins carried out a simple computer experiment about how many generations it would take for a randomly generated sequence of letters to spell out a particular phrase of Shakespeare. Each "offspring generation" consisted of the parent sequence, but with a single change in a single letter. Suppose the change, the "mutation," were at position 17. Suppose that at position 17, the "correct" letter were r, the randomly generated parent letter were an m, and the "mutant" letter at that position were a t. Because t is closer to r than m is, the sequence with t at position 17 would "survive" to replicate, whereas the sequence with m at position 17 would not. How many "generations" would be required to reproduce the goal phrase? If the sequences were generated completely at random, the number of generations would be incomprehensibly huge. To generate them, even a high-speed computer would use more time than has occurred in the history of the universe! But if the sequences were "selected," generation by generation, according to the strategy above, then a remarkably small number of generations would be required—less than 100. Moreover, no matter how many times the experiment was repeated, only a small number of generations were required.

In this example, the "goal" phrase was a given at the beginning. This provided the strategy for the selection. According to evolutionary theory, however, the only goal is survival itself, which is to say, the protection and propagation of genes via bodies. Modern-day Darwinians emphasize that genetic variation and natural selection, operating over the eons, can explain organized complexity, without imputing an overall goal or design. Indeed, Dawkins has argued that the theory of evolution is the *only* theory in principle capable of doing so. This means that the complexity of the universe does not of itself imply a design, a Creator.

What are the "goals" of body systems? Does the body "want" to regulate the temperature of its blood, the concentrations of glucose and oxygen, and so forth? Teleology is the doctrine that an overall design or purpose determines natural phenomena. Bernard's theory of the *milieu intérieur* contains an element of teleology, not in the sense of asserting the application of a Creator's supernatural will, but in the sense of imputing an overall purpose for the operations of body systems. Continuing this tradition, Walter B. Cannon wrote, in his *The Way of an Investigator:*

> My first article of belief is based on the observation, almost universally confirmed in present knowledge, that what happens in our bodies is directed toward a useful end.

The themes of compensatoriness, adaptiveness, and purposiveness of stress responses correspond roughly to mechanistic, Darwinian, and teleological views. Purposiveness, although helpful in deriving testable hypotheses, cannot constitute the essence of a rigorously scientific stress theory, since all the elements of such a theory should be both necessary and testable, and how does one prove the necessity and existence of purposiveness? Compensatoriness alone, while possibly adequate for a parsimonious definition of stress, seems inadequate to explain why and how stress responses evolved, as evidence discussed below suggests they did. A scientific theory of stress therefore should avoid including the notion of purposiveness and should transcend the notion of compensatoriness to include the survival advantage of adaptiveness.

Darwin and Ethology

Charles Darwin proposed the inheritance not only of physical characteristics but also of emotional behaviors. In fact, in his *The Expression of the Emotions in Man and Animals*, he used the latter to support his theory of the descent of man:

> I have endeavored to show in considerable detail that all the chief expressions exhibited by man are the same throughout the world. This fact is interesting, as it affords a new argument in favor of the several races being descended from a single parent-stock, which must have been almost completely human in structure, and to a large extent in mind, before the period at which the races diverged from each other.

The naturalistic studies of the ethologists Lorenz and Tinbergen largely confirmed Darwin's views about the evolution of instinctive behaviors. Indeed, Darwin provided much of the conceptual foundation for the field of ethology, the branch of zoology that deals with instinctive animal behaviors. He wrote:

> My object is to show that certain movements were originally performed for a definite end, and that, under nearly the same circumstances, they are still pertinaciously performed through habit when not of the least use. That the tendency in most of the following cases is inherited, we may infer from such actions being performed in the same manner by all the individuals, young and old, of the same species.
>
> As far as we can judge, only a few expressive movements . . . are learnt by each individual. . . . The far greater number of the movements of expression, and all the more important ones, are, as we have seen, innate or inherited; and such cannot be said to depend on the will of the individual.

Geographically diverse societies do indeed appear to have essentially the same forms of emotional expression. For instance, members of the Minangkabau culture in Bukittingi, western Sumatra, express fear, anger, sadness, and disgust similarly to Americans, and production of facial expressions of fear or anger produce immediate increases in heart rate in both cultures.

Darwin recognized that the autonomic concomitants of emotion have proved advantageous not only in preparing the organism for emergency responses but also for providing the basis for visible signs that serve important, universally understood communication functions within the species:

The movements of expression in the face and body, whatever their origin may have been, are in themselves of much importance for our welfare. They serve as the first means of communication between the mother and her infant; she smiles approval, and thus encourages her child on the right path, or frowns disapproval. We readily perceive sympathy in others by their expression; our sufferings are thus mitigated and our pleasures increased; and mutual good feeling is thus strengthened. The movements of expression give vividness and energy to our spoken words. They reveal the thoughts and intentions of others more truly than do words, which may be falsified.

Research about primates in the wild has suggested that in everyday life, most "stress" system activation accompanies instinctive social behaviors— for example, dominance displays, sexual pursuit, and submissive escape— rather than mitigating threats to physiological or metabolic homeostasis.

Darwin was acquainted with the work of Claude Bernard but had only a vague understanding of the role of the autonomic nervous system in producing the observable signs of distress. Darwin did recognize, however, the origin of these signs in the nervous system:

> Certain actions which we recognize as expressive of certain states of mind, are the direct results of the constitution of the nervous system, and have been from the first independent of the will, and, to a large extent, of habit. When the sensorium is strongly excited nerve-force is generated in excess, and is transmitted in certain directions, dependent on the connection of the nerve-cells, and, as far as the muscular system is concerned, on the nature of the movements which have been habitually practiced. . . . Claude Bernard also repeatedly insists, and this deserves especial notice, that when the heart is affected it reacts on the brain; and the state of the brain again reacts through the pneumo-gastric nerve on the heart; so that under any excitement there will be much mutual action and reaction between these, the two most important organs of the body.
>
> Any sensation or emotion, as great pain or rage, which has habitually led to much muscular action, will immediately influence the flow of nerve-force to the heart, although there may not be at the time any muscular exertion.

The homeostatic theory of stress and distress relies heavily on concepts Darwin introduced: Autonomic changes that accompany emotional experiences and their behavioral manifestations evolved, because they were advantageous in natural selection. One advantage of autonomic arousal is rapid or anticipatory adjustments in cardiovascular function, and another is provision of universally understood means of intraspecific communication.

The Selfish Gene

Stress responses have important genetic components. Selective pressures that guided the evolution of physical characteristics probably also guided the evolution of stress responses. Richard Dawkins has presented a comprehensive "selfish gene" theory about the evolution of behavior, with the following propositions.

1. The fundamental unit of selection is not the species, nor, strictly speaking, the individual, but the gene, the unit of heredity. A gene is any portion of genetic material that potentially lasts for enough generations to serve as a unit of natural selection. A gene is not a single physical piece of DNA but all replicas of that piece, distributed throughout the world. Groups of genes can be selected as units.
2. The body is an integral agent for preserving and propagating genes—a "survival machine."
3. Behavior, which is mediated by skeletal muscles, evolved because it enabled rapid movement. Generating complex, timed movements requires coordination by a computer, the brain. The genes control behavior indirectly, like a computer programmer controls a computer's functions indirectly. The genes set up the machine but cannot control it, because of time-lag problems. Instead, genes work by controlling protein synthesis, which is powerful but slow. They provide strategies, preprogrammed behavioral policies.
4. Genes influence behavioral strategies by incorporating a capacity for learning, which requires memory and feedback. Simulations represent vicarious trial-and-error predictions of future events. The evolution of the capacity to simulate culminated in subjective consciousness.

Applying the selfish gene theory, natural selection would have favored the evolution of stress responses, the body's means for preserving a stable inner world. Continual adjustments in activities of homeostatic systems reflect the operation of genetically determined algorithms, learning by combinations of classical and operant conditioning, and conscious simulations of likely future events.

The mystery, and the challenge for stress research, is not to explain why stress responses evolved but how they work. Research has begun to elucidate the molecular events underlying classical conditioning, such as in the sea snail, *Aplysia*. The genetic instructions dictating these events, and therefore the bases for evolution of stress responses, exist in our genomic encyclopedias. Identifying and interpreting those instructions are crucial aspects of scientific integrative medical research.

Hal

For centuries scientists and philosophers have argued over a definition of consciousness. By extension from Dawkins's selfish gene theory, one may propose that consciousness entails simulation where the individual is part of the simulation, predicting and anticipating consequences of externally sensed, internally perceived, or even ruminated situations for the individual's own survival or well-being.

You may remember Hal, the mutinous supercomputer in the science fiction movie and book by Arthur C. Clarke, *2001: A Space Odyssey*. If you saw the movie or read the book, you probably felt that Hal was conscious.

> He might have handled it—as most men handle their own neuroses—if he had not been faced with a crisis that challenged his very existence. He had been threatened with disconnection; he would be deprived of all his inputs, and thrown into an unimaginable state of unconsciousness.
>
> To Hal, this was the equivalent of Death. For he had never slept, and therefore he did not know that one could awake again.
>
> So he would protect himself, with all the weapons at his command. Without rancor—but without pity—he would remove the source of his frustrations.
>
> And then, following the orders that had been given to him in case of the ultimate emergency, he would continue the mission—unhindered, and alone. (New York: Penguin Books, 1993, 152)

The Price of Complexity Is Eternal Stress

One can trace the evolution of the adrenaline family to primordial challenges all higher organisms have faced as a consequence of complex structure. Single-celled organisms normally are surrounded by the nutrient medium they need, but higher organisms must use internal systems to maintain cellular temperature, take in and distribute oxygen, ingest and deliver fuels and water, and rid themselves of metabolic wastes. The evolution of increasingly complex and increasingly energy-requiring systems to deliver fuel and remove waste paralleled the evolution of the organized complexity that afforded resistance to the vicissitudes of the external environment. The price we pay to maintain our physical integrity is a continuous requirement to acquire and expend energy. Eventually these efforts produce wear and tear and, via self-reinforcing degeneration of internal systems, disorders, diseases, and death.

Ascending the phylogenetic scale, organisms have depended increasingly on complex, energy-requiring systems and on close coordination of behavioral, neural, hormonal, and physiological responses. For instance, reef corals, relatively simple animals, live a fragile existence, surviving only in unusual, suitable niches within a small range of salinity, turbulence, and temperature. Although they benefit from the lack of energy expenditure to maintain cellular temperature, they cannot live in water colder than 18°C. More versatile cold-blooded reptiles and other lower vertebrates survive a larger range of external temperatures by using the sun and shade instinctively and probably by adjusting cardiovascular system performance, but this requires more organization and more energy. Warm-blooded mammals require and use much more fuel than do reptiles or fish, simply to maintain body temperature. As in reptiles, mammals possess not only physiological but also instinctive behavioral means to regulate temperature. Ecological niches determine the adaptive value of this inheritance. Humans spend most of their lives wrapped in protective clothing or in environments where the external temperature itself is regulated.

Mechanisms for preserving body water and providing a continuous supply of essential metabolic fuels—oxygen and glucose—must also have developed early in evolution. The remarkably large repertoire of glucose "counterregulatory" systems indicates the importance of appropriate adjustments in blood glucose levels in different situations, including exercise, emotion, and the postprandial state. So many behaviors increase glucose utilization in different organs, a variety of means to maintain glucose levels evolved with those behaviors. Because all cells require glucose, these situations often call for generalized metabolic responses, elicited by hormones reaching all tissues of the body. Conversely, cellular deprivation of glucose poses a generalized threat, where no patterned neural response or readjustment of blood volume distribution can suffice. Low glucose levels therefore evoke marked hormonal responses, including large, rapid increases in secretion of adrenaline. Generalized threats such as glucose deprivation often elicit distress. In insulin-induced hypoglycemia, the patient's anxious, pale, and sweaty appearance constitutes an important clinical sign. Drugs that block effects of adrenaline mask this protective response and can render the patient and those caring for him unaware of the life threat.

Other stress responses are behaviors that are phylogenetically very old. Even relatively simple organisms such as *Aplysia* have withdrawal or escape responses to physical or chemical manipulation. Agonistic behavior, such as attack and dominance displays, also includes strong genetically determined components that evolved. Aggression facilitates predation, reproduction, social organization, and the division of ecological space. Because unchecked aggression would also threaten gene propagation, however, instinctive means to limit aggression within a species have also evolved.

In mammals, internal sensations and perceptions of changes in the body's orientation in space during orthostasis lead to patterned neural discharges that result in constriction of blood vessels in the legs and gut, increased pulse rate, and increased total peripheral resistance to blood flow, all tending to redistribute blood volume toward the heart and brain. Skeletal muscle pumping contributes to this redistribution. Ordinarily, these rapid and effective concerted responses, mediated mainly by the sympathetic nervous system, counter the stressor unconsciously.

The importance of these mechanisms for human well-being is illustrated by several clinical autonomic nervous system disorders, discussed later, and the effects of weightlessness in space flight. Weightlessness is, of course, a novel stressor in human evolution. Several manifestations of "space sickness" result from the lack of evolution of physiological and neuroendocrine mechanisms to counter the absence of gravitational force. During exposure to zero gravity, the absence of gravitational blood pooling increases venous return to the heart, in turn altering activities of several systems that maintain cardiac filling. Excretion of water and salt increases, probably because of decreased sympathetic nervous system outflow to the kidneys, decreased activity of the renin-angiotensin-aldosterone system, increased atrial natriuretic factor release by the heart, and decreased vasopressin release by the pituitary gland. A new state of equilibrium is reached, and overall sympathetic nervous system activity, as indicated by norepinephrine levels, returns to about baseline during prolonged space flight. When the astronauts return to earth, however, gravitational pooling of blood, combined with the low blood volume, evoke symptomatic orthostatic hypotension and a tendency to faint.

Catecholamine systems seem to have evolved in sequence, with dopamine the most primitive catecholamine. For instance, sea anemones contain the catecholamine precursor, dihydroxyphenylalanine (DOPA), but do not contain catecholamines or the enzyme that speeds up the conversion of DOPA to catecholamines. In most invertebrates, dopamine is the dominant catecholamine; concentrations of norepinephrine, when detected, are less than those of dopamine; and adrenaline is absent. In organs or plasma of amphibians, adrenaline is the dominant catecholamine; in reptiles, either norepinephrine or adrenaline may predominate; and in mammals norepinephrine predominates.

Theoretically, autocrine/paracrine systems can meet the needs of simple organisms that lack mechanisms of neurocirculatory regulation, whereas more sophisticated organisms use hormones to coordinate organ functions, and in the most complicated organisms, including humans, autonomic nervous system networks enable complex central neural regulation of regional resistances to blood flow and of glandular secretion. The regulation of nerve networks by the brain also fosters a close association between learned skeletal muscle movements and autonomic nervous system outflows to smooth muscle that support those movements. These principles may help to comprehend the evolution of catecholamine systems.

Autocrine/paracrine catecholamine systems still appear to operate, at least in the kidneys and adrenal glands. In the kidneys, locally formed dopamine contributes to regulation of sodium balance. In the adrenal cortex, locally formed dopamine inhibits aldosterone secretion. In both organs, however, more powerful hormonal and neuronal systems now predominate.

Selective factors favoring the evolution of coordination of activities of hormonal stress systems may explain the architectural arrangement of the adrenal cortex and adrenal medulla. In mammals, the adrenal cortex envelops the medulla. The two components of the adrenal gland have entirely different embryological sources. Because blood flow in the adrenal gland flows from the outside in, this architectural arrangement produces very high local concentrations of adrenocortical steroids in blood passing through the adrenal medulla. Glucocorticoids contribute importantly to regulation of adrenaline synthesis.

The sympathetic nervous system is immature at birth. Maturation of the sympathetic nervous system after birth allows a degree of plasticity of development based on experiences of the individual early in life. In contrast, the adrenal medulla forms in utero in mammals, adrenaline participates in embryological development, and low and unchanging basal tissue concentrations of adrenaline persist in sympathetically innervated organs throughout the life span.

Primitive Specificity

Patterns of responses of effector systems have a primitive specificity that one can comprehend in terms of the evolution of adaptively advantageous adjustments (fig. 40). During orthostasis or cold exposure, sympathetic nervous system activation predominates; during manipulations of dietary salt intake, renin-angiotensin-aldosterone system responses predominate; during manipulations of water availability, vasopressin responses predominate; and during manipulations of glucose availability, responses of insulin, glucagon, and the adrenomedullary hormonal system predominate. Small amounts of acute blood loss elicit mainly unconscious sympathetic nervous system responses, which maintain the output of blood by the heart and the flow of blood to the brain by redistributing blood volume; large amounts of acute blood loss, sufficient to decrease blood pressure, elicit a very complex and dynamic pattern of responses.

Stresses associated with adrenomedullary hormonal system activation usually evoke distress. Stressors that pose global, metabolic challenges or are perceived as threats to well-being elicit adrenomedullary hormonal system activation, even when the intensity of the stressor is mild. Adrenomedullary hormonal system activation is prominent in hypotensive hemorrhage, hypoglycemia, asphyxiation, circulatory collapse, and emotional distress. Stresses eliciting adrenomedullary hormonal system activation typically also elicit hypothalamic-pituitary-adrenocortical system activation, as indicated by circulating levels of ACTH or cortisol, and increases in release of endogenous opioids, as indicated by plasma levels of beta-endorphin, with small increases or even decreases in sympathetic nervous system outflows.

Sympathetic nervous system activation is prominent in orthostasis, mild to moderate exercise, regulation of core temperature, and the situation after eating a meal. Stresses associated with sympathetic nervous system activation often include a component of active movement. Patterned sympathetic nervous system activation during stress produces adaptive shifts in the distribution of blood volume or in glandular secretion. When these changes suffice to maintain homeostasis, they are not consciously experienced, but

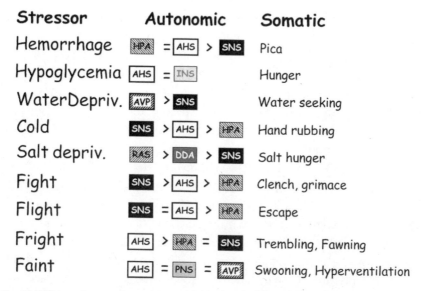

Stressor	Autonomic	Somatic
Hemorrhage	HPA = AHS > SNS	Pica
Hypoglycemia	AHS = INS	Hunger
WaterDepriv.	AVP > SNS	Water seeking
Cold	SNS > AHS > HPA	Hand rubbing
Salt depriv.	RAS > DDA > SNS	Salt hunger
Fight	SNS > AHS > HPA	Clench, grimace
Flight	SNS = AHS > HPA	Escape
Fright	AHS > HPA = SNS	Trembling, Fawning
Faint	AHS = PNS = AVP	Swooning, Hyperventilation

Fig. 40. Different forms of stress are associated with different, but relatively specific, patterns of responses of both the autonomic and somatic nervous systems.

when the organism senses that these responses are not or will not mitigate the effects of the stressor, the situation reaches consciousness, and adrenomedullary hormonal system activation ensues.

The character and intensity of response patterns during distress depend on the perceptions of the organism both about the stressor and about the available repertoire of coping responses. Hypothalamic-pituitary-adrenocortical and adrenomedullary hormonal system activation accompanies unanticipated distress. At least three patterns of experiential, behavioral, hormonal, and physiological responses occur during emotional distress— anger, which can develop into rage and fighting; fear, which can develop into terror and flight; and passivity, which can develop into "giving up," decreased blood pressure, decreased blood flow to the brain, and even heart stoppage.

Physiological distinctions between fear and anger reflect differential changes in contraction of skeletal muscle, skin blood vessel and gastrointestinal smooth muscle, and smooth muscle in glands. The extent of skeletal muscle contraction, and the extent of recruitment of sympathetic nervous system activation to redistribute blood flows appropriately, generally varies with the intensity of the emotional experience. Adrenomedullary hormonal system activation accompanies fear and sympathetic nervous system activation anger.

For each stress, neuroendocrine and physiological changes are coupled with behavioral changes. For instance, the regulation of total body water in humans depends on an interplay between behavior (the search for water and drinking), an internal experience or feeling (thirst), and the elicitation of a neurohormonal response pattern (in this case dominated by AVP, the antidiuretic hormone; and to a lesser extent angiotensin II, a potent stimulator of drinking). Evoked changes in homeostat function often produce not only neuroendocrine and physiological effects but also behavioral responses; however, because of traditional boundaries among physiology, endocrinology, and psychology, interactions producing integrated patterns of response remain incompletely understood. For instance, studies about vasopressin and activity of the renin-angiotensin-aldosterone system during blood volume depletion rarely have included controls for or monitoring of thirst and salt hunger.

This situation developed partly because of the long-held view that acts of skeletal muscle—the province of neurology and psychology—mediate the voluntary, conscious responses of the organism to the external environment, whereas the autonomic nervous system and hormonal changes—the province of physiology and endocrinology—mediate the involuntary, unconscious responses of smooth muscle and glands to maintain the internal environment. Findings in neuroendocrinology have by now refuted this distinction. Compelling evidence has accrued that the external environment, via the central nervous system, in particular, the hypothalamus, affects autonomic and hormone system activity. Biofeedback and conditioning studies have suggested learned modifications of some autonomic functions. The state of physiological arousal affects behavior by, among other things, intensifying emotions and communicating external signs of internal states. Finally, recent findings involving circumventricular organs, sites in the brain that are devoid of a blood-brain barrier, have introduced the possibility that hormones can reach central nervous system sites, eliciting various behaviors and altering outflows to the autonomic nervous system and endocrine glands.

The notion of stressor-specific response patterns disagrees with the theories of both Cannon and Selye. In his *The Wisdom of the Body*, Cannon, largely ignoring other systems, asserted that sympathicoadrenal system activation would meet most or all important threats to the internal environment.

The amazing feature of the role played by the sympathico-adrenal system is its applicability to the widespread range of possible disturbances that we have just noted. As stated earlier, the system commonly works as a unit. It is very remarkable indeed that such unified action can be useful in circumstances so diverse as low blood sugar, low blood pressure, and low temperature. . . . The appearance of inappropriate features in the total complex of sympathico-adrenal function is made reasonable, as I pointed out in 1928, if we consider, first, that it is, on the whole, a unitary system; second, that it is capable of producing effects in many different organs; and third, that among these effects are different combinations which are of the utmost utility in correspondingly different conditions of need. (298–299)

According to Cannon, the neuronal and hormonal components of the sympathicoadrenal system would function as a unit. This book emphasizes the opposite—separate regulation of the sympathetic nervous system and adrenomedullary hormonal system, with if anything a closer association between adrenomedullary responses and responses of the hypothalamic-pituitary-adrenocortical system. Differential regulation of the sympathetic nervous system and adrenomedullary hormonal system during different forms of stress supports the concept of primitive specificity.

This differential regulation also argues against Selye's doctrine of non-specificity. Selye, as Cannon, overemphasized responses of a single system—in Selye's case, the hypothalamic-pituitary-adrenocortical system. Activation of this system may produce the pathological triad of the general adaptation syndrome—thymicolymphatic degeneration, adrenal hypertrophy, and gastrointestinal ulceration—but only glimpses at the spectrum of systemic responses to stress.

Deriving a concept based on heterogeneous responses during stress would require measures of several endogenous substances indicating activities of different effectors, and descriptions of assays for these measurements appeared only long after Cannon and Selye had published their unitary theories.

The Swedish physiologist, Björn Folkow, has proposed that patterns of nervous system activity associated with stress are always expressed in closely linked, situation-specific patterns, with behavioral, experiential (emotional), and automatic (autonomic and hormonal) facets. In terms of stress and distress, these facets would correspond to externally observable and instinctively communicated movements and behaviors, mediated by the somatic nervous system; emotional feeling, resulting from cognitions about both the outside and inner worlds, along the lines of Schachter and Singer's hypothesis; and automatic, unconscious, involuntary changes in the inner world, mediated by the autonomic nervous system and by hormones.

One may speculate that stressor-specific triadic patterns of behavioral, experiential, and automatic activities during stress became intertwined so tightly in evolution that, by now, these patterns are expressed as units. In the discussion of the "selfish gene" theory, Dawkins indicated that groups of genes can be selected as a unit. If so, then maybe groups of genes associated with these three facets of primitively specific stress responses evolved as units.

8 | Dysautonomias

In dysautonomias, altered activity of one or more components of the autonomic nervous system adversely affects health. Dysautonomias can manifest as occasional episodes or chronic, persistent neurodegeneration. They occur in all age groups, from inherited genetic diseases in children to functional disorders in adults to autonomic failure in the elderly. Some entail observable macroscopic or microscopic abnormalities or quantifiable chemical or physiological changes, while others remain mysterious and controversial because of a lack of consistent objective findings. Some are rare and some common, but all involve more than one body function, and all negatively impact a person's sense of well-being. Dysautonomias also involve multiple disciplines of medicine—cardiology, neurology, endocrinology, physical medicine, and psychiatry. Predictably, relatively few cardiologists, neurologists, endocrinologists, rehabilitation medicine specialists, or psychiatrists feel comfortable in diagnosing dysautonomias or managing the patients.

Three factors have made the area of dysautonomias especially difficult. They are multidisciplinary, integrative, and mind-body disorders.

First, the disorders are multidisciplinary. Specialists certified in programs in single disciplines often cannot serve the patients, because of inadequate curriculum in medical schools and specialty training. Because of the multidisciplinary nature of dysautonomias, scientific peer-review committees tend to view as somewhat foreign applications for research funding and assign relatively low-priority scores to the grant applications. Because of the structure of scientific review procedures, scientific research about dysautonomias has in several ways lagged behind research into other clinical problems.

Second, the disorders are integrative. Many factors determine levels of pulse rate, blood pressure, body metabolism, pain, fatigue, and the sense of psychological well-being. These factors interact with each other, and they change over time, depending on development and circumstances of life, and they are themselves regulated as parts of complex feedback systems. Scientific theories have lagged behind in terms of taking into account this complexity.

Third, dysautonomias are virtually always "mind-body" disorders. Scientific theories have continued the old philosophical distinction between physical and mental body processes. I do not think that dysautonomias or the patients suffering with them can or should be classified as "medical" or "psychiatric." The many symptoms of dysautonomias reflect real biological or chemical changes. When clinicians cannot identify the causes of the symptoms, that ignorance should not lead to dismissing the patients as having a psychiatric rather than a "real" problem.

The "Mind-Body" Problem

Disorders involving the adrenaline family are, possibly more than any other ailments, mind-body disorders. In many ways the autonomic nervous system operates exactly at the border of the mind and body.

This is a difficult subject for both doctors and patients. The problem is the old notion that the body and mind are separate and distinct in a person, and so diseases must be either physical or mental. If the disorder were physical, it would be "real," something imposed on the individual, whereas if it were mental, and "in your head," it would not be real, but something created in and by the individual.

These notions date from the teachings of the Renaissance philosopher Descartes. They are outdated by now. Distinctions between the "body" and the "mind," the physical and mental, problems imposed on the individual and those in the mind of the individual, are unhelpful in trying to understand disorders that involve adrenaline (fig. 41). This is because the mind deals with both the inner and outer worlds simultaneously, continuously, and dynamically in life.

Conversely, both worlds affect the mind, and each individual filters and colors perceptions of the inner and outer world. For instance, there is no such thing as a person exercising without "central command" to tense and relax specific muscles. At the same time, and as part of the same process, the brain automatically directs changes in blood flow to the muscles. The exercising muscle and changes in blood flow lead to information, feedback, to the brain about how things are going both outside and inside the body.

It is also true that virtually every emotion a person feels includes changes

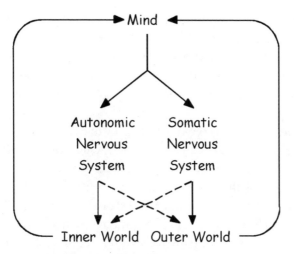

Fig. 41. A systems approach to the mind-body issue.

in these same body functions. For instance, when you are enraged, the blood flow to the skin and muscle increases, the heart pumps more blood, you sweat, your nostrils flare, and you move more air. From the point of view of the bodily changes, it would matter little whether these changes resulted from the physical experience of exercise or the mental experience of rage. Both situations involve alterations in the activity of components of the autonomic nervous system. Both situations involve changes in the inner and outer worlds, and if your autonomic nervous system were to malfunction, your reactions to *either* situation would not be regulated correctly; in either situation you could feel sick, look sick, and be sick.

A "systems" approach helps to understand conditions in which altered functions of components of the autonomic nervous system adversely affect health. According to the systems approach, the mind simultaneously directs changes in the somatic nervous system and the autonomic nervous system, based on perceptions about what is going on in the inner world and the outside world.

Note that the autonomic nervous system affects both the inner and outside worlds. For instance, if a person looked pale, because the blood quite literally had drained from the face, and were sweaty, trembling, and mumbling incoherently, other people would likely react to these signs of distress and ask, "Are you OK?" and it is well known that strong emotions, probably via adrenaline release, can energize an individual. In fact, one of the entries under weight lifting in *Guinness World Records* (e.g., in the 1976 edition,

p. 669) referred to a 123-pound mother who summoned the strength to lift the a 3,600-pound car after a jack had collapsed and the car had fallen on her child. Analogously, the somatic nervous system can affect the inner world. For instance, you can voluntarily increase your blood pressure any time you want by tightly clenching a fist or by dunking your hand in cold water.

How would a systems approach help to understand a dysautonomia? Malfunction at any station in a homeostatic system would lead to an alteration in activity of one or more components of the autonomic nervous system. For instance, if there were no feedback to the brain about the state of the blood pressure (part of the inner world), then there would be an inability to keep the blood pressure within bounds by changing the activity of the autonomic nervous system. If there were no feedback about the extent of physical exercise, there would also be an inability to adjust the blood pressure and blood flows appropriately. Of course, if there were a failure of the autonomic nervous system itself, this failure would interfere with regulation of the inner world, and there would also be difficulty in dealing with the outside world, manifested by problems like exercise intolerance or an inability to tolerate standing for a prolonged period (orthostatic intolerance). Finally, if the person had a psychiatric disorder such as panic/anxiety, then the inappropriate emotional experience of fear would be linked to both autonomic nervous system and somatic nervous system changes. A clinician's ability to treat a dysautonomia successfully would also benefit from a systems approach. Treatments at any of several steps might help, but the best place in the system to insert a treatment would be the step closest to the problem. Returning to the analogy of home temperature control, environmental exposures would correspond to open windows; genetic predispositions would correspond to design flaws in the HVAC system.

Primary versus Secondary Dysautonomias

In secondary dysautonomias, a change in autonomic function worsens another disease. In primary dysautonomias, a harmful change occurs in the autonomic nervous system itself.

Most dysautonomias are secondary; that is, the alteration in autonomic nervous system function would itself be appropriate, adaptive, and helpful, but for an independent pathological state that renders the same alteration maladaptive, harmful, or even lethal. The old man who suffers a heart attack while shoveling snow exemplifies a patient with a secondary dysautonomia. Shoveling snow usually takes place in the morning, when plasma levels of catecholamines are highest in their daily cycle; the person is standing, and sympathetic nervous system outflows approximately double with simply standing up; shoveling involves a great deal of isometric exercise, which potently stimulates the sympathetic nervous system; and so does cold exposure. Distress from a variety of sources can accompany shoveling snow. The combination of all these factors, by way of activation of catecholamine systems, greatly increases the work of the heart. Normally this would be appropriate and even necessary for continued toleration of vigorous, sustained exercise, by preserving and generating body heat and by delivering more blood to the exercising muscles. The blood pressure and pulse rate increase, the work of the heart increases, and the blood flow to the heart muscle by the coronary arteries normally increases. In the setting of an independent pathological state, however—severe coronary artery disease—the increase in the work of the heart could exceed the limited ability to increase delivery of oxygen to the heart muscle by way of the narrowed coronary arteries. The imbalance between supply and demand of this vital fuel could lead rapidly to abnormal heart rhythms, decompensated heart failure, or coronary artery occlusion, causing heart attack or sudden death.

Changes in autonomic nervous system function can also be harmful when activity of the system changes to compensate for abnormal functioning of a different body system. For instance, in heart failure, the heart fails to deliver an appropriate amount of blood to body organs. As part of compensation to improve the pump function of the heart, the sympathetic nervous system is activated. At the same time that this can improve the pump function of the heart, the activation of the sympathetic nervous system also increases the risk of fatal abnormal heart rhythms, increases the work of the heart, and promotes overgrowth of heart muscle, which can stiffen the heart walls and worsen the heart failure.

Secondary Dysautonomias
The Case of Dr. John Hunter

The case history of Dr. John Hunter illustrates beautifully the most common type of dysautonomia, a secondary dysautonomia, in which an alteration in autonomic nervous system function adversely affects health because of worsening of an independent pathological state. Understanding Hunter's story and appreciating its remarkable and historic irony require that you first learn about angina pectoris. The term is derived from the Latin for "breast choking." Angina pectoris, sometimes simply called angina, is a disagreeable, pressurelike, squeezing sensation, usually in the center of the chest, brought on by exercise, emotion, exposure to cold, or a large meal, and relieved by rest. Angina pectoris usually results from an excess of oxygen consumption by heart muscle compared with the amount of oxygen supplied by the coronary arteries that deliver blood to the heart muscle. It is a symptom complex, not a disease. The experience of angina therefore does not necessarily indicate permanent damage to heart muscle, just as leg cramping during overexertion does not necessarily indicate permanent damage to skeletal muscle.

Hunter was a renowned eighteenth-century surgeon. By all accounts he was an extraordinarily hard worker, customarily arising before dawn. He was also notoriously prone to defensive argument, irrational outbursts, obstinateness, and impatience—epitomizing what today you might call a hostile type A personality. In 1785, he began to experience angina pectoris. His friend, William Heberden, had only recently described this exact syndrome. In fact, Hunter himself had actually conducted the autopsy of one of the first described cases, a patient with angina pectoris who had collapsed and died while in a violent fit of anger.

Hunter never admitted his own condition for what it was. He did acknowledge, however, the relationship between emotional upset and his symptoms. Because arguing frequently brought them on, he admitted, "My life is at the mercy of any rogue who chooses to provoke me." This proved to be one of the most ironic statements in the history of medicine. On October 16, 1793, Hunter became incensed at critical, insolent remarks against him at a meeting of the Board of Governors of Saint George's Hospital. He left the room, collapsed, and dropped dead.

His brother-in-law and colleague, Everard Home, published Hunter's book, *A Treatise on the Blood, Inflammation, and Gun-Shot Wounds*. In the preface Home described Hunter's condition and death. The description is a classic of cardiology:

> The first attack of these complaints was produced by an affection of the mind, and every future return of any consequence arose from the same cause; and although bodily exercise, or distention of the stomach, brought on slighter affections, it still required the mind to be affected to render

them severe; and as his mind was irritated by trifles, these produced the most violent effects on the disease. His coachman being beyond his times, or a servant not attending to his directions, brought on the spasms, while a real misfortune produced no effect. . . .

On October 16, 1793, when in his usual state of health, he went to St. George's Hospital, and meeting with some things which irritated his mind, and not being perfectly master of the circumstances, he withheld his sentiments, in which state of restraint he went into the next room, and turning around to Dr. Robertson, one of the physicians of the hospital, he gave a deep groan and dropt down dead.

Angina pectoris, while it is not necessarily damaging, is a well-known risk factor for sudden death. One explanation for the increased risk is a positive feedback loop. Suppose someone had a limited ability to dilate the coronary arteries because of stiffening of the arterial walls. A stimulus such as emotional distress would increase the secretion of adrenaline into the bloodstream and the release of norepinephrine from sympathetic nerves in the heart. These would increase the rate and force of heart contraction and consequently increase the rate of oxygen consumption by the heart muscle. Ordinarily, this would relax the coronary artery walls, and coronary blood flow would increase, meeting the increased need, but this would not happen in the patient with rigid coronary arteries. An imbalance would develop between oxygen demand and supply. Moreover, high circulating adrenaline levels intensify any emotional experience, so the patient could feel more distress. This would elicit further adrenaline release. Eventually, the imbalance would become severe enough that, by unknown mechanisms, the patient would experience angina pectoris. When the patient became aware of this disagreeable, oppressive sensation, and especially if the patient recognized that sensation for the important sign that it is, the patient might become even more distressed. A vicious cycle of distress, catecholamine release, increased oxygen consumption, and imbalance between oxygen consumption and supply would ensue. Positive feedback loops are inherently unstable. Activation of a positive feedback loop in an organism, unless effectively and immediately limited, leads inevitably to a new equilibrium condition—which could be death.

This is probably what happened to Hunter. However, the story does not end here. After his death, Hunter's body was autopsied, and among the findings were coronary arteries that like "bony tubes, were with difficulty divided by the knife." Hunter's coronary arteries were rigid, but not narrowed or blocked. To this day, the issue remains open about whether hostile type A individuals have an increased risk of coronary artery blockage.

According to the theory of the "type A coronary prone behavior pattern," introduced by Ray H. Rosenman and Meyer Friedman, the type A individual's style of reaction to stress constitutes an independent coronary risk factor. The theory shifts emphasis from stressors that might accelerate development of atherosclerosis to aspects of the individual's personality that increase coronary risk—from the "seed" to the "soil." Although Friedman and Rosenman introduced and popularized the type A theory, the renowned physician William Osler presaged it more than a half-century earlier, in 1910, when he characterized the typical coronary patient as "not the delicate neurotic but the robust, the vigorous in mind and body, the keen ambitious man, the indicator of whose engine is always full speed ahead." The type A behavior pattern, as originally described, includes time urgency, competitiveness, and aggressiveness. Studies in the 1970s indicated that type A people had a twofold greater risk of developing overt ischemic heart disease than did people without type A behavior.

Several studies subsequently failed to support the type A theory. If only a portion of the type A pattern actually were related to coronary risk, this would help to explain the inconsistent findings. Redford B. Williams, Jr., and coworkers began to concentrate on the specific component of anger or hostility. Whether hostility, lack of social support, or joyless striving constitute "toxic" components of the type A pattern remains unresolved.

Eliot, Buell, and coworkers suggested that patterns of blood vessel and heart responses during emotional stress, rather than the type A pattern itself, could explain the association between cardiovascular morbidity and stress. These investigators categorized patients as "hot reactors" or "cold reactors," based on the occurrence of excessive hemodynamic responses to a panel of tests, including mathematical problems, competitive video games, and the cold pressor test. No published study has tested scientifically the predictive value of the "hot reactor" categorization.

A related view holds that stress-related risk of coronary heart disease results from excessive responses of catecholamine systems that elicit harmful effects. Type A individuals respond with excessive increases of plasma catecholamine levels and blood pressure during challenges perceived as personally threatening. An analysis based on 33 different published experiments concluded that type A individuals have about threefold larger plasma norepinephrine responses and about fourfold larger adrenaline responses during exposure to various laboratory and clinical stressors than type B individuals do. These findings are consistent with the "neuroendocrine mediator hypothesis," according to which excessive or inappropriate catecholamine responses increase coronary risk in people with the hostile type A pattern. The long-term, pathophysiological role of such responses in the future development of coronary heart disease, however, remains unproven.

Inadequate blood flow or death of heart muscle tissue decreases thresholds for lethal abnormal heart rhythms. About half of the patients with heart attacks die of this complication. It may be that, for these processes to take place, not only is inadequate blood flow required but also superimposed activation of sympathetic nervous system outflow to the heart. Many studies of laboratory animals have shown that sympathetic nervous or adrenomedullary hormonal activation contributes to the occurrence of arrhythmias in the setting of acute myocardial infarction. Sympathetic activation often precedes sudden death from the most common lethal arrhythmia, ventricular fibrillation, in patients with heart attack. This activation probably acts in several ways to increase the likelihood of arrhythmias. In addition, adrenaline decreases serum potassium levels, which may add to the effects of diuretics and digoxin in predisposition to arrhythmias. Moreover, even isolated premature heartbeats, which momentarily decrease blood pressure, almost immediately evoke reflexive increases in sympathetic activity. Because release of norepinephrine in the heart increases ventricular "automaticity," the tendency of electricity-conducting heart cells to fire spontaneously, a neurocardiological positive feedback loop might lead to rapid degeneration of cardiac rhythm in patients with heart attack.

These considerations help explain why in laboratory animals surgical removal of the ganglia that are the source of the sympathetic nervous system supply of the heart, treatment with drugs that block catecholamine effects, and treatment with a neurotoxin that selectively destroys sympathetic nerves all decrease the likelihood of fatal arrhythmia associated with sudden coronary occlusion. High plasma levels of norepinephrine and adrenaline indicate a poor 18-month prognosis in patients who have survived a heart attack.

Scared to Death

Literature since antiquity has noted an association between acute distress and sudden cardiovascular collapse. In the New Testament, in the Acts of the Apostles, Ananias and his wife Sapphira "fell down and gave up the ghost" after being chastised by Peter. Josephus, in his *Antiquities of the Jews*, wrote about the circumstances of the death of the murderous king Aristobulus:

> But Aristobulus instantly repented the slaughter of his brother. Guilt aggravated a disease and so disturbed his mind that his entrails were wracked by intolerable pain and he vomited blood. Once, a servant carrying away this blood slipped and shed some of it—by divine providence, as I cannot but think—at the very spot where stains of Antigonus' blood still remained . . . he shed many tears and gave a deep groan: "I am not, I see, to escape God's detection of the impious and hideous crimes I have been guilty of. Unforeseen punishment threatens me for shedding the blood of my kin, and now, most impudent body of mine, how long will you retain a soul that, to appease the ghosts of my brother and my mother, ought to die?" . . . With these words he died. (Glatzer NN. *Jerusalem and Rome. The Writings of Josephus.* New York: Meridian Books, 1960, 58–59)

Pathological studies about how distress actually can produce sudden death were not done until the past century. In 1907, about twelve years after the discovery of the cardiovascular stimulatory effects of adrenaline, Josue demonstrated that infusion of adrenaline can lead to death of heart muscle. The heart muscle cells rupture and die of overstraining, and a particular microscopic change called contraction band necrosis develops. An autopsy study of victims of homicidal assault who had died without sufficient evidence of internal or external injury revealed contraction band necrosis in about three quarters of the cases. Patients with stroke from bleeding inside the brain also can have death of heart muscle cells, with the extent of cell loss related to the extent of increase in plasma levels of catecholamines. Because of this phenomenon, emergency room physicians and hospital intensivists occasionally have difficulty in distinguishing cardiac effects of a stroke from brain effects of a heart attack. The same phenomenon occurs in rats subjected to immobilization, overcrowding, restraint, water immersion, repeated, small electric shocks, and other noxious laboratory stressors that have in common their ability to evoke marked activation of catecholamine systems.

The finding of contraction band necrosis helped convict a bank robber of felony murder, without physical trauma to the victim, who died soon after being presented with a paper bag and a note announcing the robbery. Autopsy examination of the heart showed changes indicating the acute pathological effects of catecholamines. Even a piece of paper and a paper bag can be lethal weapons.

Heart Failure

Normally, expansion of a chamber of the heart immediately increases the force of heart muscle contraction in that chamber. This phenomenon has been called Starling's law of the heart. Activation of sympathetic nerves to the heart shifts the Starling curve upward, so that for a given amount of cardiac filling, there is an augmented ejection of blood by the heart. During exercise, cardiac filling changes little because of the improved efficiency of heart muscle contraction exerted by the cardiac sympathetic nerves.

Heart failure can go on for many years—a condition termed "compensated heart failure." The heart muscle has intrinsically decreased pumping ability, but compensatory activation of the sympathetic nervous system outflow to the heart maintains normal cardiac function. The patient may have limited exercise tolerance. Eventually, however, the heart failure worsens in an accelerated manner—"decompensated heart failure." This situation involves positive feedback loops, which if not rapidly aborted kill the patient.

1. In patients with heart failure who already have an enlarged heart, for a given further increment in chamber size, the increment in contractile performance decreases; that is, the slope of the relationship between performance and volume flattens. If the slope were to become negative, then, with further enlargement of the ventricular chamber, ventricular performance would decrease rather than increase, rapidly resulting in a fatal backup of blood into the lungs. Most patients with heart failure die before reaching the descending portion of the Starling curve.

2. Patients with heart failure have markedly increased sympathetic nerve traffic to the heart and so have increased delivery of norepinephrine to the heart muscle cells. High levels of catecholamines such as norepinephrine not only increase the force of the heartbeat but also increase the size of heart muscle cells and predispose patients to develop abnormal heart rhythms (arrhythmias). Both increased wall stiffness and arrhythmias worsen the heart's pumping efficiency, in turn reflexively evoking further increases in sympathetic nerve traffic to the heart.

3. Heart failure recruits increased sympathetic nervous system outflows to the heart and to other organs. By way of the catecholamine release, the work of the heart increases. In a patient with narrowed coronary arteries, the rate of use of oxygen may exceed the rate of delivery of oxygen by way

of the coronary arteries. This imbalance can precipitate a heart attack or sudden cardiac death. Moreover, lack of oxygen delivery to the sympathetic nerves themselves in the heart tends to make them "leaky," augmenting norepinephrine release even for the same rate of sympathetic nerve traffic.

4. Increased sympathetic nervous system outflows to the heart and to other body regions augment cardiac filling because of constriction of veins and direct and indirect sodium-retaining effects of sympathetic nervous system stimulation in the kidneys. Increases in sympathetic nervous system outflows also increase the total peripheral resistance to blood flows because of the constriction of arterioles. Cardiac overfilling also leads to accumulation of fluid in the lungs, producing low blood oxygen levels, a buildup of acidity in the bloodstream, and respiratory distress, all of which exaggerate the responses of catecholamine systems. The combination of these factors accelerates cardiac decompensation.

Are Hypertensives "Hyper-Tense"?

I spent a dozen years in the Hypertension-Endocrine Branch of the National Heart, Lung, and Blood Institute, trying to find out whether increased overall activity of the sympathetic nervous system causes chronic high blood pressure (hypertension). The multiplicity of effectors determining blood pressure made it extremely unlikely that evidence would accrue for a direct relationship between blood pressure and sympathetic nervous system outflows, without monitoring or controlling for the activities of the other effectors (fig. 42). Compounding this difficulty, multiple homeostats share the same effectors that determine blood pressure; long-term secondary changes as a consequence of hypertension alter feedback loops over time; and instincts, conditioning, and simulations modulate the translation of genetic predispositions into disease manifestations.

A major, still unresolved, issue about blood pressure regulation relates to the baroreceptors. Release of a monitored variable from restraint by negative feedback might not only increase the variability of the monitored variable around its average level but also allow values for that variable to drift to a new average level, a level that may be pathophysiological. Researchers have debated for many years whether baroreceptor "debuffering" increases "resting" blood pressure, that is, whether debuffering produces a form of neurogenic hypertension.

In contrast with hypertension, a largely statistical disease of modern

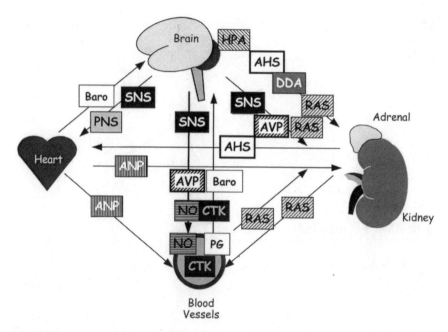

Fig. 42. Many effectors determine blood pressure. Their contributions vary, depending on genetic predispositions, learning, effector sharing by other homeostatic systems, environmental exposures, and time. This complexity has frustrated attempts to identify causes of high blood pressure in most individual patients.

man, hypotension due to traumatic hemorrhage has always posed an immediate threat to survival. Natural selection must have favored the evolution of systems to support blood pressure during emergencies. In humans, baroreflexes buffer decreases in blood pressure more effectively than they buffer increases in blood pressure. As Cannon demonstrated repeatedly, activation of catecholamine systems increases blood pressure by increasing the force and rate of the heartbeat and constricting blood vessels. One might expect that release of these effectors from baroreceptor restraint would bias blood pressure upward.

Interference with homeostatic regulation of blood pressure exaggerates increments in blood pressure in response to various stressors. In humans, baroreceptor "debuffering" by surgical denervation or local anesthesia of the carotid sinus area increases blood pressure acutely and concurrently increases values for indices of sympathetic nervous system activity. Chronic hypertension is another matter. For instance, irradiation-induced arterial

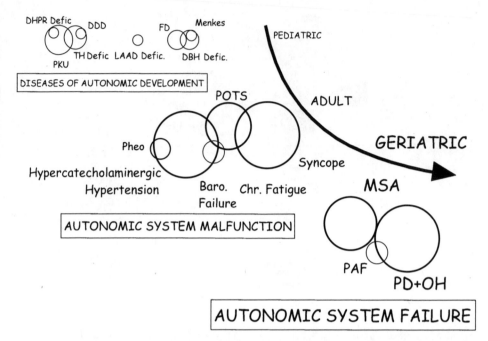

Fig. 43. The dysautonomias "universe." Dysautonomias occur in all age groups. In children there are genetic disorders of development; in adults, functional disorders in which the autonomic nervous system behaves inappropriately; and in the elderly, degenerative disorders in which autonomic nervous system components fail.

baroreceptor denervation, while predisposing patients to episodes of paroxysmal hypertension and very high plasma norepinephrine levels, does not necessarily produce sustained hypertension.

Primary Dysautonomias

When doctors think about dysautonomias, they usually don't think about altered function of the autonomic nervous system aggravating another disease or about the harmful effects of compensatory activation when another system fails, but about abnormalities of the autonomic nervous system itself. It is to these forms of primary dysautonomia that we now turn.

Different types of dysautonomia occur in different stages of life (fig. 43). In infants and children, dysautonomia often reflects a genetic change, a mutation, which is like a "typo" in the genetic encyclopedia. One type of mutation that runs in the family of people of east European Jewish extraction causes familial dysautonomia. Another mutation that produces dysautonomias in children causes a type of phenylketonuria (PKU). Another causes "kinky hair disease" (Menkes disease). In general, dysautonomias from genetic mutations are rare.

In adults, dysautonomia usually reflects a functional change in a generally intact autonomic nervous system. Examples are neurocardiogenic syncope (in which the person has frequent episodes of fainting or near-fainting), postural tachycardia syndrome (in which the person cannot tolerate standing up for long periods and has a rapid pulse rate during standing), and hypernoradrenergic hypertension (in which overactivity of the sympathetic nervous system causes a form of high blood pressure). Less commonly, there is a loss of nerve terminals, such as caused by a toxic substance, viral infection, or the body attacking itself (autoimmune autonomic failure). Dysautonomia in adults rarely reflects a genetic mutation, the one-in-a-million "typo" in the genetic encyclopedia, or a polymorphism, which is a genetic change that is more common than a mutation.

In the elderly, dysautonomia usually reflects degeneration of the autonomic nervous system, often in association with other evidence of degeneration of the brain. Examples are multiple system atrophy and Parkinson disease.

FEE-Yo

The clearest evidence for a role of high levels of catecholamines in the development of clinical hypertension comes from patients with a rare tumor called pheochromocytoma, the slang for which is "pheo," pronounced FEE-yo. Pheos usually arise in the adrenal gland. They produce all the members of the adrenaline family.

Despite their rarity, pheos are important in clinical medicine, for two reasons. First, the tumors typically are benign, so that removal of a pheo constitutes one of the unusual situations in which hypertension can be cured by surgery. Second, in response to seemingly minor perturbations such as induction of general anesthesia before an operation, pheos can release their catecholamine contents into the bloodstream, resulting in a marked and dangerous paroxysm of high blood pressure that can be lethal. Many patients with hypertension have findings that theoretically could reflect a pheo, such as hypertension that is difficult to control, headache, anxiety, pallor, sweating, fast pulse rate, and palpitations. Because of the commonness and nonspecificity of these symptoms and signs, coupled with the potentially catastrophic consequences of missing the diagnosis, doctors frequently attempt to "rule out" pheo, despite its rarity.

Pheos release their catecholamine contents directly into the bloodstream. Patients with pheo provide a highly educational "experiment of nature," for learning about the long-term consequences of high catecholamine levels. Some of these consequences are immediate, such as a hypertensive paroxysm. Some are more chronic, such as heart muscle enlargement and heart failure from the increased work of the heart. In patients who seem at death's door from heart failure because of high catecholamine levels from a pheo, removal of the tumor can be lifesaving. Some effects remain incompletely understood, such as a fall in blood pressure when the patient stands up.

Most patients in whom pheo is suspected eventually are shown not to have the tumor. Then what do they have? Once pheo is excluded in a patient with headache, anxiety, pallor, sweating, fast pulse rate, palpitations, and so forth, the patient usually is relegated to the large group labeled "essential hypertension," meaning that the cause is unknown. It seems likely that in these patients with "pseudopheochromocytoma," functional, rather than neoplastic, abnormalities of catecholamine systems will eventually come to light.

Autonomic Failure

A variety of disorders feature primary dysautonomia from failure of one or more components of the autonomic nervous system. Whether the problem is in the brain, in the nerve traffic from the brain, in the ganglia that act like transfer stations on the nervous system highway, in the nerve terminals that release the chemical messenger, or in the receptors for that messenger in the target tissue, the effects in terms of the way the patient feels and looks are about the same. Many different mechanisms can result in the same symptoms. Underactivity of the parasympathetic nervous system manifests as constipation, retention of urine in the bladder, a tendency to fast pulse rate, decreased salivation, and impotence in men. Several drugs can cause this combination of problems, but sometimes they result from failure of the parasympathetic nervous system or inappropriate regulation of parasympathetic outflows. Parasympathetic functions tend to decrease also with normal aging.

Failure of the sympathetic noradrenergic system causes a fall in blood pressure when the patient stands up—orthostatic hypotension. Sympathetic noradrenergic system failure also produces a tendency to slow pulse rate and, in men, the inability to ejaculate. This form of sympathetic nervous system failure occurs in several types of dysautonomia, including Parkinson disease with orthostatic hypotension, pure autonomic failure, and multiple system atrophy. Acute sympathetic noradrenergic system failure also appears to play a key role in episodes of fainting.

Acetylcholine is the main chemical messenger used by the sympathetic nervous system for sweating, whereas norepinephrine is the main chemical messenger used by the sympathetic nervous system to tighten blood vessels and maintain blood pressure during standing. Accordingly, a patient with a specific problem in the production, release, or receptors for norepinephrine could have orthostatic hypotension and yet sweat normally, whereas a patient with parasympathetic and sympathetic cholinergic failure would have symptoms of parasympathetic failure and also a decreased ability to sweat.

Underactivity of the adrenomedullary hormonal system produces much more subtle effects than underactivity of the parasympathetic or the sympathetic nervous system, because when you are at rest, the adrenal glands release very little adrenaline into the bloodstream. Failure of the adrenomedullary hormonal system can cause a tendency to low glucose levels— hypoglycemia. This can be a major problem in patients who have diabetes and take injections of insulin; in these patients failure of the adrenomedullary hormonal system can result in vulnerability to severe insulin reactions. Because of the "bonbon" arrangement of the adrenal gland, and the trophic effect of steroids of the adrenal cortex on adrenaline production in the adrenal medulla, attenuated adrenaline responses might contribute to some of the features of adrenocortical failure, such as fatigue, hypoglycemia, and susceptibility to circulatory collapse.

Orthostatic Hypotension and Orthostatic Intolerance

If the systolic blood pressure falls by more than 20 mm of mercury between lying flat and standing up, and the diastolic blood pressure also falls, this is called orthostatic hypotension. Inability to tolerate standing up, or orthostatic intolerance, is a symptom, a complaint about something abnormal a person notices that provides subjective evidence of a disease. Orthostatic hypotension is a sign, something a doctor observes or measures that provides objective evidence of a disease. Neither orthostatic intolerance nor orthostatic hypotension is a diagnosis, which is a decision about the cause of a specific case of disease.

Tolerating standing up requires appropriate function at all the stations of the baroreflex arc. When a person stands up, the force of gravity tends to pool blood in the legs and pelvis. This decreases the return of blood to the heart in the veins, and the heart ejects less blood. When the heart ejects less blood, the arteries stretch less, and information to the brain about these changes travels in nerves from the baroreceptors to the brain. The brain responds by directing an increase in the activity of the sympathetic nervous system. The sympathetic nerves release norepinephrine, and the norepinephrine activates receptors on cells in the blood vessel walls. This tightens the blood vessels, and so the total resistance to blood flows in the body increases. Even though the total amount of blood ejected by the heart per minute (cardiac output) has decreased, the average blood pressure normally is maintained because of the increase in total peripheral resistance.

Many factors besides sympathetic neurocirculatory failure can cause orthostatic hypotension. Prolonged bed rest for virtually any reason can do this. Orthostatic hypotension can also result from conditions that cause depletion of blood volume, such as heavy menstrual periods, gastrointestinal hemorrhage from a bleeding ulcer, or dehydration. Elderly, frail, osteoporotic women are vulnerable to a positive feedback loop, where the patient falls and breaks a bone, followed by prolonged bed rest in a cast. Upon recovery, the patient has orthostatic hypotension and therefore a high risk of another traumatic fall.

Just as there are many causes of orthostatic hypotension besides sympathetic nervous system failure, there are many causes of orthostatic intolerance besides orthostatic hypotension. Orthostatic hypotension can produce orthostatic intolerance, but orthostatic intolerance can occur without orthostatic hypotension. In the evaluation of a patient with chronic orthostatic intolerance, where the patient does not have evidence of sympathetic neurocirculatory failure, doctors often prescribe a diagnostic tilt-table test. Chapter 9 discusses this test.

In unusual cases orthostatic intolerance reflects failure of the baroreflex. In this situation, the sympathetic nervous system is not activated appropriately in response to a decrease in blood pressure or in response to a decrease in venous return to the heart. Baroreflex failure does not always cause orthostatic hypotension, but it does always cause large swings in blood pressure, both high and low, because of the inability of the baroreflex to keep the blood pressure within limits.

The remaining sections of this chapter describe several specific dysautonomias.

Pure Autonomic Failure

Pure autonomic failure (PAF) features persistent falls in blood pressure when the patient stands—orthostatic hypotension—in the absence of signs of central nervous system disease and in the absence of other known causes of orthostatic hypotension. The orthostatic hypotension results from sympathetic neurocirculatory failure. No one knows what causes pure autonomic failure. It is not inherited, and no known environmental toxin causes it. The disease occurs in middle-aged or elderly people of either sex and any race. It is not inherited or infectious and can go on for many years. Although chronic and disabling, it is not thought to be lethal. Patients report progressively worsening dizziness standing up or after a large meal. Sometimes they have decreased sweating. Because of severe orthostatic hypotension, patients with pure autonomic failure often learn to sit or stand with their legs twisted pretzel-like, because this decreases pooling of blood in the legs. In men, impotence can be an early symptom. Orthostatic hypotension, at first diagnosed as PAF, can be an early manifestation of Parkinson disease.

The sympathetic neurocirculatory failure and orthostatic hypotension in pure autonomic failure usually result from a generalized loss of sympathetic nerves in the body. Blood pressure responses to the Valsalva maneuver show the abnormal pattern that indicates sympathetic neurocirculatory failure, as discussed in chapter 9. Drug tests can confirm a diagnosis of pure autonomic failure. Because of the loss of sympathetic nerve terminals, drugs that release norepinephrine from sympathetic nerves, such as tyramine, yohimbine, amphetamine, and ephedrine, produce relatively small increases in blood pressure. In contrast, drugs that directly stimulate norepinephrine receptors, such as midodrine and phenylephrine (NeoSynephrine) constrict blood vessels and increase blood pressure. Because of the phenomenon of "denervation supersensitivity" (first demonstrated by Claude Bernard), where receptors for norepinephrine increase and other adaptive processes probably occur that exaggerate constriction of blood vessels, patients with pure autonomic failure can have surprisingly large increases in blood pressure in response to the receptor-stimulating drugs.

As a result of loss of sympathetic nerve terminals, plasma norepinephrine levels typically are low in PAF, even with the patient lying down. Another way to identify PAF is from sympathetic neuroimaging. In this type of test, the patient receives an injection of a radioactive drug that gets taken up by sympathetic nerve terminals. The sympathetic nerves in organs such as the heart become radioactive, and the nerves can be visualized by scans that depict where the radioactivity is. Because in PAF the sympathetic nerve terminals usually are absent in the organs, scanning after injection of one of these drugs usually fails to visualize the sympathetic innervation. Sympathetic neuroimaging tests such as fluorodopamine PET scanning of the chest can produce remarkably graphic results in PAF, with a failure to visualize the heart at all in the patient's chest.

Multiple System Atrophy

Multiple system atrophy (MSA) is a progressive neurodegenerative disease of middle-aged or elderly people that involves failure of components of the autonomic nervous system. Symptoms and signs include slurred speech, limb rigidity, tremor, poor coordination, urinary retention, constipation, and in men erectile failure. The disease progresses relentlessly over the years. Median survival is about six years after the diagnosis is made. MSA differs from multiple sclerosis, which is characterized clinically by remissions and exacerbations and by relatively few changes in functions of the autonomic nervous system. No one knows what causes MSA. It is not inherited or infectious, and in most cases there is no known exposure to an environmental toxin. According to one view, MSA results from a form of autoimmune process, in which the patient's immune system attacks and destroys particular brain cells.

MSA always involves one or more symptoms or signs of failure of the autonomic nervous system. Failure of the sympathetic nervous system produces a fall in blood pressure when the patient stands up (orthostatic hypotension) or after a meal (postprandial hypotension), resulting in symptoms such as dizziness, weakness, or faintness upon standing or after eating.

MSA with orthostatic hypotension is also known as the Shy-Drager syndrome. Some investigators have equated MSA with the Shy-Drager syndrome. Others have considered MSA as an umbrella diagnosis that includes the Shy-Drager syndrome when orthostatic hypotension figures prominently in the clinical presentation but also includes forms in which signs of cerebellar atrophy or of Parkinson disease stand out. A recent proposal has recommended discarding using the Shy-Drager syndrome as a diagnosis.

Symptoms and signs of parasympathetic failure in MSA include constipation and decreased urinary bladder tone, resulting in urinary incontinence and the need for self-catheterization. Symptoms and signs of other brainstem degeneration include particular abnormalities in eye movements ("progressive supranuclear palsy"), slurred speech, poor coordination of swallowing, abnormal breathing, and repeated aspiration, where swallowed food goes into the airway. These problems can occur in patients with MSA who do not have orthostatic hypotension, although most MSA patients have orthostatic hypotension.

The autonomic failure in MSA probably reflects loss of the ability to regulate sympathetic and parasympathetic nerve traffic to intact nerve terminals. This appears to be a major difference between MSA and the usual form of pure autonomic failure, in which the autonomic failure includes a loss of sympathetic nerve terminals.

The dietary supplement or herbal remedy, *ma huang*, is ephedrine, which releases norepinephrine from sympathetic nerves. Because patients with MSA and sympathetic neurocirculatory failure have intact sympathetic nerves, and they also have failure of the brain to regulate sympathetic nerve traffic appropriately via baroreflexes, taking *ma huang* can evoke a dangerous increase in blood pressure in MSA patients.

Patients with MSA have approximately normal sympathetic nerve traffic to intact sympathetic nerve terminals when the patients are resting, and so, MSA patients usually have normal plasma levels of norepinephrine, in contrast to patients with pure autonomic failure. As a result of baroreflex failure, MSA patients typically have deficient increases in sympathetic nerve traffic when they stand up and therefore have subnormal increases in plasma norepinephrine levels.

Scanning the chest after injection of a sympathetic neuroimaging agent visualizes the normal innervation of the heart in MSA. In contrast, in pure autonomic failure (and in Parkinson disease, discussed later), where the sympathetic nerve terminals typically are lost, sympathetic neuroimaging fails to visualize the cardiac sympathetic innervation.

Parkinson Disease with Orthostatic Hypotension

Parkinson disease occurs in elderly people of either sex and any race. Classic Parkinson disease involves a triad of slow movement (bradykinesia), a particular type of limb rigidity called cogwheel rigidity, and a type of rhythmic, "pill-roll" tremor that is most noticeable when the limb is at rest and that decreases or disappears when the limb is moved intentionally. These movement problems usually improve with treatment by drugs that increase occupation of dopamine receptors in the brain; the most frequently used such drug is the levodopa-carbidopa combination called Sinemet. The disease can be inherited, although most patients do not report a positive family history, and it progresses slowly over the years.

Orthostatic hypotension, a fall in blood pressure when the patient stands up, occurs fairly commonly in Parkinson disease. Orthostatic hypotension may have contributed to the repeated episodes of "fainting" suffered by the former Attorney General, Janet Reno. Neurologists have presumed that orthostatic hypotension results from treatment with levodopa, or else the patient doesn't really have Parkinson disease but has a different disease, such as "striatonigral degeneration" or MSA. Numerous studies during the past decade, however, have reported that all patients with Parkinson disease and orthostatic hypotension—even patients off levodopa or never treated with levodopa—have failure of regulation of the heart and blood vessels by the sympathetic nervous system. In other words, in Parkinson disease, orthostatic hypotension at least partly reflects sympathetic neurocirculatory failure and therefore is a form of dysautonomia.

In patients with Parkinson disease and orthostatic hypotension, the sympathetic neurocirculatory failure appears to result partly from loss of sympathetic nerves in the body as a whole. Because of the sympathetic denervation, there is a decreased amount of norepinephrine available for release in response to standing up. In addition, the patients have failure of baroreflexes, explaining their typically constant pulse rate during performance of the Valsalva maneuver (baroreflex-cardiovagal failure) and blunted increases in plasma norepinephrine levels when the patients stand up (baroreflex-sympathoneural failure). The combination of sympathetic denervation, baroreflex-cardiovagal failure, and baroreflex-sympathoneural failure may constitute a "triple whammy" that can explain the orthostatic hypotension attending Parkinson disease.

Many patients with Parkinson disease who do not have a fall in blood pressure when they stand up still have a loss of sympathetic nerves in the heart. Parkinson disease, in general, therefore appears to be not only a movement disorder but also a dysautonomia. The functional significance of cardiac sympathetic denervation in Parkinson disease is unknown.

Patients with Parkinson disease also often complain of constipation and urinary urgency and incontinence. These symptoms might reflect dysregulation of reflexes that use the parasympathetic nervous system as an effector.

Postural Tachycardia Syndrome

Patients with the postural tachycardia syndrome (postural orthostatic tachycardia syndrome, POTS) have an excessive increase in pulse rate during standing. The condition occurs predominantly in young or middle-aged, Caucasian women. Although POTS can be a lifelong problem, it can also resolve over the years. It does not appear to progress to a neurodegenerative, lethal disease.

The orthostatic tachycardia in POTS usually occurs without orthostatic hypotension. The finding of orthostatic hypotension does not exclude a diagnosis of POTS, however, as delayed orthostatic hypotension can occur in this condition.

The occurrence of a rapid pulse rate when a person stands is necessary but is not sufficient to diagnose POTS. The key word in postural tachycardia syndrome is the word *syndrome*. A syndrome is a set of symptoms that occur together. Patients with POTS not only have a rapid pulse rate when they stand up but also have several other nonspecific symptoms, such as orthostatic intolerance, chronic fatigue, heat intolerance, exercise intolerance, headache, chest pain, palpitations, disturbed sleep, and a tendency to experience panic or anxiety in threatening situations. Many of these symptoms probably reflect increased effects of catecholamines both inside and outside the brain.

Because POTS is a syndrome and not a single disease, POTS has many potential causes. Some investigators view POTS as synonymous with chronic orthostatic intolerance. Other terms have also been used, such as "hyperadrenergic orthostatic intolerance," "hyperdynamic circulation syndrome," "inappropriate sinus tachycardia," and "neurasthenia," probably reflecting different emphases by different research groups and gaps in knowledge about the underlying mechanisms. Trying to identify a specific cause in a particular patient with POTS can be a great challenge to clinicians. There are probably as many causes of a fast pulse rate as there are of a fever, and all the symptoms of POTS are not specific for any single disease.

Researchers have thought that usually in POTS sympathetic nerve traffic to the heart is increased as a compensation for a decrease in the amount of blood returning to the heart or a decrease in the total peripheral resistance to blood flow when the patient stands up. Either situation could alter information from the baroreceptors to the brain, leading to a reflexive increase in sympathetic nervous system activity directed by the brain. There are many potential causes for a decrease in venous return to the heart when a patient stands up. The possibility of blood volume depletion or excessive pooling of blood in the legs has drawn particular attention. Indeed, low blood volume was noted in the first case report of POTS. Low blood volume in turn can result from blood loss, from failure of the bone marrow to make an adequate number of red blood cells, or from failure of hormone systems such as the renin-angiotensin-aldosterone system. Blood volume can also fall while a person stands, because of leakage of fluid out of the blood vessels into the tissues (extravasation). Finally, an "effective" low blood volume can occur when the blood pools excessively in the veins after a person stands, such as due to a lack of muscular "tone" in the vein walls. Consistent with excessive blood pooling in the legs or lower abdomen during orthostasis, inflation of a military antishock trousers (MAST) suit reduces substantially the increase in heart rate in response to orthostasis in patients with POTS.

In "partial dysautonomia," or "neuropathic POTS," it is thought that there is a patchy loss of sympathetic innervation, such as in the legs or abdominal organs. When the patient stands up, the blood would pool because of failure of the arterioles or veins to constrict, and the sympathetic nervous system supply to the heart would be stimulated reflexively. POTS can also result from failure of a key system regulating salt balance in the body—the renin-angiotensin-aldosterone system.

Rarely, POTS can result from failure to inactivate norepinephrine by reuptake via the cell membrane norepinephrine transporter. Normally, most of the norepinephrine released from sympathetic nerve terminals is "recycled," by being taken back up into the nerve terminals. When the transporter is underactive, more norepinephrine is delivered to its receptors in the heart and blood vessel walls for a given amount of norepinephrine release, producing an exaggerated increase in pulse rate and blood pressure when the sympathetic nervous system is activated.

In baroreflex failure, the brain does not respond appropriately to information from the cardiovascular system, and the sympathetic nervous system is activated as a result of release from baroreflex restraint. In acute baroreflex failure, orthostatic intolerance is associated with large swings in blood pressure, because of the inability of the baroreflexes to keep the blood pressure in check, with episodes of extreme high blood pressure and fast pulse rate. Because of this failure, relatively minor stimuli can produce large increases in the activity of the sympathetic nervous system.

In "hyperadrenergic orthostatic intolerance," the problem is thought to be a primary abnormality in the functioning or regulation of the autonomic nervous system itself. In a related syndrome, the "hyperdynamic circulation syndrome," the patients have a fast pulse rate all the time, variable high blood pressure, increased heart rate responses to the drug isoproterenol, and increased plasma norepinephrine and adrenaline levels at rest and during provocative maneuvers. Beta-adrenoceptor blockers such as Inderal or benzodiazepines such as Valium improve the syndrome. It is unclear whether patients with this syndrome have an increased frequency of later development of established hypertension.

"Neurasthenia," a term introduced in the late 1860s, refers to a syndrome initially described in Civil War soldiers. Also called neurocirculatory asthenia, the syndrome consists of a large number of symptoms, including breathlessness, palpitations, chest pain, dizziness, shortness of breath on exertion, fatigue, excessive sweating, trembling, flushing, dry mouth, numbness and tingling feelings, irritability, and exercise intolerance. Most modern research about neurocirculatory asthenia has been conducted in Russia. Western cardiovascular researchers rarely use this term. Injection of adrenaline can evoke these symptoms, and beta-adrenoceptor blockers often normalize the cardiovascular findings without affecting the other symptoms and signs.

In "inappropriate sinus tachycardia," the heart rate is increased substantially, even during resting lying down. Radiofrequency ablation of the sinus node, the heart's pacemaker area, is considered for patients with inappropriate sinus tachycardia who are resistant to treatment with medications.

Patients with POTS often have high plasma levels of norepinephrine during standing up. Indeed, according to one suggestion, criteria for diagnosing chronic orthostatic intolerance include a high plasma norepinephrine level while the patient is upright. Whether increased sympathetic nervous outflows constitute a primary abnormality or compensatory response usually remains unknown in individual patients. In general, one would predict that if the orthostatic tachycardia were primary, then treating it would help the patient, but if the orthostatic tachycardia were secondary, then treating the tachycardia would not help the patient. Keeping this principle in mind can help one understand how a patient with POTS may feel better during treatment with a beta-blocker, which forces the pulse rate to go down, while another patient may not feel better at all, even though the pulse rate has decreased to the same extent.

Over the course of months or years, patients with POTS can improve, or else they can learn to cope with this chronic, debilitating, but not life-threatening disorder.

Neurocardiogenic Syncope

Neurocardiogenic syncope is fainting. Neurocardiogenic presyncope is near-fainting without actual loss of consciousness. Syncope is defined medically as sudden loss of consciousness (blackout) that is associated with loss of muscle tone (you go limp) and that reverses rapidly (you wake up spontaneously within seconds to minutes). Neurocardiogenic syncope is also called vasovagal syncope, vasodepressor syncope, neurally mediated syncope, and the common faint. It is by far the most common cause of sudden loss of consciousness in the general population. Neurocardiogenic syncope is most common in young adult women and in children. Most patients with frequent episodes of neurocardiogenic syncope recognize early warning signs and are able to abort the episode before syncope actually occurs.

In middle-aged or elderly adults, syncope is more likely to be a sign of a heart problem (abnormal heart rhythm, abnormal conduction of electrical impulses in the heart, or heart valve problem) or orthostatic hypotension.

In patients in whom neurocardiogenic syncope is a frequent problem, even between episodes the patients often feel unwell, with an inability to tolerate prolonged standing, chronic fatigue, headache, and heat intolerance, as in POTS. Both disorders also mainly involve young adult women. As in POTS, the outlook is variable, and the condition can improve over the years. Unlike in POTS, in neurocardiogenic syncope the patients have a normal pulse rate during standing.

Neurocardiogenic syncope typically involves a particular pattern in which adrenaline levels are high at the time of the acute episode, and the sympathetic nervous system shuts down. This pattern has been called sympathoadrenal imbalance. The combination of loss of sympathetic vasoconstrictor tone and adrenaline-induced relaxation of blood vessels in skeletal muscle could decrease vascular resistance in skeletal muscle and in the body as a whole, without a compensatory increase in the ejection of blood by the heart, the cardiac output. The proximate cause of neurocardiogenic syncope would then be decreased delivery of blood to the brainstem.

9 | Tests for Dysautonomias

There are four types of tests to diagnose dysautonomias: physiological, neuropharmacological, neurochemical, and neuroimaging. Physiological tests involve measurements of a body function in response to a manipulation such as standing, tilt-table testing, or a change in room temperature. Neuropharmacological tests involve giving a drug and measuring its immediate effects. Neurochemical tests involve measuring levels of body chemicals, such as the catecholamines norepinephrine and adrenaline, either under resting conditions or in response to physiological or neuropharmacological manipulations. Neuroimaging tests involve visualizing parts of the autonomic nervous system—in particular, the sympathetic nerves in the heart.

Each testing modality has advantages and disadvantages. Most centers that carry out autonomic function testing use more than one type of test, but few if any use all the tests described in this section. Physiological tests usually are simple, quick, painless, and safe. The main problem with these tests is that several steps always take place between the brain's directing a change in nerve traffic in the autonomic nervous system and the physiological changes that are supposed to measure the autonomic changes. As a result, the results of physiological tests are indirect, and they may or may not identify a problem correctly.

Neuropharmacological tests are relatively simple and quick, but they depend on drug effects, on how the patient feels, or on how the body functions. This means that there always is at least some risk of side effects. In addition, neuropharmacological test results can be complex and indirect. For instance, a neuropharmacological test of the role of the sympathetic nervous system in a person's high blood pressure might include measuring the effects of a drug that blocks sympathetic nerve traffic on blood pressure, because a large fall in blood pressure would suggest an important role of the sympathetic nervous system in keeping the blood pressure high. But if blocking the sympathetic nerve traffic activated another system compensatorily, then the sympathetic blocking drug might not decrease the pressure, and the doctor might mistakenly infer that the sympathetic nervous system played no role in the patient's high blood pressure.

Neurochemical tests involve measurements of levels of compounds such as norepinephrine in body fluids such as plasma. These tests can be done while the patient is at rest lying down, during a physiological manipulation such as exercise or tilting on a tilt table, or during a neuropharmacological manipulation such as blockade of sympathetic nerve traffic by a drug. Neurochemical tests themselves are safe, but the type of body fluid sampling, such as arterial blood sampling or cerebrospinal fluid sampling after a lumbar puncture, can involve some risk. A major disadvantage of neurochemical testing is no test of parasympathetic nervous system activity exists. This is because acetylcholine, the chemical messenger of the parasympathetic and sympathetic cholinergic systems, is broken down by the enzyme acetylcholinesterase almost as soon as the acetylcholine enters body fluids. Neurochemical testing based on plasma norepinephrine levels also can be problematic, because those levels are determined not only by the rate of entry of norepinephrine into the plasma but also the rate of removal (clearance) of norepinephrine from the plasma. In addition, plasma norepinephrine levels are determined complexly by a variety of processes in the sympathetic nerve terminals. Neurochemical testing by plasma norepinephrine levels requires a carefully controlled testing situation and expert technical analysis and interpretation. Few laboratories can measure adrenaline at the levels normally seen in plasma of healthy people at rest. Laboratories also vary in the validity, reliability, and sensitivity of the assay methods.

Neuroimaging tests, which are relatively new, enable visualizing the autonomic nerve supply in body organs such as the heart. As yet there is no accepted neuroimaging test to visualize parasympathetic nerve terminals. Sympathetic neuroimaging is done in relatively few centers. This type of testing can produce striking images of the sympathetic innervation of the heart. Neuroimaging provides anatomic information about whether sympathetic nerve terminals are present, but it is less clear whether neuroimaging can provide information about whether those terminals are functioning normally or not.

Physiological Tests

The Valsalva Maneuver

The Valsalva maneuver test is one of the most important clinical physiological tests of autonomic function. In the Valsalva maneuver, the patient blows against a resistance (30–40 mm Hg, depending on the medical center) for 12–20 seconds and then relaxes.

The instant the patient begins to blow, the sudden increase in chest and abdominal pressure forces blood out of the chest and down the arms. This increases blood pressure briefly (phase I of the maneuver). The increase in blood pressure in phase I is mechanical and not part of a reflex (fig. 44). Soon afterward, however, the amount of blood ejected by the heart with each beat (stroke volume) plummets, because the straining decreases entry of blood from the veins into the heart. Blood pressure progressively falls (phase II). The brain immediately senses this fall because of decreased input to the brain from stretch receptors (baroreceptors) in the walls of the heart and major blood vessels. The brain directs a rapid increase in outflows of the sympathetic nervous system to the blood vessels and a rapid decrease in outflow of the parasympathetic nervous system to the heart. The increase in sympathetic nerve traffic leads to more release of norepinephrine from the nerve terminals, and the released norepinephrine tightens blood vessels throughout the body. The total peripheral resistance to blood flow in the

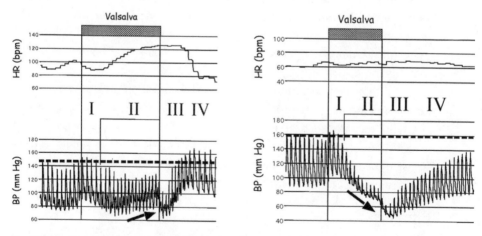

Fig. 44. Heart rate and blood pressure during and after the Valsalva maneuver normally change in four phases. The recording on the left is from a healthy subject; the recording on the right is from a patient with primary chronic autonomic failure.

body goes up, just like tightening the nozzle at the end of a garden hose increases the pressure in the hose. Therefore, normally, at the end of phase II the blood pressure increases from its minimum value, even though the amount of blood ejected by the heart remains low. When the patient relaxes at the end of the maneuver, the blood pressure falls briefly (phase III)—a mirror image of the brief increase in phase I. Blood rushes back into the chest, and the heart ejects this blood. The blood pressure increases (phase IV). Since the blood vessels are constricted, the normal amount of filling of the constricted vessels produces an overshoot of blood pressure, just as pressure in a garden hose attains higher levels if one opens the faucet with the nozzle tightened. Finally, in response to this phase IV overshoot of blood pressure, sympathetic nervous system outflow to blood vessels falls and parasympathetic nervous system outflow to the heart increases. This causes a rapid return of blood pressure and heart rate to normal.

In a patient with sympathetic nervous system or baroreflex-sympathoneural failure, during phase II the blood vessels fail to constrict reflexively, and so the blood pressure falls progressively and does not increase toward baseline at the end of phase II. During phase IV, because of the lack of tightening of blood vessels, there is no rapid increase in blood pressure and no phase IV overshoot of pressure. Instead, the blood pressure gradually increases slowly back to the baseline value.

The responses of pulse rate to the Valsalva maneuver depend mainly on changes in parasympathetic nervous system outflow to the heart via the vagus nerve. In phase II, the pulse rate increases, and in phase IV the pulse rate returns rapidly to baseline. In baroreflex-cardiovagal failure, the pulse rate remains unchanged both during and after performance of the maneuver.

Note that one must monitor the beat-to-beat blood pressure changes to diagnose sympathetic neurocirculatory failure based on the Valsalva maneuver. Until recently, such monitoring required insertion of a catheter into an artery. The recent introduction of special testing devices has provided noninvasive means to monitor blood pressure beat-to-beat and detect sympathetic neurocirculatory failure.

Forearm Blood Flow

This noninvasive test measures the rate of blood flow in the forearm. The forearm vascular resistance (FVR) can be estimated from the forearm blood flow (FBF) and the blood pressure (mean arterial pressure, MAP). In the garden hose analogy, the FVR would correspond to the extent of tightening of the vascular nozzle in the forearm.

To measure forearm blood flow, a blood pressure cuff is attached around the upper arm, and a special braceletlike device called a strain gauge is attached around the upper forearm. The strain gauge measures stretch very sensitively. For a measurement of forearm blood flow, the blood pressure cuff is inflated to just above the venous pressure but below the arterial pressure. This is like tightening a tourniquet around the upper arm for obtaining a blood sample. Because the cuff pressure is above the venous pressure, blood in the forearm and hand can't get past the cuff, and because the cuff pressure is below the arterial pressure, blood can still enter the forearm and hand. In this situation, the volume of the forearm increases slightly, and the strain gauge senses the increase in volume. If the rate of blood flow into the forearm is high, then the volume of the forearm increases rapidly after the cuff is inflated; and if the rate of blood flow is low, then the volume of the forearm increases slowly. By a simple calculation one can estimate the blood flow into the forearm from the rate of increase in the volume of the forearm after the cuff is inflated.

Once the rate of FBF is known, the FVR can be calculated from the average blood pressure (MAP) divided by the FBF. This calculation is similar to that for measuring total peripheral resistance (TPR) from the MAP divided by the cardiac output (CO). When a person stands up or is tilted on a tilt table, the FVR normally increases. Failure of the FVR to increase during standing can indicate a problem in the baroreflex arc or local loss of sympathetic nerves.

Power Spectral Analysis of Heart Rate Variability

This test is much simpler than the fancy name suggests. A healthy person's heart rate is not constant. The pulse rate increases when the person inhales slowly and then decreases when the person exhales. The pulse rate normally oscillates in a wavelike pattern. The change in pulse rate from breathing is called respiratory sinus arrhythmia. This sounds like an abnormal heart rhythm, but it actually is a sign of a healthy heart. Respiratory sinus arrhythmia mainly reflects changes in parasympathetic nervous system influences on the heart.

If you were to graph the size of the oscillation as a function of its frequency, then at the frequency of breathing (the respiratory frequency) there would be a peak of "power." Patients with inhibition of the parasympathetic cardiovagal system have a reduced or absent peak of power at the respiratory frequency. The power spectral analysis often reveals a second peak of power at a lower frequency than the respiratory frequency. Researchers have thought that this low-frequency power is related to sympathetic nervous system influences on the heart but exactly how remains unclear. Power spectral analysis of heart rate variability offers the advantages of safety, technical ease, and speed. The main disadvantages are that the meaning of low-frequency power as an index of sympathetic nervous system activity in the heart remains in dispute and that a much less expensive way to assess parasympathetic cardiovagal function is to measure the amount of heart rate change during deep breathing or the Valsalva maneuver.

Tilt-Table Testing

Tilt-table testing is done to see if standing up (orthostasis) provokes a sudden fall in blood pressure (neurally mediated hypotension), an excessive increase in pulse rate (as in postural tachycardia syndrome, POTS), or fainting (neurally mediated syncope).

The testing itself is simple. The patient lies on a stretcherlike table, strapped in place with safety belts; the patient is then tilted upright at an angle. The exact angle varies from center to center and may be from 60 degrees to 90 degrees. The tilting goes on for up to 45 minutes, the duration also varying among centers. If the patient tolerates the tilting for this period, then the patient may receive a drug, such as isoproterenol or nitroglycerine, which might provoke a sudden fall in blood pressure or loss of consciousness. As soon as the test becomes positive, the patient is put back into a position lying flat or with the head down; sometimes fluid is given by vein. Consciousness returns within a minute or two.

In general, there are two types of positive tilt-table test results. An excessive, progressively more severe increase in pulse rate during the tilting would be compatible with a diagnosis of postural tachycardia syndrome, or POTS. A decrease in the level of consciousness and finally losing consciousness (syncope) would be compatible with a diagnosis of neurocardiogenic syncope. Loss of consciousness evoked by tilt-table testing virtually always is associated with a fall in blood pressure, sometimes called neurally mediated hypotension. A tilt-table test can yield results compatible with both POTS and neurocardiogenic syncope, such as when the patient has a large increase in pulse rate, followed by a sudden fall in pulse rate back to normal that is accompanied by neurally mediated hypotension and syncope.

Tilt-table testing is a form of provocative test, with the goal to reproduce the patient's problem in a controlled laboratory situation. The testing is safe when done by experienced personnel, in a setting where emergency backup is available. A limitation of tilt-table testing is false-positive results, especially when a drug such as isoproterenol is used. In a false-positive test, the results of the test are positive, but enough healthy people can have a positive test result that a positive test result might not actually mean that anything really is "wrong." A positive tilt-table test can give a false sense of assurance that the patient does not have serious heart disease. Reggie Lewis was a basketball star for the Boston Celtics. He collapsed and lost consciousness during a game. After several cardiology tests, including a tilt-table test, it was decided that he had a relatively benign condition such as neurocardiogenic syncope, and he was cleared to return to playing basketball. Before he played another game professionally, during a pickup game, he collapsed again and died.

Sweat Tests

Sweating is important for regulating body temperature. In response to exposure to a hot environment, the brain increases sweating by directing an increase in sympathetic nervous system traffic to sweat glands in the skin. The chemical messenger, acetylcholine, is released, and the acetylcholine acts on the sweat glands to stimulate production of sweat.

There are several ways to assess sympathetic cholinergic sweating in response to external heat (thermoregulatory sweat test, TST). One is based on sprinkling starch with iodine all over the body. When the starch-iodine combination is wetted, the powder turns brown. One can then photograph the body and see which parts sweated. Sometimes other powder-dye combinations are used. Sweat increases local humidity, and one can monitor the humidity in a chamber attached to the skin. When the skin becomes sweaty, the ability to conduct electricity increases dramatically, because of the salt and water in the sweat, and one can also monitor the skin electrical conductance. The galvanic skin response (GSR), or skin sympathetic test (SST), is often part of polygraphic "lie detector" testing. When a person is startled or distressed acutely, or a small electric shock is delivered to the skin, increased activity of the sympathetic cholinergic system evokes sweating.

These sweat tests, in general, are safe, simple, and quick. They only measure physiological changes, mainly from effects of acetylcholine. Decreased sweating provides little or no information about the site of the lesion in the thermoregulatory reflex arc. Sweating is normal in dysautonomias specifically of catecholamine systems.

QSART stands for quantitative sudomotor axon reflex test. This is a form of sweat test. Sweating in response to altered environmental temperature results from the effects of the chemical messenger, acetylcholine, released from sympathetic nerve terminals near sweat glands in the skin. In the QSART, dried nitrogen (or dried air, or air with a known amount of humidity) is pumped at a controlled rate through a small plastic capsule placed on the skin. When the person sweats, the humidity in the chamber increases as sweat droplets evaporate, providing a measure of sweat production. For QSART testing, a drug that stimulates acetylcholine receptors (for instance, acetylcholine itself) is applied to a nearby patch of skin, by a special procedure called iontophoresis. The locally applied acetylcholine evokes sweating at the site where it is given, but in addition, by way of a type of reflex called an axon reflex, sympathetic nerve terminals under the nearby plastic capsule release the body's own acetylcholine, resulting in sweat production measured by increased humidity in the capsule.

If a person had a loss of sympathetic nerve terminals that release acetylcholine (loss of cholinergic terminals), then applying acetylcholine to the patch of skin near the test capsule would not lead to increased sweating or increased humidity in the test capsule. On the other hand, if the person had intact sympathetic cholinergic nerve terminals, then applying acetylcholine to a patch of skin near the test capsule would increase the humidity in the capsule. If the person had a brain disease that prevented increases in sympathetic nerve traffic during exposure to increased environmental temperature, the person would not be able to increase the humidity in the capsule in response to an increase in the room temperature, but the person would have a normal QSART response. By this sort of neuropharmacological test, doctors can distinguish sympathetic cholinergic failure due to loss of cholinergic terminals from failure due to abnormal regulation of sympathetic nerve traffic to intact cholinergic terminals.

In general, the QSART is safe, quick, quantitative, and easy for a technician to perform. The equipment required is expensive, and relatively few centers have QSART testing available. The key factor measured is physiological (in this case, sweat production) and therefore nonspecific. If a patient had a problem with the ability to make acetylcholine in the nerve terminals or with the ability of acetylcholine to bind to its receptors in the sweat glands, the same abnormal QSART result would be obtained as if the sympathetic cholinergic terminals were lost. QSART results also do not allow inferences about the status of other components of the autonomic nervous system.

The Cold Pressor Test

In the cold pressor test, the patient dips a hand into ice-cold water. This rapidly increases the blood pressure by increasing activity of the sympathetic nervous system. Because the test involves not only cold but also pain, the cold pressor test can only be done for about a minute. A similar limitation applies for the isometric handgrip exercise.

Neuropharmacological Tests

Different centers apply different drug tests in autonomic nervous system testing. The following are examples.

Ganglion Blockade

Trimethaphan and pentolinium are of a type of drug called a ganglion blocker. In the autonomic nervous system, control signals from the brain and spinal cord are relayed through the ganglia, and nerves from the ganglia, postganglionic nerves, deliver those signals to the nerve terminals near or in the target tissues. The control signals are relayed in the ganglia by release of the chemical messenger, acetylcholine, which binds to specific receptors called nicotinic receptors on the postganglionic cells.

Stimulation of the nicotinic receptors, such as by nicotine itself, increases postganglionic nerve traffic in both the parasympathetic nervous system and the sympathetic nervous system. Trimethaphan and pentolinium do just the opposite. They block nicotinic receptors in the ganglia, thereby blocking the transmission of nerve impulses in the ganglia to the postganglionic nerves of the sympathetic nervous system and parasympathetic nervous system. The rates of sympathetic nerve traffic and parasympathetic nerve traffic fall to virtually zero. Because of the blockade of transmission of nerve impulses in ganglia, ganglion blockers affect a variety of body functions. The drugs always produce orthostatic hypotension. If the person is lying down, blood pressure falls by relatively little, but as soon as a ganglion-blocked person stands up, the blood pressure plummets. Probably the most noticeable effect of ganglion blocker is a dry mouth, due to inhibition of the parasympathetic nervous system, which is responsible for production of watery saliva. Other effects include decreased urinary bladder and gastrointestinal functions.

If a patient had autonomic failure due to a loss of sympathetic nerve terminals, such as in pure autonomic failure, norepinephrine would not be released from the nerve terminals. Ganglion blockers in such a patient would not affect the blood pressure. But if a patient had autonomic failure due to a brain disease, such as the Shy-Drager syndrome, there might be ongoing, unregulated release of norepinephrine from the nerve terminals, in which case ganglion blockade would decrease the blood pressure substantially. Measuring cardiovascular responses to ganglion blockade therefore can provide information about whether autonomic failure is associated with a loss of sympathetic nerve terminals or from failure of the brain to regulate sympathetic nerve traffic appropriately.

In some patients with long-term high blood pressure (hypertension), the hypertension seems to reflect an overall increase in the rate of nerve traffic in the sympathetic nervous system. This increases delivery of norepinephrine to its receptors in the heart and blood vessels, causing an increase in the output of blood by the heart and tightening of the blood vessels. By either or both mechanisms, the blood pressure would be high because of the high rate of delivery of norepinephrine to its receptors. Some investigators have called this hypernoradrenergic hypertension. In a patient with hypernoradrenergic hypertension, ganglion blockade would be expected to decrease the rate of norepinephrine release from the sympathetic nerve terminals, and the extent of the fall in the plasma norepinephrine level would be related to the extent of fall in the blood pressure. In a patient with the same severity of hypertension but with a normal rate of nerve traffic in the sympathetic nervous system, ganglion blockade would not be expected to decrease the blood pressure by as much.

Yohimbine Challenge Test

Yohimbine is a type of drug called an alpha-2 adrenoceptor blocker. Alpha-2 adrenoceptors are receptors for norepinephrine that exist at high concentrations in certain parts of the brain, on sympathetic nerve terminals, and in blood vessel walls.

When alpha-2 adrenoceptors in the brain are blocked, sympathetic nerve traffic increases. Alpha-2 adrenoceptors on sympathetic nerve terminals act like a brake on norepinephrine release from the terminals. When alpha-2 adrenoceptors on sympathetic nerves are blocked, the amount of norepinephrine release for a given amount of sympathetic nerve traffic increases. Yohimbine, by blocking alpha-2 adrenoceptors in the brain and on sympathetic nerves, therefore releases norepinephrine from the nerve terminals. The released norepinephrine binds to alpha-1 adrenoceptors in blood vessel walls, causing an increase in blood pressure.

Because of the blockade of alpha-2 adrenoceptors in the brain, yohimbine can produce any of several behavioral or emotional effects, which vary from person to person. Yohimbine can cause an increase in alertness or feelings such as anxiety or sadness, or, on the other hand, happiness or a sense of energy. Yohimbine sometimes evokes a panic attack.

In the yohimbine challenge test, the drug is given by vein for several minutes or given by mouth as a single dose. Yohimbine given by vein is currently an investigational drug. The blood pressure and pulse rate are monitored frequently or continuously, and blood may be sampled from an indwelling catheter in an arm vein for measurement of plasma norepinephrine levels or levels of other neurochemicals.

If a patient had autonomic failure because of a loss of sympathetic nerve terminals, such as in pure autonomic failure, there would be decreased release of norepinephrine from the nerve terminals, regardless of the nerve traffic. Yohimbine in such a patient would increase the blood pressure by relatively little. But if a patient had autonomic failure because of a brain disease, such as the Shy-Drager syndrome, yohimbine would increase the blood pressure, and because of the inability to regulate sympathetic nerve traffic, the brain would not reflexively decrease the sympathetic nerve traffic to compensate for the increased blood pressure. The infusion would increase blood pressure substantially.

In patients with hypernoradrenergic hypertension, some of the released norepinephrine binds to the alpha-2 adrenoceptors on the sympathetic nerve terminals, putting a brake on the norepinephrine release. Infusion of yohimbine into such patients blocks this restraint and increases both the blood pressure and the plasma norepinephrine level. The finding of a large increase in blood pressure coupled with a large increase in the plasma norepinephrine level provides support for a diagnosis of hypernoradrenergic hypertension.

In patients who have decreased activity of the cell membrane norepinephrine transporter, or NET, when yohimbine releases norepinephrine from the sympathetic nerve terminals, "recycling" of the norepinephrine back into the nerve terminals does not inactivate the released norepinephrine. This results in excessive delivery of norepinephrine to its receptors, both in the brain and outside the brain. In patients with NET deficiency, yohimbine therefore produces a large increase in the plasma norepinephrine level and large increases in the pulse rate and blood pressure. Yohimbine can also evoke panic or chest pain or pressure that can mimic symptomatic coronary artery disease.

The yohimbine challenge test therefore can provide information about whether autonomic failure is associated with a loss of sympathetic nerve terminals or with failure of the brain to regulate sympathetic nerve traffic appropriately. The test can also be used to identify hypernoradrenergic hypertension or NET deficiency.

Clonidine Suppression Test

Clonidine stimulates alpha-2 adrenoceptors in the brain, on sympathetic nerve terminals, and in blood vessel walls. When alpha-2 adrenoceptors in the brain are stimulated, sympathetic nerve traffic decreases, and when alpha-2 adrenoceptors on sympathetic nerve terminals are stimulated, the amount of norepinephrine release for a given amount of sympathetic nerve traffic decreases. Released norepinephrine binds to both alpha-2 adrenoceptors and alpha-1 adrenoceptors in blood vessel walls. Even though clonidine stimulates alpha-2 adrenoceptors, which would constrict blood vessels, the drug is so powerful in decreasing release of norepinephrine that normally after a dose of clonidine the blood pressure falls. Clonidine is an approved drug for the treatment of long-term high blood pressure (hypertension). By stimulating alpha-2 adrenoceptors in the brain, clonidine usually produces some sedation. It can cause a decrease in alertness or a decrease in the sense of energy. Clonidine is effective in relieving symptoms of withdrawal from alcohol or opiate-type narcotics.

In the clonidine suppression test, the drug is given by mouth, usually at a dose of 300 µg, which would be the total amount of the drug given in divided doses in a day. The blood pressure and pulse rate are monitored over the course of a few hours, and blood is sampled from an indwelling catheter in an arm vein for measurements of plasma norepinephrine levels.

The rationale for the clonidine suppression test is about the same as that for the ganglion blockade test. If a patient had autonomic failure due to a loss of sympathetic nerve terminals, there would be no release of norepinephrine from the terminals. Clonidine would not affect the blood pressure, or it might actually increase the blood pressure because of stimulation of alpha-2 adrenoceptors in the blood vessel walls. In a patient with auto-nomic failure from a brain disease, clonidine would decrease the blood pres-sure; and because of the inability to regulate sympathetic nerve traffic, the brain would not reflexively increase the sympathetic nerve traffic to com-pensate for the decreased pressure. This means that clonidine might pro-duce a large decrease in pressure.

By stimulating alpha-2 adrenoceptors on sympathetic nerve terminals, clonidine puts a brake on the norepinephrine release. Clonidine given to patients with hypernoradrenergic hypertension therefore decreases both blood pressure and the plasma norepinephrine level. The finding of a large decrease in blood pressure coupled with a large decrease in the plasma nor-epinephrine level provides support for the diagnosis of hypernoradrenergic hypertension.

Rarely, hypernoradrenergic hypertension results from a tumor that pro-duces catecholamines such as norepinephrine and epinephrine. The tumor is called a pheochromocytoma. The clonidine suppression test is an accepted diagnostic test for pheochromocytoma. If the hypernoradrenergic hyper-tension resulted from a high rate of sympathetic nerve traffic, then cloni-dine would decrease the elevated plasma norepinephrine level. But if the patient had a "pheo," which would produce catecholamines independently of the rate of sympathetic nerve traffic, clonidine would fail to decrease the plasma norepinephrine level. In other words, in a positive clonidine suppres-sion test for pheochromocytoma, the plasma norepinephrine level fails to decrease after a dose of clonidine, despite the presence of hypernoradren-ergic hypertension.

Isoproterenol Infusion Test

Isoproterenol (brand name Isuprel) stimulates beta-adrenoceptors. Beta-adrenoceptor stimulation has several important effects in the body. In par-ticular, stimulation of beta-adrenoceptors in the heart increases the rate and force of the heartbeat and therefore increases the output of blood by the heart per minute (cardiac output). Stimulation of beta-adrenoceptors in the liver converts stored energy in the form of glycogen to immediately avail-able energy in the form of glucose. Stimulation of beta-adrenoceptors in blood vessel walls of skeletal muscle relaxes the blood vessels, decreasing the resistance to blood flow in the body as a whole (total peripheral resistance). Stimulation of beta-adrenoceptors on sympathetic nerve terminals increases the release of norepinephrine.

In the hyperdynamic circulation syndrome, the patient has a relatively fast pulse rate, high cardiac output, a variable blood pressure that tends to be increased, a tendency towards panic or anxiety attacks, excessive increases in pulse rate in response to isoproterenol given by vein, and improvement by treatment with the beta-adrenoceptor blocker propranolol. The same holds true for many relatively young patients with early, borderline hypertension. Patients with the postural tachycardia syndrome (POTS) also can have a fast pulse rate, even when lying down, excessive increases in pulse rate during isoproterenol infusion, and sometimes panic evoked by the infusion.

Isoproterenol is also occasionally infused as part of tilt-table testing in patients with chronic fatigue syndrome or chronic orthostatic intolerance. After prolonged upright tilting, infusion of isoproterenol can bring on a rapid fall in blood pressure or loss of consciousness, converting a negative tilt-table test to a positive test.

Neurochemical Tests

Neurochemical tests of autonomic nervous system function mainly involve the sympathetic noradrenergic and adrenomedullary hormonal systems. This is because the main chemical messengers of these systems, norepinephrine and adrenaline, are relatively stable in the plasma, whereas the main chemical messenger of the parasympathetic nervous system, acetylcholine, undergoes rapid breakdown and cannot be measured in the plasma.

Plasma Norepinephrine

Because norepinephrine is the main chemical messenger of the sympathetic nervous system, doctors have often used the plasma norepinephrine level as an index of sympathetic nervous system "activity" in the body as a whole.

The relationship between the rate of sympathetic nerve traffic and the concentration of norepinephrine in the plasma is complex, indirect, and influenced by many factors such as commonly used drugs and activities of daily life. The blood sample therefore should be obtained under carefully controlled or monitored conditions, and the plasma norepinephrine level should be interpreted by an expert.

Here is a brief description of some of the complexities involved. First, only a small proportion of the norepinephrine released from sympathetic nerve terminals actually reaches the bloodstream. Most is recycled back into the nerve terminals by uptake-1, via the cell membrane norepinephrine transporter (NET). This means that a person might have a high plasma norepinephrine level, despite a normal rate of sympathetic nerve traffic, if the NET were blocked by a drug or weren't working correctly. Second, the plasma norepinephrine level is determined not only by the rate of entry of norepinephrine into the plasma but also by the rate of removal of norepinephrine from the plasma. Norepinephrine is cleared from the plasma extremely rapidly. This means that a person might have a high plasma norepinephrine level because of a decrease in the rate of removal of norepinephrine from the plasma, such as in heart or kidney failure. Third, norepinephrine is produced in sympathetic nerve terminals by the actions of multiple enzymes, cofactors, and transporters. A problem with any of these can result in decreased norepinephrine production and low plasma norepinephrine levels, regardless of the rate of sympathetic nerve traffic. Fourth, plasma norepinephrine usually is measured in a blood sample drawn from a vein in the arm. Because the skin and skeletal muscle in the forearm and hand contain sympathetic nerves, the plasma norepinephrine level in blood from an arm vein is determined not only by the rate of norepinephrine release from sympathetic nerve terminals in the body as a whole but also by the rate of release locally in the forearm and hand. Fifth, the plasma norepinephrine level varies depending on the posture of the person at the time of blood sampling (the level doubles within minutes of standing up from lying down), the time of day (highest in the morning), whether the person has been fasting, the temperature of the room, dietary factors such as salt intake, and any of a large number of commonly used over-the-counter and prescription drugs or herbal remedies.

Plasma Adrenaline

Compared with the plasma norepinephrine level, which is complexly and indirectly related to sympathetic nervous system "activity" in the body as a whole, the plasma adrenaline level is a fairly direct indicator of activity of the adrenomedullary hormonal system.

Nevertheless, some of the same factors that complicate interpreting plasma norepinephrine levels apply to plasma adrenaline. Numerous common and difficult-to-control life experiences influence activity of the adrenomedullary hormonal system. These include drugs, alterations in blood glucose levels (such as after a meal), body temperature, posture, and emotional distress. Distress increases adrenaline levels proportionately even more than it does norepinephrine levels.

An additional problem is technical. Adrenaline is a very powerful hormone, and correspondingly plasma adrenaline levels normally are very low, straining the sensitivity of available assay methods. Other chemicals besides adrenaline can interfere with the measurement, especially in coffee drinkers, because plasma from such individuals contains high levels of dihydrocaffeic acid, which can mimic adrenaline in the assay results. It is important that blood sampling for plasma adrenaline be carried out under controlled conditions and the assay performed by expert personnel.

Neuroimaging Tests

Compared with other types of testing for dysautonomias, testing using neuroimaging is new. Neuroimaging visualizes nervous system tissue, such as in the brain. In testing for dysautonomias, the neuroimaging visualizes the sympathetic innervation of organs outside the brain—especially the heart, which possesses dense sympathetic innervation.

Sympathetic nerves in the heart travel with the coronary arteries that deliver blood to the heart muscle. The nerves then dive into the muscle and form meshlike networks that surround the heart muscle cells. Because neuroimaging tests have a limited resolution of a few millimeters, the imaging does not show individual nerves. Since the nerves are distributed throughout the heart muscle, the image looks very much like a scan of the heart muscle.

The radioactive drugs used for imaging the sympathetic nerves in the heart are given by vein and delivered to the heart muscle by way of the coronary arteries. This means that one must distinguish decreased radioactivity in the scan due to loss of sympathetic nerves from decreased radioactivity due to coronary artery blockage; either abnormality would lead to the same lack of radioactivity in the heart muscle. Centers that carry out sympathetic neuroimaging therefore often do two scans in the same test, one scan to see where the blood is going and one to see where the sympathetic nerves are.

In the United States, sympathetic neuroimaging is available in relatively few centers, whereas it is more readily available in European countries and Japan. Worldwide, probably the most commonly used sympathetic neuroimaging agent is ^{123}I-metaiodobenzylguanidine (^{123}I-MIBG). ^{123}I-MIBG is not a catecholamine, but it is taken up by sympathetic nerves via the cell membrane norepinephrine transporter, and once inside the nerves it is taken up by storage vesicles via the vesicular monoamine transporter.

At the National Institutes of Health our group developed another sympathetic neuroimaging agent, which is 6-[^{18}F]fluorodopamine. This is a radioactive form of the catecholamine dopamine. After injection of 6-[^{18}F]fluorodopamine by vein, the drug is taken up by sympathetic nerve terminals, and the radioactivity is detected by a special type of scanning procedure called positron emission tomographic scanning, or PET scanning. A positron emitter is a type of radioactive substance that releases a short-lived form of radiation that can penetrate the body and reach detectors outside it, enabling construction of a PET scan. Other PET-imaging agents for visualizing sympathetic nerves include ^{11}C-hydroxyephedrine, [^{18}F]fluorometaraminol, and ^{11}C-adrenaline.

Different forms of dysautonomia result in different pictures of the sympathetic nerves in the heart by fluorodopamine PET scanning. Probably the most striking images are obtained in diseases in which there is a loss of sympathetic nerve terminals, such as in pure autonomic failure and in Parkinson disease. To such patients, even when the blood flow to the heart muscle is normal, there is no heart visible in the PET scan! A much more difficult issue is whether analysis of the amount of radioactivity in the heart can provide information about how the sympathetic nerve terminals are functioning. This is a matter of research now.

Treatments for
Dysautonomias

Successful treatment of dysautonomias requires an individualized program, which can change over time. Because the underlying disease mechanisms often are not understood well, treatment is likely to involve some trial and error.

Nondrug Treatments

Several nondrug treatments are used for different types of dysautonomias. The reasons for a treatment depend on the particular dysautonomia. Sometimes, the responses of a patient to a treatment help the doctor determine the diagnosis. Patients with dysautonomias can feel differently from day to day, even without any clear reason. This means that if a treatment is tried, it may take several days to decide whether the treatment has helped.

Elevation of the Head of the Bed

In patients who have a fall in blood pressure every time they stand up (orthostatic hypotension), elevation of the head of the bed at night, by a variety of ways, improves the ability to tolerate standing up in the morning.

Salt Intake

High salt intake tends to increase the volume of fluid in the body. A small percent of this volume is in the bloodstream. Doctors usually recommend a high salt diet for patients with an inability to tolerate prolonged standing (chronic orthostatic intolerance) or a fall in blood pressure during standing (orthostatic hypotension). When a person takes in a high salt diet, the kidneys increase the amount of salt in the urine, and this limits the increase in blood volume. Drugs that promote retention of sodium by the kidneys, such as Florinef, are usually required for high salt intake to increase body fluid volume effectively.

Meals

Eating a big meal leads to shunting of blood toward the gut. In people with orthostatic intolerance or orthostatic hypotension, it is usually advisable to take frequent small meals.

Compression Hose

Compression hose or other compression garments decrease the amount of pooling of blood in veins when a person stands. This can decrease leakage of fluid from the veins into the tissues and decrease swelling of the feet. In patients with veins that fill up or leak excessively during standing, compression garments can improve toleration of prolonged standing. In patients with orthostatic hypotension, the problem may be less with the veins than with the arteries and arterioles, the vessels that carry blood under pressure to the organs and limbs. Wearing compression garments therefore may be disappointing in the management of orthostatic hypotension.

Coffee

Some patients with dysautonomias feel better drinking caffeinated coffee frequently. Others feel jittery or anxious and avoid caffeinated coffee. Still others notice no effect.

Temperature

Patients with dysautonomias often have an inability to tolerate extremes of external temperature. When exposed to the heat, patients with failure of the sympathetic nervous system may not sweat adequately to maintain the core temperature by evaporation of the sweat. Patients with chronic orthostatic intolerance, such as from postural tachycardia syndrome (POTS), can have heat intolerance because of loss of blood volume by sweating or shunting of blood away from the brain. When exposed to cold, patients with sympathetic nervous system failure may not constrict blood vessels adequately in the skin, so that the body temperature falls (hypothermia).

Exercise

Patients with dysautonomias can benefit from an exercise-training program. Often, however, the training does not decrease the sense of fatigue. As a person exercises, the blood vessels carrying oxygen-rich blood to the exercising muscle (arteries and arterioles) tend to relax, at least in part because of the accumulation of by-products of metabolism. The sympathetic nervous system normally counters this tendency by increasing the tone of the blood vessel walls. The blood flow to the exercising muscle therefore is in a dynamic state of balance. Activation of sympathetic nerves to the heart during exercise increases the force and rate of the heartbeat, and the total amount of blood pumped by the heart in one minute (cardiac output) increases. Meanwhile, muscle pumping during exercise promotes movement of blood from the limbs back to the heart. Increased metabolic activity tends to increase body temperature, and sweating, stimulated by the sympathetic nerves to sweat glands, increases evaporative heat loss, helping maintain appropriate body temperature. If a patient had failure of the sympathetic nervous system, excessive production of the by-products of metabolism, or a form of heart disease involving an inability to increase the force or rate of the heartbeat, then the blood pressure would fall during exercise, producing fatigue or exhaustion.

After exercise, when muscle pumping ceases, the blood can pool in the legs or abdomen, while the rate of sympathetic nerve traffic falls to the resting rate. If the decline in sympathetic nerve traffic did not balance the decline in production of by-products of metabolism, the blood pressure would fall after exercise. At the same time, loss of body fluid via evaporative sweating decreases the blood volume. Patients with a dysautonomia therefore often feel especially bad after exercise. It is important to stay hydrated and to avoid activities like eating a large meal after exercise, because this can divert already limited blood volume to the gut.

Perhaps surprisingly, even vigorously healthy, muscular, lean people can have a susceptibility to faint (neurocardiogenic syncope), and it is unclear if exercise training helps them. On the other hand, some patients can improve by isometric calf muscle training, where the patient learns to tense calf muscles when standing, because this tends to decrease blood pooling in the legs.

Pacemakers and Sinus Node Ablation

Insertion of a pacemaker in the heart can help patients with neurocardiogenic syncope or POTS. This is an area of active research and controversy. In some patients with neurocardiogenic syncope, having a pacemaker inserted may not be curative, because the low pulse rate at the time of fainting might not cause and might even be the result of low blood flow to the brain. On the other hand, a sudden absence of electrical activity in the heart produces loss of consciousness within seconds, and in this setting a pacemaker could be curative. Some patients who have a very fast pulse rate undergo destruction of the sinus node pacemaker cells in the heart (sinus node ablation). The doctor must be sure that the fast pulse rate results from a problem with the heart and not from a compensation by the sympathetic nervous system for another problem such as low blood volume, because eliminating this compensation could make the patient worse.

Neurosurgery

Some patients with chronic orthostatic intolerance have a type of change in the brainstem called Chiari malformation. This is an anatomic abnormality in which part of the brainstem falls below the hole in the skull between the brain and spinal cord. Neurosurgery can correct the malformation, but the orthostatic intolerance does not necessarily disappear. This is a controversial topic; patients should seek a second opinion before agreeing to this procedure.

Constipation or Urinary Retention

Patients with failure of the parasympathetic nervous system have constipation and retention of urine in the bladder. The constipation is treated nonspecifically, with stool softeners, bulk laxatives, milk of magnesia, magnesium citrate, senna, or cascara. Urinary retention can be associated with urinary urgency and incontinence. Drugs that stimulate receptors for acetylcholine, such as urecholine, might be tried. Often patients with autonomic failure must learn to self-catheterize to empty the bladder, by inserting a plastic or rubber tube into the urethra and then into the bladder to obtain relief.

Water Drinking

A relatively recently described tactic to increase blood pressure in patients with autonomic failure is to drink 16 ounces of water or other fluid. Why and how water drinking increases blood pressure in patients with autonomic failure remains unclear. Patients with chronic orthostatic intolerance, neurocardiogenic syncope, or POTS often keep a water container with them and sip from it frequently during the day—the "water bottle sign." One may speculate that this practice reflects a tendency to dehydration or low blood volume.

Table 3. Drugs used to treat dysautonomias

Drug	Goals of treatment
Florinef Fludrocortisone	Increase blood volume Increase blood pressure
Proamatine Midodrine	Tighten blood vessels Increase blood pressure Prevent fainting
Beta-blocker	Decrease heart rate Decrease blood pressure Decrease adrenaline effects Prevent fainting
Procrit Erythropoietin	Increase red blood cell count Increase blood pressure
Amphetamines	Tighten blood vessels Increase alertness
Desmopressin	Tighten blood vessels
NSAID	Tighten blood vessels
Octreotide	Tighten blood vessels in gut
SSRI	Improve mood, allay anxiety
Tricyclic	Improve mood
Xanax Alprazolam	Increase sense of calmness Improve sleep
Catapres Clonidine	Decrease blood pressure Improve sleep
Urecholine Bethanechol	Increase salivation Improve gut action Improve urination
Yohimbine	Increase blood pressure

Abbreviations: NSAID, nonsteroidal anti-inflammatory drug; SSRI, selective serotonin reuptake inhibitor; tricyclic, antidepressant drug that blocks catecholamine reuptake.

Drug Treatments

Several drug treatments are used for dysautonomias (table 3). Some of them are powerful and can produce harmful effects, so dysautonomia patients should take medications only under the supervision of a doctor with relevant expertise and experience.

Fludrocortisone (Florinef)

Florinef is a synthetic salt-retaining steroids, or mineralocorticoid. This drug closely resembles the body's main salt-retaining steroid, aldosterone. For Florinef to work it must be taken with a high-salt diet and liberal water intake. Florinef forces the kidneys to retain sodium in exchange for potassium. Water follows the sodium, and Florinef is thought to increase the extracellular fluid volume. The extracellular fluid volume includes the blood volume. The patient gains "fluid weight," and blood pressure increases because of the increased volume. Florinef tends to waste potassium, causing a fall in the serum potassium level. Patients taking Florinef should have periodic checks of their serum electrolytes.

Florinef given to patients with chronic autonomic failure worsens their high blood pressure when they are lying down. Sometimes the doctor faces a difficult dilemma, balancing the long-term increased risk of stroke, heart failure, or kidney failure from high blood pressure against the immediate risk of fainting or falling from orthostatic hypotension.

Beta-Adrenoceptor Blockers

Norepinephrine and adrenaline produce their effects by binding to specific receptors on target cells such as heart muscle cells. There are two types of receptors for norepinephrine and adrenaline—alpha-adrenoceptors and beta-adrenoceptors. Adrenaline stimulates both alpha- and beta-adrenoceptors, eliciting vasoconstriction in most organs of the body such as the skin because of stimulation of alpha-adrenoceptors, but with the important exception of the skeletal muscle, where the blood vessels relax because of stimulation of beta-2 adrenoceptors. Stimulation of beta-adrenoceptors tends to decrease the total peripheral resistance to blood flow and potently increases the force and rate of the heartbeat. The amount of blood pumped by the heart per minute (cardiac output) increases, and so does the blood pressure when the heart is contracting (systolic blood pressure).

There are three types of beta-adrenoceptors: beta-1, beta-2, and beta-3.

The human heart contains abundant beta-1 and beta-2 adrenoceptors; stimulation of these receptors produces about the same cardiac effects. In contrast, skeletal muscle blood vessels contain mainly beta-2 adrenoceptors. This difference may be relevant to the mechanism of neurocardiogenic syncope, as explained below.

Beta-adrenoceptor blockers decrease the pulse rate, the force of heart contraction, and the systolic blood pressure. In patients with postural tachycardia syndrome (POTS), the value of treatment with beta-adrenoceptor blockers depends on whether the rapid pulse rate when the patient stands up reflects a primary abnormality or a compensatory response. If the rapid pulse rate were a compensation for another problem, such as low blood volume due to bleeding, then blocking that compensation would not help the patient; but if the rapid pulse rate were the result of an inappropriate, excessive rate of sympathetic nerve traffic to the heart, then blocking the effects of the excessive nerve traffic would help the patient.

There are two types of beta-adrenoceptor blockers, selective and nonselective. Selective beta-adrenoceptor blockers block beta-1 adrenoceptors, and nonselective beta-adrenoceptor blockers block both beta-1 adrenoceptors and beta-2 adrenoceptors. A potentially important difference between these drugs is that nonselective beta-adrenoceptor blockers block the beta-2 adrenoceptors in blood vessel walls of skeletal muscle, whereas beta-1 adrenoceptor blockers do not. In patients with neurocardiogenic syncope and high levels of epinephrine in the bloodstream, the epinephrine might stimulate beta-2 adrenoceptors on blood vessels in skeletal muscle. This would relax the blood vessels, decreasing the resistance to blood flow. This in turn could shunt blood away from the brain and toward the limbs, contributing to lightheadedness or loss of consciousness. In such patients, nonselective beta-adrenoceptor blockers might be preferable to selective blockers.

Midodrine (Proamatine)

Midodrine (Proamatine) is a relatively new drug that constricts blood vessels throughout the body by stimulating alpha-adrenoceptors in blood vessel walls. Midodrine acts like an artificial form of norepinephrine; it stimulates alpha-adrenoceptors directly. In patients with orthostatic hypotension due to a loss of sympathetic nerve terminals, so that there is little or no norepinephrine release, the alpha-adrenoceptors in the blood vessel walls accumulate on the cell surface, and the blood vessels become supersensitive. In this setting, midodrine can be very effective in raising the blood pressure. Stimulation of alpha-adrenoceptors can worsen symptoms of prostate problems in elderly men. Alpha-1 adrenoceptor blockers are effective in treating benign prostatic hypertrophy (BPH), and alpha-1 adrenoceptor blockers interfere with the actions of midodrine.

Clonidine

Clonidine stimulates alpha-2 adrenoceptors in the brain, which decreases the rate of sympathetic nerve traffic, and stimulates alpha-2 adrenoceptors on sympathetic nerve terminals, which decreases the amount of release of norepinephrine for a given amount of sympathetic nerve traffic. Therefore, even though clonidine stimulates a type of alpha-adrenoceptor, clonidine normally decreases blood pressure. There are several uses of clonidine in the diagnosis and treatment of dysautonomias. In the clonidine suppression test, discussed in chapter 9, the drug is used to differentiate high blood pressure due to increased sympathetic nervous system activity from high blood pressure due to a pheochromocytoma tumor that produces norepinephrine and adrenaline. In patients with long-term high blood pressure caused by excessive release of norepinephrine from sympathetic nerve terminals (hypernoradrenergic hypertension), clonidine can be very effective in lowering the blood pressure. It is also effective in treating withdrawal from some addictive drugs. Clonidine usually causes drowsiness and often causes a dry mouth. Sedation often limits its use.

Yohimbine

Yohimbine acts in a mirror image fashion to clonidine. Yohimbine blocks alpha-2 adrenoceptors in the brain and on sympathetic nerves and therefore releases norepinephrine from sympathetic terminals. The released norepinephrine binds to alpha-1 adrenoceptors in blood vessel walls, causing the blood vessels to constrict and the blood pressure to increase. Even though yohimbine blocks alpha-2 adrenoceptors in blood vessel walls, the drug releases so much norepinephrine, and there are so many alpha-1 adrenoceptors in blood vessel walls, that normally yohimbine increases the blood pressure. In patients with chronic autonomic failure and an inability to regulate sympathetic nerve traffic to intact terminals, such as in the Shy-Drager syndrome, yohimbine releases norepinephrine from the terminals and effectively increases the blood pressure. In patients with neurocardiogenic syncope, yohimbine can prevent tilt-induced fainting. Yohimbine can cause trembling, paleness of the skin, goose bumps, hair standing out, an increase in salivation, and emotional changes. Oral yohimbine is approved as a prescription drug to treat impotence from erectile dysfunction in men. Yohimbine, in the form of yohimbe bark, can be purchased in health food stores.

Intravenous Saline

Inability to tolerate prolonged standing can result from low blood volume, excessive pooling of blood in the veins of the legs during standing, or exit of fluid from the blood vessels into the tissues during standing (extravasation). In these situations, infusion of physiological saline solution can temporarily improve the ability to tolerate standing up. This is also useful for diagnostic purposes. Some patients with chronic orthostatic intolerance benefit from intravenous saline infusion given repeatedly by way of a permanent intravenous catheter. Saline infusion temporarily increases blood volume.

Amphetamines

Amphetamines are chemicals that resemble the drug, dextro-amphetamine or d-amphetamine. Amphetamines are in a class of drugs called indirectly acting sympathomimetic amines. They produce their effects at least partly by increasing delivery of norepinephrine to its receptors, both inside and outside the brain. By way of effects in the brain, amphetamines increase the state of arousal and attention, prevent or reverse fatigue, decrease appetite, and at high doses increase the rate and depth of breathing. By way of effects on the sympathetic nervous system, they increase the blood pressure.

Pseudephedrine (Sudafed) is structurally a mirror image (stereoisomer) of ephedrine. This difference changes the properties of the drug, producing much less central nervous system stimulation. By releasing norepinephrine from sympathetic nerve terminals in the mucous membranes of the nasal airways, pseudephedrine tightens blood vessels, making them less leaky and thereby relieving nasal congestion. Methylphenidate (Ritalin), another sympathomimetic amine, is used commonly to treat attention-deficit hyperactivity disorder. Phenylpropanolamine (PPE), until relatively recently, was used in over-the-counter diet pills until the discovery of serious adverse effects such as severe high blood pressure and stroke. Phentermine prescribed with fenfluramine (Phen-Fen) was an effective combination to decrease weight, until serious adverse effects of this combination came to light.

In treating patients with dysautonomias, amphetamines should be used sparingly, because of the potential for tolerance, dependence, and abuse. In patients with sympathetic neurocirculatory failure from abnormal regulation of sympathetic nerve traffic to intact sympathetic nerve terminals, this type of drug releases norepinephrine from the terminals and increases the blood pressure. Some patients with chronic orthostatic intolerance, such as neurocardiogenic syncope, can improve during treatment with an amphetamine.

Selective Serotonin Reuptake Inhibitors (SSRIs)

SSRIs inhibit a key process required for inactivating and recycling the chemical messenger, serotonin. The process is reuptake of released serotonin back into the nerve terminals that store it. SSRIs are widely used to treat depression, anxiety, and other psychiatric or emotional problems. They have also been used to treat some forms of dysautonomia, with occasional beneficial results.

Erythropoietin (Procrit)

Erythropoietin is a hormone that is used as a drug (Procrit or Epogen). Erythropoietin is released into the bloodstream by the kidneys and stimulates the bone marrow to increase production of red blood cells. Erythropoietin is helpful to treat low red blood cell counts (anemia), such as in kidney failure. Patients with anemia look pale and feel tired. By mechanisms that remain incompletely understood, erythropoietin tends to increase the blood pressure. Some doctors prescribe erythropoietin to treat low blood pressure in patients with chronic fatigue syndrome who have a low red blood cell count.

L-Dihydroxyphenylserine (L-DOPS)

L-DOPS is an amino acid very closely related chemically to L-dihydroxyphenylalanine (Levodopa, L-DOPA), the drug used to treat Parkinson disease. Just as L-DOPA is converted to the catecholamine, dopamine, L-DOPS is converted to the closely related catecholamine, norepinephrine. L-DOPS can provide norepinephrine even in the absence of sympathetic nerve terminals. L-DOPS has promise to treat orthostatic hypotension, prevent fainting, and treat disorders involving decreased norepinephrine biosynthesis.

A problem with L-DOPS to treat orthostatic hypotension in patients with

Parkinson disease is that the patients often are treated with Sinemet. Sinemet is a combination of L-DOPA and carbidopa. The carbidopa in Sinemet interferes with the conversion of L-DOPS to norepinephrine. This would be expected to prevent or blunt the hoped-for increase in blood pressure by L-DOPS treatment.

Bethanechol (Urecholine)

Bethanechol stimulates muscarinic receptors for acetylcholine, the chemical messenger of the parasympathetic nervous system. Urecholine is a brand name for bethanechol. The drug increases production of saliva, increases gut activity, and increases urinary bladder tone. Bethanechol may be useful to treat urinary retention or constipation in patients with chronic autonomic failure, but no formal study of this has been reported yet.

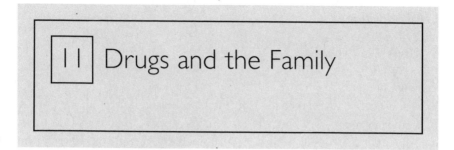

Catecholamines as Drugs

All three members of the adrenaline family are powerful drugs. Adrenaline itself is the most potent. In current algorithms of the American Heart Association for Advanced Cardiac Life Support (ACLS), adrenaline is the drug of first choice for sudden death from asystole, when the heart goes "flatline." No other drug has such an ability to restore the electrical activity of the heart. The most common cause of sudden cardiac death is ventricular fibrillation, in which the heart muscle fibers begin to contract independently of each other. The heart becomes a "can of worms" and stops pumping blood. For ventricular fibrillation, delivering an electrical shock can restore heart rhythm. This is why busy areas like elevator lobbies and airport terminals increasingly prominently display automatic electrical defibrillators (AEDs). When electrical shock has failed three times to reinitiate heart rhythm, the ACLS protocol calls for adrenaline injection, followed by further attempts at electrical defibrillation. Adrenaline plays a role in other ACLS algorithms, such as for pulseless electrical activity, where the electrocardiogram shows a heart rhythm but the heartbeat is too weak to generate a pulse, and for complete heart block, where the electrical activity fails to follow the proper sequence from the atria to the ventricles, and the ventricles begin to beat at a low intrinsic rate. In other potentially life-threatening conditions, such as severe asthma attack, and anaphylactic shock after a bee sting, adrenaline injection can be lifesaving. For all these causes of sudden death, injection of adrenaline as a drug can be truly "biogenic."

Norepinephrine, the chemical messenger of the sympathetic nervous system, also is a clinically indicated drug, to constrict blood vessels and thereby raise the blood pressure of patients in shock. Dopamine acts in the kidneys to promote excretion of salt and water; dopamine infusion can alleviate congestive heart failure.

Legal Addictions

Chances are you are addicted to one or more drugs. Drinking coffee, smoking cigarettes, and drinking alcohol are all addictive behaviors because caffeine, nicotine, and ethyl alcohol are all addictive drugs. As you would expect, addictive drugs pass through the blood-brain barrier and act in the brain to alter mood, emotion, motivation, perception, memory, or alertness.

All addictive drugs also exert important effects, directly or indirectly, on catecholamine systems in the brain. This is part of the reason that for decades researchers have considered—and debated—whether these effects on catecholamine systems cause or contribute to addiction itself. For instance, drugs that produce a "high" tend to release dopamine in a particular pathway of the brain; the positive reinforcement produced by dopamine might motivate an individual to acquire the addictive behavior.

There is no such thing as an addictive drug that does not in some way also affect the autonomic nervous system—especially the adrenomedullary hormonal system and sympathetic nervous system, which use members of the adrenaline family as the main chemical messengers. This chapter presents some drugs whose effects on the functions of catecholamine systems help explain the drug effects, side effects, and toxicity.

Nicotine

Smoking cigarettes is harmful to health and doggedly addictive, at least partly because of the high nicotine content of cigarettes. It is by way of the release of adrenaline evoked by nicotine that the heart pounds and blood pressure and the work of the heart increase after smoking a cigarette. Sweating also increases, but the sweating probably results not from nicotine-evoked release of adrenaline as a hormone so much as from release of acetylcholine, the chemical messenger released from sympathetic nerves innervating sweat glands.

Once I collaborated in a study of adrenaline responses to cigarette smoking. In cigarette smokers, who by definition are addicted to nicotine, plasma adrenaline levels increased after the subjects smoked but by a disappointingly small amount. The question arose whether nonsmokers would have brisker adrenaline and cardiovascular responses to smoking a cigarette. The institution's ethical review board disallowed extending the study to nonsmokers, however, on the grounds that nonsmoker normal volunteers could become addicted to nicotine after smoking even a single cigarette.

The U.S. Food and Drug Administration has decided that Ariva, a brand of mint-flavored lozenges consisting of 60% compressed and powdered tobacco, is not a drug and can be sold without regulation or restriction over the counter. Because of an effective "gut-blood barrier" for adrenaline and other members of its small chemical family, swallowing adrenaline itself exerts no important effects in the body; however, the nicotine in Ariva bypasses the gut-blood barrier and enters the bloodstream. The nicotine in the bloodstream could easily evoke release of the body's own adrenaline from the adrenal glands and produce potentially harmful effects. Of particular concern would be patients with coronary heart disease, who might take Ariva to help quit cigarette smoking, the same behavior that spurred development of their disease in the first place.

Nicotine is a potent stimulator of the transmission of nerve impulses in ganglia of the autonomic nervous system. At low doses, nicotine stimulates ganglionic transmission; at high doses the drug does just the opposite and blocks ganglionic transmission. This finding of the early 1900s helped Henry Dale to delineate two types of effects of acetylcholine, nicotinic and muscarinic (the latter referring to muscarine, derived from a type of poisonous mushroom). These discoveries about chemical mechanisms of nerve impulse transmission led to knighthood for Sir Henry in 1932 and a Nobel Prize in 1936.

Several years ago, my brother, to celebrate the birth of his newborn daughter, offered me a cigar. My wife wouldn't let me smoke in the house, so I decided to walk around the block and smoke the cigar. I was puffing away, walking proudly with my hands clasped behind me and my chin in the air, looking like a rooster, when about half-way around the block, I came to the sudden realization that I was about to die. I had what in medicalese is called the "feeling of impending doom," which occurs in all situations associated with drastic release of adrenaline. I broke out in a sweat and noticed my heart pounding. I knew these were effects of nicotine, but even so I immediately sought a safe haven. By the time I reached home, I could do nothing but fling myself on the couch in our family room, where I lay prostrate until the nicotine effects wore off. This was a morbid reminder that nicotine stimulates the adrenal medulla to release catecholamines. I still find it hard to believe that the Thompson Cigar Co. has advertised the Macanudo Baron de Rothschild cigar as a "stress management tool."

Caffeine

As a coffee drinker, I am addicted to caffeine. Each year, on the Jewish fast day of Yom Kippur, that addiction becomes painfully obvious. I always develop a caffeine withdrawal headache. As far as I know, the bases for caffeine addiction, and of the headache brought on by caffeine withdrawal, remain unknown.

Caffeine, like nicotine, stimulates the adrenal gland to release adrenaline. Whereas in nicotine addicts, smoking a cigarette still increases adrenaline levels, in caffeine addicts drinking a cup of coffee does not increase adrenaline levels.

A chemical called caffeic acid constitutes a substantial component of coffee beans and coffee, whether decaffeinated or not. Caffeic acid is not related chemically to caffeine. Instead, it is a catechol. In the gut, bacteria convert caffeic acid to dihydrocaffeic acid, which also is a catechol. The plasma of coffee drinkers (as well as of drinkers of decaffeinated coffee) therefore contains extra catechols besides those made in the body normally. These can lead to erroneous values for levels of adrenaline measured in clinical laboratories. Whether caffeic acid or dihydrocaffeic acid exerts effects in the human body remains unknown. Because they are catechols, they should be broken down by the enzyme, catechol-O-methyltransferase (COMT), just as adrenaline and other catechols in the bloodstream are broken down. It is possible that competition between caffeic acid or dihydrocaffeic acid with dopamine for COMT might explain the unexpected finding from population studies that coffee drinkers have a decreased risk of developing Parkinson disease.

Alcohol

Ethyl alcohol ingestion produces a wealth of acute and chronic metabolic effects that are beyond the scope of this book. A few aspects do merit comment. One is "the shakes." This refers not to the acute effects of alcohol but to the withdrawal from it. Alcohol withdrawal features trembling, goose bumps, anxiety, a tendency to seizures, fast pulse rate, and increased blood pressure. These changes probably reflect adrenaline release. Consistent with this view, treatment with benzodiazepine sedatives, such as diazepam (Valium), which are known to attenuate plasma adrenaline responses to a variety of stressors; treatment with beta-adrenoceptor blockers, which antagonize adrenaline effects; and treatment with clonidine, which decreases

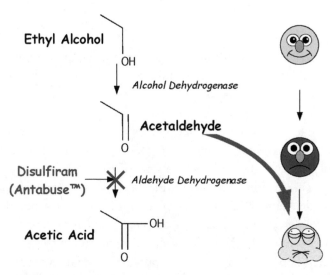

Fig. 45. Disulfiram (Antabuse) works by causing a buildup of a toxic chemical called acetaldehyde if the patient drinks alcohol.

sympathetic nervous system outflows, are all effective drugs in treating alcohol withdrawal.

Disulfiram (Antabuse) is used to prevent alcoholics from drinking by making them feel terrible afterward (fig. 45). Alcohol normally is broken down in the liver by an enzyme called alcohol dehydrogenase. In the process, an intermediate metabolite, acetaldehyde, is formed. Acetaldehyde is in turn broken down by another enzyme, called aldehyde dehydrogenase (sometimes called acetaldehyde dehydrogenase). Acetaldehyde is a noxious chemical. It produces flushing and headache, followed by pallor, sweating, fast pulse rate, anxiety, nausea, vomiting, and, in severe cases, shock. Disulfiram blocks aldehyde dehydrogenase. This means that if a patient taking disulfiram were to imbibe alcohol, acetaldehyde would build up rapidly in the bloodstream, and the patient would rapidly feel awful. By classical conditioning, described previously in this book, a person taking disulfiram could learn to associate even previously neutral cues, such as the smell in a tavern or the sound of ice tinkling in a glass (conditioned stimulus) with feeling terrible (unconditioned response), thereby motivating avoidance of situations that would lead to alcohol ingestion.

Cocaine

Cocaine rapidly enters the brain and produces a reinforcing and addictive "high." Outside the brain, cocaine has a local anesthetic effect. It also is a classic, potent inhibitor of uptake of norepinephrine by sympathetic nerves. You may recall that this process, uptake-1, involves movement of norepinephrine molecules from the outside nerve cells into the cells, by way of the cell membrane norepinephrine transporter (NET). The heart stands out among all organs of the body in terms of the extent of its dependence on uptake-1 for inactivating norepinephrine. Because cocaine blocks uptake-1, without concurrently inhibiting norepinephrine release, cocaine drastically increases delivery of norepinephrine to its receptors in the heart. This helps explain why people who die after cocaine administration die of heart problems, such as abnormal rhythms, heart attack, heart failure, or sudden cardiac death.

Other drugs besides cocaine block uptake-1. All tricyclic antidepressants, for instance, do this. Unlike cocaine, tricyclic antidepressants markedly decrease sympathetic nervous system outflows from the brain. This decreases the rate of release of norepinephrine from sympathetic nerves in the heart. The decrease in release is large enough that the rate of delivery of norepinephrine to its receptors in the heart is only increased statistically rather than massively as with cocaine.

Speed Kills

Catecholamines in the bloodstream do not enter the brain, because of the effective blood-brain barrier for these chemicals. Amphetamines do enter the brain (fig. 46).

Until relatively recently, doctors prescribed amphetamines for people who wanted to lose weight. The amphetamine, phentermine, was prescribed with fenfluramine and called Phen-Fen. The combination worked well but occasionally produced severe and sometimes fatal heart and lung problems, probably from the fenfluramine.

Countless entertainers and some politicians have taken amphetamines and become addicted to these drugs. Elvis Presley may have been the most well-known entertainer with amphetamine addiction. Dr. George Nichopoulos ("Dr. Nick"), Elvis's personal physician, prescribed large amounts of amphetamines for him until the rock star's death. The Tennessee Board of

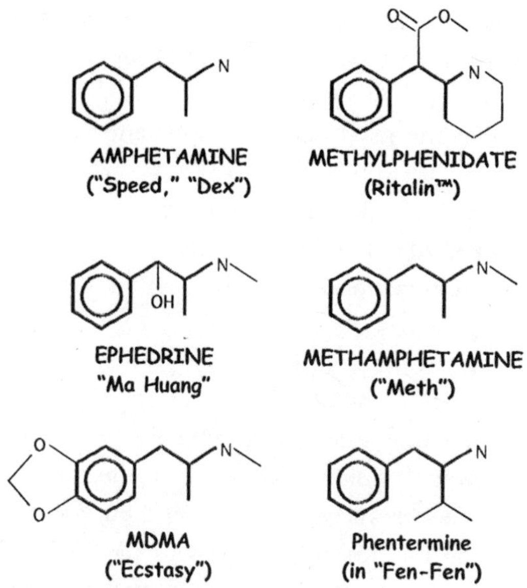

Fig. 46. Some amphetamines.

Medical Directors charged Dr. Nick with inappropriately prescribing more than 5,000 pills and vials for Elvis in the months before Elvis died and suspended Dr. Nick's medical license for three months. A jury subsequently acquitted him of malpractice or unethical conduct.

The country music singer Johnny Cash admitted many years of amphetamine abuse, before quitting in the late 1960s. In 1997 he became dizzy during a performance in Flint, Michigan, after bending down to retrieve a guitar pick. Shortly afterward, he was diagnosed with the Shy-Drager syndrome (multiple system atrophy with orthostatic hypotension). Cash was hospitalized many times for pneumonia, but, in general, he fared better than most patients with this disease do. Because amphetamines are toxic to central nervous system cells that produce catecholamines, one wonders whether chronic neurotoxic effects of amphetamines might have led to a disorder that mimicked the Shy-Drager syndrome.

Since World War II, military services have used amphetamine and methamphetamine as "awakening drugs." Indeed, as recently as the war against the Taliban in Afghanistan, U.S. fighter pilots flew combat missions under the influence of these drugs.

Inhabitants of Yemen and Africa have for centuries chewed Khat (also spelled qat, for Scrabble aficionados), from leaves of a shrub, *Catha edulis*.

The active ingredient is cathinone, which is converted by maturation and decomposition of the leaves to cathine, or d-norisoephedrine, an amphetamine.

Some people become psychotic on amphetamines. Possibly the most notorious example of this phenomenon was Peoples Temple leader Jim Jones, who convinced his followers in Guyana to commit mass suicide in 1978, the largest mass suicide in modern history. Animals allowed to self-inject methamphetamine without limit do so until it kills them.

Morphine

Morphine and chemically similar drugs are called opiates, because of the historical connection with opium, derived from the poppy plant. Opiates work by binding to specific receptors inside and outside the brain. Opiate receptors are quite distinct from receptors for catecholamines. In general, opiates produce sedation and anesthetic effects, whereas amphetamines do not. Withdrawal from amphetamines produces listlessness, depression, and increased appetite, whereas withdrawal from opiates produces tremor, anxiety, and loss of appetite.

Just as amphetamines work via effects on the body's catecholamine systems, opiates work via effects on the body's own opioid system. In essence, you make your own "morphine" in the form of enkephalins and endorphins, just as you make your own adrenaline. Both amphetamines and opiates produce a reinforcing positive feeling—euphoria—at least partly by releasing dopamine in a particular chemical pathway in the brain.

Barbs and Benzos

Barbiturates (Barbs) and benzodiazepines (Benzos) are classic "downer" drugs, which alleviate anxiety but also decrease vigilance. Benzodiazepines are used clinically to treat anxiety disorder, induce sedation, relieve muscle spasm, reverse certain types of seizures, and alleviate symptoms of alcohol withdrawal. Some of the more common brand names are Valium, Xanax, Klonopin, Librium, Ativan, and Halcion.

Barbiturates are used rather uncommonly clinically today, because they have a smaller margin of safety than do benzodiazepines and have attained more notoriety as drugs of abuse. Their street names often go by their pill colors, "blue devils" for amobarbital, "yellow jackets" for pentobarbital, "purple hearts" for phenobarbital, "red devils" for secobarbital, and "rainbows" or "reds and blues" for tuinal.

Both types of drugs depress respiration and the level of consciousness, but benzodiazepines taken alone are rarely fatal, in contrast with barbiturates, where even a small overdose can cause respiratory arrest. Both types of drugs are thought to work by promoting effects of gamma-aminobutyric acid (GABA), a major inhibitory neurotransmitter in the brain. In general, these drugs produce a calming effect, rather than the euphoria typical of cocaine, amphetamines, and opiates. They tend to decrease, rather than increase, release of dopamine in the dopamine pathway thought to underlie positively reinforcing feelings. They also blunt norepinephrine release in multiple brain centers during exposure to different stressors. Outside the brain, both types of drug attenuate adrenaline responses to a variety of experimental perturbations, such as to drugs that deprive cells of glucose.

When barbiturates are administered in the usual therapeutic doses for clinical indications, addiction does not occur, even though the patients may take the drugs for many months. On the other hand, taking large amounts of barbiturates for long periods can result in true addiction, where abrupt withdrawal produces seizures, high core temperature, and delirium.

Benzodiazepines produce a well-known amnesic effect. I did a study years ago about effects of Valium treatment on responses of healthy people to wisdom tooth extractions. At the time of the surgery, the subjects seemed to experience discomfort, as judged by body readjustments and sometimes moaning. Nevertheless, upon recovery they did not recall having experienced pain or distress during the surgery. During the surgery, which in subjects treated only with local anesthetic caused about a tripling of plasma adrenaline levels, in subjects treated with Valium adrenaline levels did not increase at all. According to the characterization in chapter 6 about distress, if the patients had no adrenaline response to the surgery, then they would not have experienced distress.

You Aren't What You Eat, Luckily

Ma Huang

The Chinese herb, *ma huang*, is a naturally occurring form of ephedrine. Ephedrine is an amphetamine, in the same class of drugs as the "upper" street drug, "dex," or "speed." As such, ephedrine results in a variety of effects, including an increased sense of energy, an actual increase in the metabolic rate, an antifatigue effect, insomnia, increased vigilance, and loss of appetite.

Ma huang was a key active ingredient in Metabolife. Millions of jars of Metabolife have been sold in the United States as a dietary supplement to increase energy and lose weight. In 1990 the president and cofounder of Metabolife, Michael Ellis, pled guilty to a felony charge of illegally manufacturing and selling methamphetamine, which can be produced from *ma huang*.

In February 2003, a 23-year-old pitcher for the Baltimore Orioles, Steve Bechler, took Xenadrine RFA-1, the active ingredient of which is *ma huang*, to lose weight and help him get in shape during spring training in Florida. Soon afterward he complained of dizziness during practice, collapsed, and died within 24 hours. The Broward County medical examiner determined that Bechler had died as a direct effect of taking ephedrine. This aroused substantial media attention, and a panel of invited experts met to decide whether *ma huang* should be considered a drug rather than a dietary supplement. The U.S. FDA eventually forced *ma huang* off of "health" store shelves.

Drugs like *ma huang* work by increasing the delivery of norepinephrine (the chemical messenger of the sympathetic nervous system) to its receptors in the brain and cardiovascular system. Ordinarily, this results in a small increase in blood pressure. The increase in pressure is small, not because the drug is weak but because reflexes to regulate blood pressure are strong. Blood pressure is one of many "monitored variables" of the inner world, regulated by the brain. Normally, increased blood pressure exerts slight stretching of the walls in major arteries, including the carotid arteries that deliver blood to the brain. In the walls of the carotid arteries sit distortion receptors, called baroreceptors. The brain tracks the blood pressure from input by the baroreceptors about the amount of stretching in the walls of the arteries and heart. When the brain senses the increased stretching, it directs a powerful, rapid reflex, the baroreflex, which alters activities of several automatic systems, including the sympathetic nervous system, to decrease the rate and force of heart contraction and relax blood vessels. This effectively counters the initial disturbance.

Years ago I studied a patient who first came to medical attention because of a huge increase in blood pressure from taking *ma huang* tea. He had been noticing slowed movement, increased fatigue, decreased exercise tolerance, and lightheadedness that would come on after standing. He thought that taking *ma huang* tea would energize him and increase his sense of well-being.

Unfortunately, his symptoms were early manifestations of a neurodegenerative disease multiple system atrophy, or MSA. In MSA, because of loss of particular clusters of cells in the brainstem, the brain does not respond to the information delivered to it by the baroreceptors. This prevents the patient from "buffering" changes in blood pressure. Soon after the patient drank the *ma huang* tea, he developed a terrible headache and pain and stiffness in the back of his neck, coupled with a paroxysm of high blood pressure. This combination led the doctor in the emergency room to diagnose a form of stroke from hemorrhage in the brain that carries with it a high risk of death.

Yohimbe Bark

"Dietary supplements" are supposed to improve functions of the body or mind or increase resilience to stress, without causing harm. One such dietary supplement is yohimbe bark. Behind my desk, a container of yohimbe bark sits right next to a small jar of the chemical, yohimbine, the active ingredient in yohimbe bark. The label on the container of yohimbe bark does not mention the potentially adverse health consequences of ingesting the contents. The label on the jar of yohimbine, however, displays a skull and crossbones, because the powder inside is poisonous.

Yohimbe bark is sold to increase the sense of energy or vitality or improve mood. It also has been used as an aphrodisiac. Yohimbine administration can cause spontaneous penile erection in men, and yohimbine received approval by the U.S. Food and Drug Administration as a prescription drug for impotence, long before the introduction of Viagra and related drugs.

Yohimbine releases norepinephrine from sympathetic nerves. In the heart, norepinephrine is inactivated mainly by recycling, by reuptake back into the nerves. Any of a group of effective antidepressant drugs, called tricyclics, block norepinephrine reuptake, both inside and outside the brain. Predictably, whereas yohimbine ordinarily produces relatively small increases in blood pressure, in a person taking a tricyclic yohimbine evokes dangerously high blood pressure. I could envision a scenario in which a man with chronic high blood pressure (hypertension) becomes impotent—a common and poorly understood side effect of medication to lower blood pressure. This would make him depressed. His doctor would prescribe a tricyclic, to help lift the patient's mood, and also prescribe yohimbine, to help "lift" the patient's relevant organ. The treatment combination could precipitate a stroke or even sudden cardiac death.

Adrenal Extract

In the window alcove behind my desk, an ampule of adrenaline solution for injection sits next to a jar of "Adrenal Support" tablets, which I bought at a health store as a dietary supplement. The tablets contain an extract of adrenal gland, defatted so as not to contain steroids. When you swallow an Adrenal Support tablet, you ingest a mixture of chemicals, and a major one is adrenaline.

Why isn't ingesting adrenal gland extract dangerous? To answer this question requires thinking in terms of "Darwinian medicine." Darwinian medicine views body functions and diseases in the context of evolution. We humans are omnivorous. We eat "mountain oysters" (testes), heart, tongue, "sweetbreads" (a euphemism for the pancreas or thyroid of a young animal, soaked and then fried), feet, kidney pie, pig tripe, oxtail, and kishka (stuffed intestine). When our family toured Beijing a few years ago, we visited a restaurant that featured soup made from the freshly drained blood and bile of a snake slit live before the diners' eyes. To our ancestors, the adrenal gland would be an edible morsel embedded in the fat at the top of the kidney. We omnivores have been eating adrenal glands for millions of years. We have been able to do so without killing ourselves because of the evolution of multiple enzymes in the wall of the gastrointestinal tract and in the liver that form a virtually impenetrable "gut-blood barrier" for catecholamines. These enzymes remain important to this day, not only to detoxify ingested adrenaline but probably also to prevent numerous other poisons from reaching the bloodstream. A variety of effective drugs in modern medicine, psychiatry, and neurology, however, work by blocking the activity of one or more of these enzymes. If you were on one of these drugs, you probably could harm or kill yourself by taking Adrenal Support.

12 | The Future
Scientific Integrative Medicine

In this book you have learned a lexicon for the political science of the inner world. You have come across many new words and phrases—effectors, homeostats, allostatic load, monitored variable, dysautonomias—and new perspectives about old ones—negative feedback, the autonomic nervous system, stress, distress, fight-or-flight, and, of course, adrenaline. I have used these words and phrases to teach you about the "wisdom of the body," as Walter B. Cannon beautifully phrased it. This last chapter relies on this vocabulary to introduce what I consider to be no less than the future of medical science and practice: scientific integrative medicine.

With completion of the human genome project, medical science faces a unique and novel challenge. Now we have access to a huge fund of genetic information and to sophisticated, powerful, computerized means to assemble and analyze that information. For developmental diseases of specific, isolated body processes, abnormalities of genes or the proteins coded by them might suffice to trace the pathophysiological pathways from cause to disease. But disease has changed, even as genetic information–gathering accomplishments have accumulated. Chronic, complex, degenerative disorders, involving derangements of multiple body processes, multiple drug treatments, and myriad interactions among those processes and the drugs used to treat them, have come to the fore. A key challenge for medical science lies in understanding how genetic changes already present at birth interact with individual life experiences and time, to lead to chronic, multisystem disorders decades later, at the other side of life.

An "integrative" approach seems required for this understanding. But what does "integrative" mean? In popular parlance, the word is used interchangeably with "holistic," "complementary," or "alternative." This chapter offers a different point of view by emphasizing the *scientific* in scientific integrative medicine. What renders scientific integrative medicine new, different, and powerful is the focus on disorders of the multiple, interacting, feedback-controlled systems that regulate the monitored variables of the body. This is more than systems physiology with another name. Scientific integrative medicine recognizes that the operating characteristics of internal systems change over time, based on numerous life exposures and experiences that range from carrying out genetic instructions (especially in fetal development through adolescence) to aging-related degenerative disorders and interactions between medications and those disorders.

Rather than "complementary" or "alternative," scientific integrative medicine is entirely mainstream. Expert clinicians apply principles of scientific integrative medicine continually and seemingly intuitively in diagnosing and treating complex diseases; however, as in any professional endeavor, ostensible effortlessness usually reflects diligent learning and long years of practice and experience. Scientific integrative medicine provides a framework for understanding what renders a clinician astute.

Return of the Getaway Car

In the analogy about the getaway car in front of the bank (in chapter 3), the car is kept idling at the curb, because you would use it when you must get away—fast. For the same reason that you would keep a getaway car in idle, the brain keeps chemical messenger systems in idle. You have to be able to release those chemicals rapidly when needed. It is no coincidence that in Parkinson disease, a neurodegenerative disease resulting from loss of the catecholamine, dopamine, in a particular brain pathway, a key manifestation is the inability to initiate movement or move quickly.

Keeping a car's engine idling eventually leads to wear and tear because of ongoing fuel combustion, which results in a buildup of harmful waste products. Keeping catecholamine systems in idle all the time eventually leads to wear and tear on those systems because of ongoing metabolic combustion of the catecholamines themselves, which results in formation of a variety of toxic metabolites.

Like all cars, getaway cars have obsolescence built in. Manufacturers don't make cars to last forever but to last long enough to convince you to buy again from the same manufacturer. Your body also has obsolescence built in, because the purpose of human bodies is not for them to last forever but to protect and propagate genes.

A manufacturing flaw in the catalytic converter of the getaway car might accelerate the accumulation of "gunk" in the idling engine, to the point that the engine fails completely over time. A manufacturing defect in the body's catalytic converters—enzymes—due to genetic mutation or polymorphism, might also accelerate the accumulation of metabolic "gunk" in the idling cells, to the point that the cells malfunction or die. Contamination of the fuel in the getaway car also could accelerate accumulation of "gunk" in the idling engine. Analogously, exposure to environmental agents, dietary factors, or medications might accelerate the accumulation of "gunk" in cells producing chemical messengers.

Is there any evidence that a chronic disease actually can develop from accumulation of metabolic "gunk" in cells? An example of such a phenomenon may be in Parkinson disease. The movement problems in Parkinson disease result from loss of dopamine cells in the nigrostriatal pathway of the brain. Patients with Parkinson disease usually also have evidence for a loss of norepinephrine cells in the sympathetic nervous system supply to the heart. In the diseased tissue, in the nigrostriatal system of the brain, the pathological hallmark of Parkinson disease is the presence of Lewy bodies. These are clumps of material in the cells that haven't completely disappeared yet. Lewy bodies are also seen outside the brain in patients with Parkinson disease, including in the ganglia, the sites of origin of the sympathetic nerves to organs such as the heart.

Lewy bodies contain high concentrations of a protein called alpha-synuclein. In patients with inherited Parkinson disease from mutation of the alpha-synuclein gene, you might think of alpha-synuclein deposits as analogous to an error in the formulation of the engine oil. In patients with inherited Parkinson disease from replicate copies of the normal alpha-synuclein gene, alpha-synuclein deposits would be analogous to engine oil that is formulated correctly but is too concentrated. Either way, cellular gunk could build up in the engine of the getaway car.

Parkinson disease is an ailment mainly of the elderly. Over time, a combination of abnormalities eventually kill catecholamine cells. There might be a faulty catalytic converter. Metabolic breakdown of dopamine results in formation of toxic by-products, which in turn normally are detoxified by enzymes. If the detoxifying enzymes malfunctioned, the toxic by-products would accumulate. A faulty catalytic converter might not process by-products quickly enough, corresponding to decreased processing of proteins by "proteosomes" in nerve cells. There might be "over-revving," corresponding to excessive turnover of catecholamines, such as by decreased efficiency of recycling via cell membrane or vesicular transporters. There might be a deviation in the oil, such as a tendency to break down at high temperature, corresponding to a hyperfunctional polymorphism of the alpha-synuclein gene. The fuel might contain a contaminant, corresponding to a harmful environmental agent such as a pesticide or a toxin converted to a harmful biochemical in the body. There might even be misprogrammed "planned obsolescence," corresponding to accelerated aging of nerve cells in general. These processes, especially if combined and operating over decades, could build up "gunk," represented by the Lewy bodies seen in the catecholamine cells of patients with Parkinson disease (fig. 47).

Allostatic Load for People Who Hate Snakes

Anyone who has had a bad cold with a low-grade fever for a few days knows from personal experience what allostasis is. Your core temperature is regulated at a higher level, your pulse rate increases, you lose your appetite, you curl up in bed, and you sleep more. You withdraw socially and become more irritable. You are "not yourself."

When you have an acute illness like this, the monitored variables of the inner world do not change in a completely uncontrolled way. For instance, your core temperature is regulated; but the virus somehow resets the thermostat. Once you recover and are back to your "old self," all the homeostatic settings return to those before the acute illness, with no damage done.

Now you are older, and you come down with the same illness. The low-grade fever and other symptoms and signs don't resolve so quickly. Maybe they persist or worsen over weeks or months. You could become enfeebled, bedridden, emaciated, disabled, disheveled, and disheartened (in the biblical sense discussed in chapter 3). You undergo blood tests, scans, biopsies, hospitalizations, surgeries, treatments, complications, and rehabilitation. Eventually you recover. But do you recover fully? Possibly not, and if not, the incomplete recovery would reflect effects of allostatic load.

As you have learned, *allostatic load* refers to effects of prolonged activation of effectors involved in allostasis. In the analogy to the HVAC system (see chapter 1), leaving a window or door open for several months would increase allostatic load on all the HVAC system components. Several clinical states can be understood by progressively accumulating allostatic load.

Allostatic load links stress with degenerative diseases. Activation of effectors to counter threats to homeostasis produces wear and tear on the organs determining the level of the monitored variable and on the effectors them-

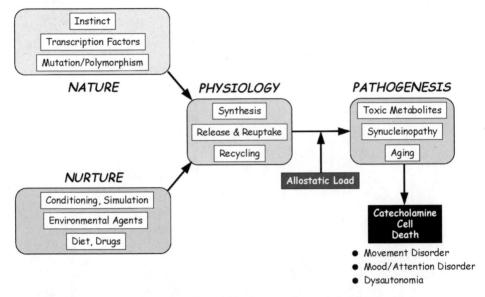

Fig. 47. Parkinson disease may reflect harmful long-term effects of allostatic load because of interactions among genetic makeup ("nature"), life experience ("nurture"), and time.

selves. Wear and tear, combined with planned obsolescence, decreases effector efficiency. The same perturbation then results in greater wear and tear and further decreases effector efficiency. Eventually, even with the effectors activated continuously, the monitored variable drifts from the allostatic setting. Finally, when the effectors fail, the organism can no longer mount a stress response at all.

One thing that has convinced me that allostasis and allostatic load are scientific concepts is the ability to create kinetic models, from which one can predict effects of various manipulations on levels of monitored variables and test the predictions experimentally. Remember that such an ability distinguishes an idea as scientific. In the homeostatic model of stress, adjusting the setting of the homeostat leads to maintenance of the monitored variable at a different steady-state value—an "other sameness." In your home, adjusting the thermostat setting changes the steady-state temperature, and adjusting the humidistat setting changes the steady-state humidity. These adjustments correspond to allostasis. By analogy, in your body, fever when you are sick is part of an "other sameness"; the temperature increases to a new steady-state level. Other examples of allostasis in the inner world or the body would be the increase in blood coagulability after

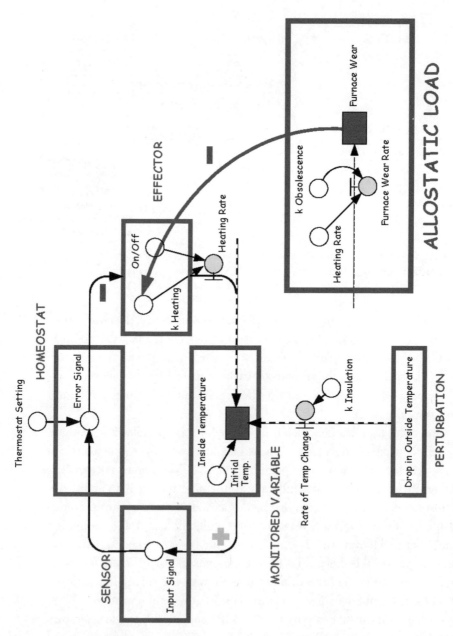

Fig. 48. A kinetic model of allostatic load.

major trauma and the increase in the blood glucose level in shock. Over the eons, temporary adjustments such as these in homeostatic settings have provided long-term survival advantages, explaining why they evolved. In a kinetic model of a homeostatic system altering the setting, or set point, for responding, always changes the steady-state level of the monitored variable.

Modern computer-modeling packages enable you to put together a complex kinetic model without knowing higher mathematics (fig. 48). The underlying calculus is almost invisible. You can put together a workable model without encountering any integration signs—my mentor, Irv Kopin, a whiz at calculus, used to call them "snakes." If you hate, fear, or panic instinctively at the sight of the snakes of integrative calculus, you can still learn to use an icon-based computer application for kinetic modeling. You place icons on the computer screen, draw lines connecting the icons, and sprinkle in some numbers. The "input" into the model can be from a "cloud" and the output also to a "cloud," yet you can generate quantitative predictions to test your idea.

Such a model can predict allostatic load. In the analogy of the home HVAC system, allostatic load would correspond to "wear and tear" on the effectors. The rate of wear and tear on each effector would depend on intrinsic factors (e.g., variability within manufacturing specifications, planned obsolescence, deterioration with time) and extrinsic factors (e.g., duration of time on, number of times cycled on and off, environmental exposures). Sophisticated systems might even incorporate self-monitoring and self-repair mechanisms or preventive maintenance procedures.

Eventually, HVAC systems break down, are replaced, or are eliminated as part of demolition of the building. A key way HVAC systems break down is by development of positive feedback loops. Wear and tear eventually decreases the efficiency with which the effector does its job. A gasket leaks from a crack in the rubber, causing more activation of the boiler, which accelerates degeneration of the gaskets, and eventually the pressure head of steam decreases. Deposits build up in the pipes, and laminar flow changes to turbulent flow, which accelerates the buildup of deposits, and eventually the pipes don't transport the steam. Electrical insulation frays, and eventually short circuits shut down the control system.

In patients with chronic diseases of almost any sort, the inner world breaks down eventually; a key way this happens is also by development of positive feedback loops. Heart failure stimulates the sympathetic nervous system and renin-angiotensin-aldosterone system, which increases fluid retention, growth of heart muscle, and the work of the heart, worsening the heart failure. Chest pain from coronary ischemia evokes distress, stimulating the adrenomedullary hormonal system and increasing the rate of consumption of oxygen by the heart, worsening the ischemia. Orthostatic hypotension from failure of the sympathetic nervous system causes lightheadedness, a fall, fracture of a hip, and prolonged bed rest in traction, worsening the orthostatic hypotension when the patient tries to get up. A footballer practicing in full uniform in the heat releases adrenaline, which constricts skin blood vessels and augments heat production in the body, producing heat exhaustion, which releases more adrenaline, bringing on heat shock and death. Loss of dopamine terminals in the nigrostriatal system in the brain increases pathway traffic to the remaining terminals, accelerating dopamine turnover and thereby production of toxic by-products of dopamine metabolism, increasing the rate of loss of dopamine terminals, eventually manifesting clinically as Parkinson disease.

The timing and rapidity of system failure from positive feedback loops depend on dynamic interactions between usage experience of the system and built-in manufacturing and design characteristics. Analogously, in the body, the occurrence, timing, and rapidity of progression of degenerative diseases would depend on interactions between environmental exposures and genetic predispositions. The kinetic model of allostasis and allostatic load provides a nice framework for linking stress, distress, allostatic load, and degenerative diseases.

The Dialectic

The past three decades have witnessed the remarkable ascendance of molecular biology and molecular genetics, outdistancing integrative physiology in the perennial competition for money and programmatic priorities in biomedical research. Yet according to Sir James Black, who shared the Nobel Prize for Physiology or Medicine in 1988, the future will see "the progressive triumph of physiology over molecular biology."

This struggle continues an ancient dispute about what medical scientific knowledge is and about how one should go about acquiring it. The resolution will not be victory for either side but merging of the two disciplines into a new one—I call it "scientific integrative medicine." More about that later; first let us analyze the strengths and weaknesses of molecular and integrative approaches, considered separately, in explaining diseases.

Table 4. Molecular and homeostatist approaches to causes and treatments of diseases

Molecular	Homeostatist
Regressive	Emergent
Linear schema	Circular schema
Serial	Parallel
Etiology	Pathogenesis
Mutation model for cause	Evolutionary model for cause
Gene therapy	Organismic treatment
Computer-aided design	Chess computer algorithm
No "goals"	Apparent purposefulness

Molecular medical science uses a stepwise, regressive, essentially linear approach to acquire knowledge about causes of disease (table 4). One identifies the proximate preceding step, then the next proximate step, and so on, in a seemingly never-ending quest to identify "first causes" of clinical phenomena. Suppose a disease has several "causes," and suppose that for the most common ones, feedback loops, modulators, and parallel pathways complicate the picture. By using molecular genetic approaches, the exact mutation associated with a rare inherited form of the disease could be identified. The search for the rare mutant gene might not only lead to identification of a first cause but also provide information about the other more complex, more common pathways.

Moreover, one might presume that, after identification of a defective gene, reversal of the steps in the discovery process might "explain" the disease. This is a key presumption based on a reductionist approach. Even if all patients with a particular disease shared the same mutation, however, this would not imply that all people with the mutation would develop the disease—exactly because of the multiple feedback loops, modulators, and parallel pathways that characterize living organisms. The mutation might lead to the disease only in the setting of another mutation, or dysfunction of a membrane ion channel, or a deformed cell structure, or failure of an organ. Until very recently, most molecular science research used a linear schema, ignoring central determinants of release of effector compounds and the consequences of cellular activation on those determinants.

With mutation, the etiological trail seems to end. The trail begins with the clinical findings, various intermediate neurochemical or enzymatic changes follow, and at the end of the trail lies the seeming first cause, the genetic defect. Of course, the medical scientific quest about how a genetic defect actually causes a clinical disease—the pathophysiological trail—only begins here, and even the etiological trail only appears to end with the identification of a mutation, because this still leaves unanswered why the mutation occurred where and when it did and why it escaped detection and correction.

The lack of a word to describe the conceptual foundation of integrative physiology has led to the proposition of a neologism: "homeostatism." Homeostatism uses a feedback-dependent (i.e., circular) approach to the apparent steady states that characterize all living things. The "circular schema" refer to loops, where afferent information about levels of monitored variables leads to centrally regulated alterations in activities of parallel effector systems.

The central idea of homeostatism is that organisms maintain their internal environment by the operation in parallel of adaptive, feedback-regulated systems. Via negative feedback regulation, comparator "homeostats," and multiple effectors, adult organisms maintain levels of monitored variables within prespecified ranges. According to the homeostatic concept, growth, senescence, disease, and, ultimately, organismic death result from instability introduced by positive feedback loops—upward and downward spirals rather than circles—leading to new apparent steady states.

A strength of the homeostatic model lies in predicting the emergence of complex phenomena, based on processes such as compensatory activation of alternative effectors, effector sharing, and homeostat resetting. The emergent phenomena can include shifts among apparent steady states, evocable even from near-random perturbations. This not only helps to explain phenomena that one might otherwise find impossible to comprehend but also can lead to otherwise underivable mechanistic hypotheses. A weakness of the model is its essential circularity, with few or no simple causal chains or cascades. The model in pure form does not incorporate the genetic determinants of the functions at each station of homeostatic systems.

Let us compare the molecular and homeostatist approaches to the causes—and treatments—of a particular disease. One cause of neurodegeneration that leads to premature death in childhood is phenylketonuria (PKU). In most cases, PKU results from lack of activity of the enzyme phenylalanine hydroxylase, producing a toxic buildup of phenylalanine. Thus, a low phenylalanine diet, begun early enough after birth, normalizes

THE FUTURE: SCIENTIFIC INTEGRATIVE MEDICINE 257

neurobehavioral development in PKU, effectively treating if not curing the disease. Some babies have an atypical form of PKU, which a low phenylalanine diet alone does not ameliorate. The patients not only have a buildup of phenylalanine but also have decreased synthesis of major neurotransmitters including catecholamines and serotonin. What causes this combination? One cause is decreased ability to hydroxylate not only phenylalanine but also tyrosine, the precursor of catecholamines, and tryptophan, the precursor of serotonin. What causes the decreased hydroxylation? One cause is absence of tetrahydrobiopterin (BH_4), a required cofactor for the hydroxylating enzymes. What causes deficiency of BH_4? One cause is mutation of the gene encoding dihydropteridine reductase (DHPR), which catalyzes the conversion of dihydrobiopterin to BH_4. Here then would be a first cause, an etiology, of at least one pediatric neurodegenerative disease.

A homeostatic explanation for the same disease might focus more on the pathophysiological changes that lead to the disease as actually manifested clinically. There are alternative pathways for generating BH_4 independent of DHPR. No amount of analysis of mutations of the DHPR gene itself could lead to the hypothesis of an alternative biosynthetic pathway for generating BH_4 to explain the actual clinical findings in the patients. That would require homeostatic thinking based on informative neurochemistry.

A gene therapy advocate might take the extreme position of asking, "Why not leapfrog directly from the genetic abnormality to gene therapy, which has the potential to cure?" Thus, for DHPR deficiency, the direct approach would bypass enzymatic and neurochemical abnormalities and focus on identifying the genetic mutation, replacing the defective gene, or setting up a factory to provide the missing protein encoded by the gene, thereby curing the disease. This seems straightforward, but so far at least, it has not worked in practice. In fact, Dr. Seymour Kaufman, the NIH scientist who discovered DHPR deficiency, wrote a letter to the Editor of the *Washington Post* in 1995, to comment on an article about how genes work:

> The article . . . did, however, contain a serious factual error that feeds into the unwarranted assumption that has been repeated so often that it is now axiomatic: The identification of an affected gene (or genes) in a disease will automatically lead to an effective treatment for that disease.
>
> In fact, there are few, if any, examples where this has proven to be true. PKU . . . is a case in point . . . the article states that "after geneticists understood the problem at the molecular level, they realized that modifying diet prevented the disease."

This chronology is incorrect! The dietary treatment for PKU . . . was introduced by Bickel in 1954, more than 30 years before it was known that mutations in the enzyme, phenylalanine hydroxylase, cause the disease.

As this bit of medical history illustrates, despite the power of molecular biology to clarify aspects of many diseases, it is not the only route to the development of effective treatments, even for genetic diseases.

To a homeostatist, the goal of treatment is to counter the pathophysiological mechanism of the disease. This also seems straightforward, and in the case of DHPR deficiency has worked, by using treatment with folinic acid, in conjunction with L-DOPA and 5-hydroxytryptophan, to maximize synthesis of neurotransmitters via the alternative pathway. We must remain skeptical, however, about the appropriateness of any mechanistic treatment, rational as that treatment might seem. This is because scientific integrative medicine attempts to explain diseases by a continuing process of formulating and testing pathophysiological theories, and theories can be proved false but never proved true. Because our understanding of mechanisms of diseases will always remain incomplete, there will always be a risk to employing rational treatments in attempting to reverse a pathophysiological mechanism. This is what actually happened to patients who underwent bloodletting, trephination, cupping, and purging in the course of medical history.

Some think that molecular genetics holds the key to future acquisition of medical knowledge, partly because of the potential to discover first causes of disease. The genotype is the disease, and pathogenetic mechanisms are secondary. This view, which ignores the myriad adaptive responses organisms express and depend on continuously in life, has arisen partly from the choice—so far—by molecular geneticists to study rare inherited diseases that seem to entail the least complexity necessitated by the multiple adaptive changes required for homeostasis. Thus, the finding that mice with genetic absence of dopamine-beta-hydroxylase die during fetal development, yet patients with absence of the same enzyme survive to adulthood, poses a problem. Others think that learning all the mechanistic pathways in a disease and predicting rational, beneficial treatments constitute all that one can learn from medical scientific research. The phenotype is the disease, and first causes lie within the province of metaphysics, not science. But during embryological development, postnatal growth, pubescence, and senescence, relatively long periods when steady states are not maintained, the genes may act fairly directly. So far, homeostatists have chosen for study complex common diseases involving "dysregulation," with mutations viewed as anomalies only distantly related to pathogenetic mechanisms.

The dialectic between molecular and integrative medicine is not new. Rather, it continues centuries-old, fundamental disputes about philosophies of science—reductionist vs. emergent, linear vs. circular, atomistic vs. organismic, phenomenological vs. purposive. Both types of concept explain phenomena in terms of relatively few basic principles, and both lead to hypotheses that observation or experimentation can test. Thus, both types of approach are scientific. Research in both traditions should continue, with the expectation that from the creative friction at their interface future breakthroughs will arise. According to Hegel's dialectic, thesis and antithesis result eventually in synthesis. These considerations lead to the hope and prediction that under the aegis of scientific integrative medicine, molecular geneticists will include feedback-regulated, interacting, adaptive systems that operate in parallel and consider not only direct genetic programming, analogous to computer-aided design, but also genetic "algorithms," analogous to the simulations encoded in a chess computer's software. Geneticists will recognize that humans depend on nervous, endocrine, and autocrine/paracrine systems to maintain apparent steady states—to keep us alive—since the time lags for transcriptional responses obviate direct genetic actions. Physiologists, in turn, will apply new genetic tools to examine the body's homeostatic systems and consider genetic constraints on the functioning of those systems.

Darwinian Medicine

You can buy overclocked computer equipment. Overclocking makes a computer's processor run faster than originally intended. This speeds up system performance and improves the sense of reality when you play a video game, at a fraction of the cost of a computer actually designed to handle so much information so quickly. Overclocking, however, also reduces the life span of the processor. The notion of increased immediate gains of overclocking, at the cost of reduced life span, provides a useful analogy for the development of chronic diseases in people. Diseases involving degeneration of multiple systems in the elderly may be a predictable consequence of the evolutionary advantages of physiological overclocking in the reproductive years.

Consider diseases of senescence. Aging-related increases in susceptibilities to cardiovascular, neurological, oncological, and immunological diseases have always limited our life span and always will. One may search for rare genetic mutations causing premature degeneration. Alternatively, however, one may recognize that our bodies have been designed to protect and propagate genes, not to live indefinitely. Accordingly, one may hypothesize that groups of genes bias toward accelerated neuronal loss in the elderly because they enhance protection and propagation of genes in the younger reproducers. Perhaps the same homeostatic systems that organisms rely on to counter acute threats early in life cause senescence by the accumulation of toxic by-products of the actions of those systems.

For instance, parkinsonism in the elderly appears to result from cumulative injury to dopamine cells over the years. In the young, enhanced release of dopamine might enable rapid initiation of locomotion or of other behaviors relevant to survival. Analogously, cardiovascular hypertrophy, and consequently susceptibility to stroke and heart failure in the elderly, could result from prolonged bombardment of adrenoceptors or continuous "reving" of vesicular engines, enhancing adaptive fight-or-flight responses in the young at the cost of chronic changes in cardiovascular architecture.

This genetic-evolutionary perspective also leads to therapeutic hypotheses. If chronic production and metabolic breakdown of dopamine led to toxic injury to the cells, then long-term decrease in that breakdown in individuals with a genetically determined high rate could prolong the average useful life of human nervous systems. Analogously, disconnecting genetically determined hyperreactivity of catecholamine systems from chronic cardiovascular hypertrophy could prolong the average useful life of human circulatory systems.

Darwin's Disease

Considering that scientific integrative medicine views chronic, multisystem disorders from an evolutionary point of view, it is ironic that for much of his life Charles Darwin himself suffered from a mysterious multisystem disease, which was never diagnosed during his life and which medical historians have argued about ever since.

From his autobiography one can glean few specific hints. Both Charles and his father, a highly successful physician but overbearing parent, abhorred the sight of blood. At his father's recommendation, Darwin began to study medicine, but he was sickened by dissection and by operations. Twice he rushed away from surgeries before they were completed, and the two cases "fairly haunted me for many a long year."

Before Darwin's famous voyage on the HMS *Beagle*, he spent two months at Plymouth, awaiting sailing weather: "I was out of spirits at the thought of leaving all my family and friends for so long a time, and the weather seemed to me inexpressibly gloomy. I was also troubled with palpitations and pain about the heart, and like many a young ignorant man, especially one with a smattering of medical knowledge, was convinced that I had heart-disease."

It seems Darwin had the insight to recognize that his symptoms resembled those of, but did not actually reflect, heart disease. According to his autobiography, while on the voyage and after his return to England in 1836, he had episodic "unwellness." He rarely specified his symptoms—remarkable given his well-known attention to detail. After his father died in 1847, Darwin neither attended the funeral nor acted as executor, due to being "out of health." *The Descent of Man*, which appeared in 1871, took three years for Darwin to write, some of this time lost by "ill health."

In the summer of 1842, when 33 years old, he took a tour by himself in northern Wales. This was the last time he felt strong enough to climb mountains or to take long walks. The same year, he moved with his family to Down House, in the countryside outside London, where he lived a largely reclusive existence for the rest of his life.

> During the first part of our residence we went a little into society, and received a few friends here; but my health almost always suffered from the excitement, violent shivering and vomiting attacks being thus brought on. . . . My chief enjoyment and sole employment throughout life has been scientific work; and the excitement from such work makes me for the time forget, or drives quite away, my daily discomfort.

Darwin did not seem to suffer loneliness or depression from this isolation. On the contrary, in a letter in 1835 to his sister during the voyage of the *Beagle*, seclusion seemed part of a life strategy: "I am convinced that it is a most ridiculous thing to go round the world, when by staying quietly, the world will go round with you."

Darwin depended on his wife for sympathy. She in turn cared for and commiserated with him: "I cannot tell you the compassion I have felt for all your suffering for these weeks past that you have had so many drawbacks. Nor the gratitude I have felt for the cheerful and affectionate looks you have given me when I know you have been miserably uncomfortable."

In sum then, we have someone with an early abhorrence of blood and operations, repeated bouts of trembling, palpitations, chest pain, vomiting, social withdrawal, frequent references to general lack of well-being, and dependence on a spouse for caretaking and sympathy. This constellation would seem to indicate a psychiatric disorder, such as panic/anxiety, with a component of social phobia; and this has been the interpretation of most medical historians on the subject.

According to a completely different interpretation, Darwin suffered from a chronic infectious disease, Chagas disease, contracted in Argentina during his voyage on the *Beagle*. Chagas disease is caused by a trypanosome parasite, *Triatoma infestans*, which could have been transmitted by the bite of an insect, as noted in Darwin's *Voyage of the Beagle:* "At night I experienced an attack (for it deserves no less a name) of the Benchuca, a species of *Reduvius*, the great black bug of the Pampas. It is most disgusting to feel soft wingless insects, about an inch long, crawling over one's body. Before sucking they are quite thin but afterwards they become round and bloated with blood."

In Central and South America, Chagas disease is also a cause of dysautonomia. The disease is associated with pathological changes not only of the cardiovascular and digestive systems but also the autonomic nervous systems, with a loss of autonomic nerves in the heart, probably from an autoimmune attack. The Chagas disease explanation would of course not account for Darwin's aversion to blood and operations in medical school, nor for his chest pain and palpitations before the *Beagle* set sail.

In 1848 and 1858, Darwin underwent "hydropathic" treatment, which temporarily made him feel better. Hydropathy, or the "water cure," consisted of treating diseases by internal and external use of copious amounts of pure water, especially at cold temperature. According to a biography by Desmond and Moore, "A third of his working life was spent doubled up, trembling, vomiting, and dousing himself in icy water."

What can be made of Darwin's temporary improvement by hydropathic treatment? Some patients with chronic orthostatic intolerance have what I call the "water bottle sign." They have learned that they feel better with frequent water ingestion, and they keep a water bottle with them. Others report temporary benefit from intravenous infusion of saline. Patients with postural tachycardia syndrome have multiple nonspecific complaints, including palpitations, trembling, atypical chest pain, chronic fatigue, inability to concentrate, abdominal bloating, and general debility. Moreover, recent studies have demonstrated that patients with dysautonomias can have substantial increases in blood pressure or improvements in orthostatic tolerance for up to a couple of hours after simply drinking 16 ounces of water. Finally, cold

THE FUTURE: SCIENTIFIC INTEGRATIVE MEDICINE   263

exposure markedly stimulates sympathetic nervous system outflows, which raises blood pressure temporarily. Perhaps there was a scientific basis for Darwin's improvement with hydropathic treatment, the net effects being increases in blood pressure and venous return to the heart and consequently increased cerebral blood flow.

The illness seems to have contained elements of both "mind" and "body"; however, proposed explanations usually have followed the dichotomous approach of Descartes, with medical historians weighing in about whether the disease was infectious or mental. The debate about the cause of Darwin's illness recalls the debate between Louis Pasteur and Claude Bernard about germs and intrinsic decomposition, about the "seed and the soil," as causes of disease. According to the germ theory, diseases would be due mainly to external threats to the well-being of the organism, such as infection by a chagasic parasite; the body's responses would be relatively unimportant. According to the homeostatic theory, diseases would be caused by inappropriate or inadequate responses of the body; the actual threats themselves would be relatively unimportant. According to the scientific integrative medical approach, Darwin's illness would have reflected an interaction of genetic predisposition with life experiences and classical and operant conditioning in childhood and early adulthood. He could have had a dysautonomia.

Tactics and Strategies of Scientific Integrative Medicine

Clinicians apply tactics of scientific integrative medicine continually in their practices (table 5). One such approach is to "exploit the lesion," where a treatment's success depends on an abnormality that occurs as part of the disease process itself. An example would be treatment of angina pectoris by nitroglycerine in patients with coronary artery disease. Nitroglycerine relaxes veins, decreasing venous return to the heart and cardiac stroke volume. Normally, decreased cardiac filling "unloads" baroreceptors, and heart rate increases reflexively. The work of the heart changes little, because while the heart rate increases, the systolic blood pressure falls from the direct effects of the drug. Patients with angina pectoris from coronary artery disease, however, typically have low baroreflex-cardiovagal gain. When they take nitroglycerine, the drug reduces systolic blood pressure, but because of the low baroreflex-cardiovagal gain, the heart rate increases relatively little. The work of the heart therefore decreases, relieving the angina pectoris.

Another adage of scientific integrative medicine is, "treat patients, not

Table 5. Tactics and strategies of scientific integrative medicine

Tactics and strategies	Examples
Tactics	
Exploit the lesion	Nitroglycerine for angina pectoris from coronary disease
Treat patients, not numbers	Transfusion for hyperglycemia in gastrointestinal bleeding
Two wrongs can make a right	Deep brain stimulation for Parkinson disease
Block harmful reflexes	Beta-adrenoceptor blockade for postoperative hypothermia
Prevent vicious cycles	Sedation for myocardial infarction
Abort vicious cycles	Fursemide, oxygen, nitroglycerine for pulmonary edema
Exploit beneficial reflexes	Cartoid sinus massage for supraventricular tachycardia
The patient: a conscious homeostat	Self-controlled morphine infusion
Strategies	
Detect compensatory activation	Timing of heart valve replacement
Prevent positive feedback loops	Carvedilol for heart failure
Minimize allostatic load	Beta-adrenoceptor blockade for heart failure
Early detection	Catecholamine terminal loss in Parkinson disease
Exploit genetic knowledge	Avoid tyramine-containing foods in MAO-A deficiency[a]
Prosthetic homeostats	Glucose sensor/insulin pump

[a]MAO-A, monoamine oxidase A.

numbers." You read about how for hyperglycemia in gastrointestinal bleeding, or hyponatremia in heart failure, astute clinicians focus on treating the underlying problem. Appropriate treatment eliminates secondary effects of effector sharing, such as hyperglycemia and hyponatremia, whereas attempting to reverse the abnormal laboratory findings directly can make matters worse.

According to the notion that "two wrongs make a right," when two effectors balance each other in regulating levels of a monitored variable, and one effector fails as part of a disease process, then the symptoms of the disease can be ameliorated by intentionally interfering with the other effector. An example would be surgical ablation of the globus pallidus of the basal ganglia (pallidotomy), which can be an effective treatment of the movement disorder in Parkinson disease.

One can also try to prevent "compensatory damages," deleterious effects of reflexive effector activation. For instance, patients awakening from general anesthesia typically have postoperative hypothermia. Sympathetic nervous and adrenomedullary hormonal system activation to counter hypothermia increases myocardial oxygen consumption. This can contribute to the relatively high frequency of morbid events in patients with coronary artery disease during the immediate postoperative period. Treatment with a beta-adrenoceptor blocker can prevent such events.

The major strategic goal of scientific integrative medicine is to treat effectively or prevent diseases before they become symptomatic (fig. 49). Beyond

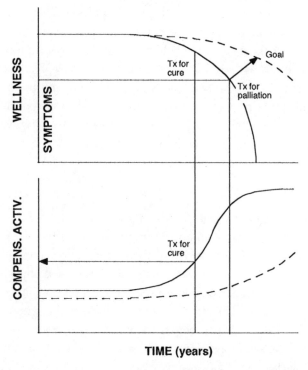

TIME (years)

Fig. 49. Model-generated trends in wellness and compensatory activation. A goal of scientific integrative medicine is to detect threats to wellness in the presymptomatic phase of disease, by accelerated compensatory activation of effectors; timely treatment (Tx) and prevention measures would then avoid premature system failures.

practices that promote health in general, such as regular exercise, dietary moderation, and refreshing sleep, the rapidly expanding availability of genetic, physiological, and biochemical information enables prevention of allostatic load and timely institution of effective treatments that are specific for the individual. For instance, a person with a "functional" heart murmur from an aortic valve with two cusps (bicuspid aortic valve), rather than the normal three cusps, can have stable health and no symptoms for many years. Over millions of heartbeats, turbulence and shear stress would lead to calcification and narrowing of the valve orifice. The heart would eject blood less forcefully, and in response to the altered afferent information from baroreceptors, the brain would reflexively increase sympathetic nervous system outflow to the heart; this could maintain cardiac function for many years. Cardiac sympathetic stimulation, however, also promotes thickening and stiffening of heart muscle, increasing the amount of wall tension required to generate the same amount of pumping. Cardiac sympathetic outflow would be recruited further—a positive feedback loop. Theoretically, by detecting increasing activation of the cardiac sympathetic nerves, one might decide to replace the heart valve, before the patient had symptoms. An even more effective strategy would be to forestall the positive feedback loop, by decreasing the force and rate of the heartbeat slightly throughout the individual's adult life, using a low dose of a beta-adrenoceptor blocker. The treatment might prolong the useful life of the valve sufficiently that symptomatic heart failure would not limit the person's life span.

What, How, and Why

A clinician always has to deal with the questions, what, how, and why. I am indebted to Dr. Basil Eldadah for his insights on this topic.

The "what" of disease consists of the manifestations the patient brings to the clinical encounter, the assemblage of complaints, physical findings, laboratory test results, personal interpretations, expressed fears, and outside professional opinions. The effective clinician sticks to the symptoms and to the assumption that when it comes to symptoms patients always tell the truth, even if the symptoms don't make sense or fit neatly into a particular diagnostic pigeonhole.

Once a positive feedback loop destabilizes a chronic disorder to the extent of clinical manifestations as a degenerative disease, there is little likelihood of successful cure or reversal of the pathogenic process. All homeostatic adjustments have already been overwhelmed. At this stage, attempts at treatment for cure or effective reversal of the disease process typically are expensive, incomplete, dangerous, or doomed. For instance, for symptomatic heart failure in aged people, clinicians rarely identify a curable cause, nor delineate a specific pathophysiological process they can reverse. Surgeries such as heart valve replacement or cardiac transplantation in such patients usually entail prohibitive morbidity and mortality. Similar considerations apply for symptomatic coronary artery disease, Parkinson disease, Alzheimer disease, liver or kidney failure, and cerebrovascular disease. Unfortunately, patients often do not seek medical help until they have symptoms, and degenerative diseases, once symptomatic, lead inexorably to death, often in a surprisingly short time.

At this stage the effective clinician emphasizes palliation, not treatment for cure. There almost always are symptoms that treatments can alleviate. A cancer causing pain may not be resectable, but the pain can be reduced. A narrowed aortic valve causing angina pectoris may not be replaceable, but the angina can be relieved. Heart muscle disease causing shortness of breath from pulmonary edema may not be reversible, but the shortness of breath can be alleviated. Disability causing depression may not improve, but the depressed mood can be lifted. Even in the absence of any treatment, understanding of the pathophysiology of the disease can provide some solace; the patient can benefit from coping strategies such as occupational and physical therapy; and there is time for getting finances in order, planning the estate, and visits, reminiscences, and reconciliations with family.

The "how" of disease is within the province of scientific integrative medicine, because here the clinician can exploit knowledge of homeostatic systems to understand their roles in disease and to devise rational treatments. Dysregulation of monitored variables accounts for the manifestations of disease. The dysregulation can result from inadequate or incorrect information, disruption of one or more homeostats, homeostat resetting, failure of one or more effectors, or effector sharing or interactions. Identifying the site of the lesion in homeostatic feedback loops constitutes much of the art of scientific integrative medicine.

An example of dysregulation from inadequate information would be chronic orthostatic intolerance, labile blood pressure, chest pain, headache, insomnia, and chronic fatigue from baroreflex failure as a consequence of irradiation of the neck. The baroreceptors in the walls of the carotid arteries would be splinted in the walls of vessels that have stiffened over time by accelerated arteriosclerosis. The treatment, ideally, would be a prosthetic baroreceptor. An example of disruption of a homeostat and failure of an effector would be fainting and orthostatic hypotension from baroreflex failure and loss of sympathetic nerves in Parkinson disease. An effective treatment would exploit the phenomenon of denervation supersensitivity of blood vessels in this condition. An example of homeostat resetting would be fever, chills, malaise, irritability, and social withdrawal from effects of a bacterial toxin or from effects of cytokines elaborated in response to the infection. Blockade of cytokine effects might be a reasonable treatment. Examples of effector sharing would be sudden worsening of diabetes in gastrointestinal hemorrhage due to sharing of the adrenomedullary hormonal system effector by both the glucostat and volustat; and delirium and collapse from low serum sodium levels in heart failure, due to sharing of the vasopressin system effector by both the barostat and osmostat. An effective treatment of the former condition would be repletion of blood volume and of the latter "unloading" the heart.

As to why there are diseases—specifically why there are chronic, degenerative diseases—the question is of course largely philosophical. An answer, based on Darwinian medicine, would be that degenerative diseases of the elderly reflect evolutionary compromises, necessary consequences of the survival advantages afforded for protection and propagation of genes in the younger reproducers. For instance, survival advantages of being able to initiate movement rapidly in the young may have led to the possibility of Parkinson disease in the elderly, along the lines of the getaway car analogy. We may not be able to avoid the consequences of evolutionary compromises, but we may be able to affect the timing at which those consequences become clinically overt. The goal would be to prolong useful life by preventing or effectively treating failures of organ systems that otherwise would cause premature death.

As noted above, scientific integrative medicine focuses on prevention and treatment in the presymptomatic phase of organ dysfunction. The goal is to prevent positive feedback loops that would cause premature system failure. In general, it is in the pediatric age group that genetic or biochemical testing would have the greatest chance of success in revealing the existence of diseases before symptoms occur. If a patient had a mutation, a typo in the genetic encyclopedia, then correcting that typo with some form of gene therapy might make sense, as in gene therapy for adenine deaminase deficiency. If a patient had absent activity of an important enzyme, replacing that enzyme could work, as in enzyme replacement therapy for Gaucher disease. In a disease such as Menkes disease, prenatal or early neonatal biochemical diagnosis offers the only hope of survival, by initiation of treatment with copper. After the neonatal period, the baby is doomed, with or without the treatment.

For adult medicine, the future of clinical science is neither in molecular genetics nor in integrative pathophysiology but in building bridges between the two. Common, but complex, modern-day diseases will be found to be mainly disorders of regulation, only indirectly related to genetic changes. Most of the genetic contribution to disease in adults will be found to result not from direct genetic orders but from subtle genetic advice, which has afforded a survival advantage in evolution.

To the end, there is hope. In the presymptomatic, stable phase, there is hope of prevention. In the presymptomatic, unstable phase, there is hope of curative treatment. In the symptomatic, unstable phase, there is hope of alleviating symptoms. Even in the terminal phase, there is hope of allaying anxiety and distress, reducing pain, and offering commiseration.

Conclusion

A person's genes link that person not only with his or her family, and not only with the family of man, but with all things that have ever lived. This surely is a basis for the fascination of genetics. As amazing as is the detail of the genetic instructions revealed by the Human Genome Project, we must now turn to the uses to which those instructions are put by living things to maintain organismic integrity so well for so long. The genes are life's blueprint; ongoing information processing and compensatory adjustments enable life to go on. Scientific integrative medicine focuses on how that processing and those adjustments go awry and on means to predict and prevent premature system failures. The future development of scientific integrative medicine will require redirection of molecular genetics, molecular biology, and integrative physiology to focus on the real first causes of many modern diseases of adults: the loss of "wellness," where both health and disease depend on genetic algorithms determining the development and adaptive regulation of homeostatic systems.

Conducting integrative medical research, especially in patients, is difficult. Studying one drug or one gene is always easier, cheaper, and more conclusive than studying more than one simultaneously. Studying the effects of a single gene knockout for an endogenous substance is always easier, cheaper, and more conclusive than studying the homeostatic systems that use that substance. Nevertheless, studying multiple homeostatic systems that operate in parallel and interact, according to influences of multiple genes, life experiences, drug treatments, and time, offers unique opportunities for early detection of presymptomatic system failure and optimal timing of interventions for prevention, cure, or effective treatment of chronic diseases of adults. Because of the availability of genomic information and computer software for database mining and kinetic modeling, the time seems ripe for development of scientific integrative medicine in research, teaching, and practice. I believe that the adrenaline family, those venerable effectors of the inner world, will lead the way.

Glossary

acetylcholine. A particular chemical that functions as the chemical messenger of the parasympathetic nervous system

ADH. An abbreviation for *antidiuretic hormone*

adrenal, adrenal gland. A gland near the top of each kidney that produces steroids such as cortisol and catecholamines such as adrenaline

adrenal cortex. The "bark" or outer layer of the adrenal gland

adrenaline. The same as *epinephrine*

adrenal medulla. The "marrow" or core of the adrenal gland

adrenoceptors. Specialized proteins in cell membranes of various tissues that bind to the catecholamines norepinephrine (noradrenaline) or epinephrine (adrenaline), resulting in changes in the state of activity of the cells

adrenocortical. Referring to the cortex or shell of the adrenal gland

adrenocorticotropic hormone. The same as *corticotropin*

adrenomedullary hormonal system (AHS). The part of the autonomic nervous system where adrenaline (epinephrine) is released from the adrenal medulla

AHS. An abbreviation for *adrenomedullary hormonal system*

alae nasi. The muscles that control the size of the nostrils. Contraction of these muscles widens the nostrils in anger.

aldosterone. The main sodium-retaining steroid produced in the adrenal gland

allostasis. A concept according to which organisms maintain stability through change. By analogy, one can keep home temperature at different but constant levels by changing the thermostat setting.

allostatic load. A concept according to which prolonged activation of effectors involved in allostasis contributes to wear and tear. This idea provides a basis for studying the long-term health consequences of stress.

alpha-adrenoceptors. One of the two types of receptors for norepinephrine (noradrenaline) and epinephrine (adrenaline)

alpha-1 adrenoceptors. A particular type of adrenoceptor that is prominent in blood vessel walls. Stimulation of alpha-1 adrenoceptors in blood vessel walls causes the vessels to tighten.

alpha-2 adrenoceptor blocker. A drug that blocks alpha-2 adrenoceptors

alpha-2 adrenoceptors. A type of adrenoceptor that is present on particular cells in the brain, in blood vessel walls, in several organs, and on sympathetic nerve terminals

alpha-methylDOPA (Aldomet). A drug that resembles levodopa and is an effective drug to treat high blood pressure

amine. A chemical that contains an ammonia (a nitrogen bonded to hydrogens) group

amino acid. A particular type of chemical that contains an amino chemical group and a carboxylic acid chemical group. It is a building block of proteins.

amphetamines. Drugs that share a particular chemical structure. Amphetamines decrease appetite, increase attention, decrease sleep, and produce behavioral activation.

anemia. A decreased amount of red blood cells. Patients with anemia look pale and feel tired.

angina pectoris. Also simply called *angina*. This is an unpleasant sensation of squeezing or pressure in the chest as a result of inadequate delivery of blood to the heart by way of the coronary arteries.

ANS. An abbreviation for *autonomic nervous system*

antidiuretic hormone (ADH). The same as *vasopressin*

aorta. The main artery carrying oxygenated blood from the heart to the body. The heart pumps blood into the aorta, which distributes the blood to the organs by way of the arteries.

aortic valve. The heart valve through which the blood is ejected into the aorta

aquaporin. A particular type of protein that enables water to enter cells via pores in the cell membrane

arginine vasopressin (AVP). The same as *vasopressin*

L-aromatic amino-acid decarboxylase (LAAAD). The enzyme that converts levodopa to dopamine in the body

arrhythmia. Lack of rhythm, such as from an abnormality of the heartbeat

arterial blood sampling. Obtaining blood from a large blood vessel that moves blood away from the heart

arterial pressure. The blood pressure in an artery

arteriole. Like "twigs" of the arterial tree, the arterioles are tiny arteries that carry blood from the heart. The overall amount of constriction of arterioles is the main determinant of the total resistance to blood flow in the body. Constriction of arterioles therefore increases the blood pressure, just like tightening the nozzle increases the pressure in a garden hose.

arteriosclerosis. Hardening of the arteries. When associated with a buildup of fatty plaque, the condition is called atherosclerosis.

artery. A muscular blood vessel that carries blood from the heart to organs. Arteries deliver blood rich in oxygen, with the exception of the pulmonary artery from the heart to the lungs.

asphyxiation. Suspended animation, such as from suffocation. *Asphyxia* comes from the Greek words for "no pulse," whereas *suffocation* comes from the Latin for choking.

aspiration. Inhalation of a foreign body into the airway

asystole. Sudden lack of the heartbeat caused by the absence of cardiac electrical activity. Asystole is a cause of sudden death.

atria. Plural of atrium

atrium. A thin-walled chamber of the heart where the blood in the great veins enters the heart

atropine. A drug derived from the plant, *Atropa belladonna*, which blocks muscarinic receptors for acetylcholine

autocrine/paracrine substance. A chemical messenger produced in, released from, and acting locally on the same type of cells within an organ

autoimmune autonomic failure. A form of autonomic failure associated with an "attack" of the immune system on a part of the autonomic nervous system

autonomic. Referring to the autonomic nervous system

autonomic failure. A condition involving failure of one or more components of the autonomic nervous system

autonomic function testing. Testing of one or more functions of the autonomic nervous system

autonomic myasthenia. Nickname for a form of chronic autonomic failure associated with an antibody to the acetylcholine receptor responsible for transmission of nerve impulses in ganglia

autonomic nerve supply. The amount of autonomic nerve fibers and terminals in a tissue or organ

autonomic nervous system (ANS). The body's "automatic" nervous system, responsible for many automatic, usually unconscious processes that keep the body going

AVP. An abbreviation for *arginine vasopressin*

axon reflex. A type of reflex in which stimulation of nerves going toward the brain leads directly to a change in nerve activity toward a nearby site

baroreceptor reflex. A rapid reflex in which an increase in blood pressure sensed by the brain leads to relaxation of blood vessels and a decrease in heart rate

baroreceptors. Stretch or distortion receptors in the walls of large blood vessels such as the carotid artery and in the heart muscle

baroreflex. The same as *baroreceptor reflex*

baroreflex failure. An unusual disorder in which the baroreceptor reflex fails, resulting in variable blood pressure and orthostatic intolerance

barostat. A homeostat that regulates blood pressure

basal ganglia. A group of brain structures that contribute importantly to regulation of movement and locomotion

benign essential tremor. A condition characterized by involuntary, rhythmic shaking of the hands

benign prostatic hypertrophy (BPH). Long-term enlargement of the prostate gland that does not result from a cancer

benzodiazepine. A type of drug with a particular chemical structure that causes sedation, an antianxiety effect, relaxation of skeletal muscle, and decreased seizure activity

beta-adrenoceptor blocker. A type of drug that blocks one or more types of beta-adrenoceptors

beta-adrenoceptors. One of the two types of receptors for norepinephrine (noradrenaline) and epinephrine (adrenaline)

beta-1 adrenoceptors. One of the three types of beta-adrenoceptors that are prominent in the heart muscle

beta-2 adrenoceptors. One of the three types of beta-adrenoceptors that are prominent in blood vessel walls in skeletal muscle, in the heart muscle, and on sympathetic nerve terminals

beta-3 adrenoceptors. One of the three types of beta-adrenoceptors that are prominent in fatty tissue

beta-endorphin. A particular type of opioid that is measurable in the bloodstream

bethanecol (Urecholine). A drug that stimulates muscarinic receptors for acetylcholine, mimicking some of the effects of stimulating the parasympathetic nervous system

biogenic amines. A particular group of chemicals made by living organisms and containing an amine component

blood-brain barrier. Something that prevents chemicals in the bloodstream from entering the central nervous system. The blood-brain barrier for catecholamines, such as adrenaline, is the result of particular cells just outside blood vessel walls that possess multiple enzymes that break down the catecholamines before they can reach the brain cells.

blood glucose. The concentration of the important metabolic fuel, glucose (dextrose), in the blood

blood pressure. The pressure in arteries. Systolic blood pressure is the maximum pressure while the heart is beating, and diastolic blood pressure is the minimum pressure between heartbeats.

blood volume. The total volume of blood in the body. Most of the blood volume is in the veins.

BPH. An abbreviation for *benign prostatic hypertrophy*

brachial artery. The artery, in the elbow crease area, that carries blood to the fore-arm and hand

brainstem. The lowest, innermost part of the brain, located just above the spinal cord. The brainstem includes the hypothalamus, midbrain, pons, and, just at the top of the spinal cord, the medulla oblongata.

caffeic acid. A particular chemical found in coffee beans that is not caffeine and has a catechol structure

caffeine. A chemical found in high concentrations in coffee beans

carbidopa. A drug that inhibits the conversion of L-DOPA (levodopa) to dopamine. Because carbidopa does not enter the brain from the bloodstream, it blocks the conversion of L-DOPA to dopamine outside the brain.

carbon. An important chemical element. Organic chemistry is the study of carbon-containing compounds.

carbon dioxide. A gas produced as a by-product of metabolism

cardiac output. The amount of blood pumped by the heart in one minute

carotid artery. The main artery delivering blood to the head

carotid body. A structure near where the common carotid artery splits into the internal and external carotid arteries in the neck. The carotid body contains chemoreceptor cells that sense blood levels of oxygen, carbon dioxide, and acidity.

carotid sinus. A region at the split-up of the common carotid artery into the internal and external carotid arteries, containing distortion receptors called baroreceptors

catecholamine. A member of an important chemical family that includes adrenaline

catecholamines. Norepinephrine (noradrenaline), epinephrine (adrenaline), and dopamine

catechols. Chemicals with a structure that includes two adjacent hydroxyl groups on a benzene ring. The catecholamines norepinephrine (noradrenaline), epinephrine (adrenaline), and dopamine are catechols, as are the noncatecholamines levodopa and carbidopa in Sinemet.

cell membrane norepinephrine transporter (NET). The transporter responsible for recycling of norepinephrine back into sympathetic nerves

central nervous system. The brain and spinal cord

central sympathetic hyperactivity. A condition in which the brain directs an increase in the rate of sympathetic nerve traffic in the body as a whole

cerebellar. Referring to the cerebellum

cerebellar atrophy. A decrease in size of the cerebellum, a part of the brain

cerebellum. A part of the brain, located above and behind the brainstem, that plays important roles in coordination of movement and the sense of orientation in space

cerebral cortex. The outermost layer of the brain, especially large and highly developed in primates such as humans

cerebrospinal fluid (CSF). The clear fluid that bathes the brain and spinal cord

chemoreceptors. Cells that sense local levels of chemicals such as oxygen, carbon dioxide, and sodium

Chiari malformation. An anatomic abnormality in which part of the brain falls below the hole between the brain and spinal cord

chronic autonomic failure. Long-term failure of the autonomic nervous system

chronic fatigue syndrome. A condition in which the patient has a sense of persistent fatigue for more than six months, without an identified cause

chronic orthostatic intolerance. Long-term inability to tolerate standing up

clearance. The volume of fluid cleared of a substance in given period of time

clonidine. A drug that stimulates alpha-2 adrenoceptors in the brain, in blood vessel walls, and on sympathetic nerve terminals. Clonidine decreases release of norepinephrine from sympathetic nerves and decreases blood pressure.

clonidine suppression test. A test based on the effects of clonidine administration on blood pressure and plasma levels of chemicals such as norepinephrine (noradrenaline)

common faint. The same as *neurocardiogenic syncope*

compensatory activation. A situation in which failure of one effector system compensatorily activates another effector system, allowing a degree of control of the monitored variable

complete heart block. A cardiac emergency situation in which the electrical activity in the heart fails to follow the proper sequence from the atria to the ventricles, and the ventricles beat at a low intrinsic rate

constipation. Infrequent and difficult bowel movements

contraction band necrosis. A particular pattern of death of heart muscle cells caused by extreme stimulation

coronary arteries. The arteries that deliver blood to the heart muscle

coronary artery disease. A disease in which the coronary arteries become narrowed or blocked by fatty deposits and thickening of the walls

cortex. The outermost layer of tissue in an organ. The cerebral cortex is the outermost layer of the brain. The adrenal cortex is the outermost layer of the adrenal gland.

corticotropin (ACTH). A hormone released by the pituitary gland that stimulates secretion of steroids by the adrenal cortex

corticotropin-releasing hormone (CRH). A particular hormone released in a part of the hypothalamus that stimulates the pituitary gland to release ACTH

cortisol. A major steroid hormone produced in the adrenal cortex cranial nerves. The twelve nerves that come through holes in the skull from the brainstem and go to many organs, from the eyes to the gastrointestinal tract

CRH. An abbreviation for *corticotropin-releasing hormone*

cytokines. A class of proteins made in blood, lymphoid, and other cells, that act as autocrine/paracrine agents affecting immunity, allergy, inflammation, and growth of particular cell types

d-amphetamine. The dextro-mirror image form of amphetamine

DBH. An abbreviation for *dopamine-beta-hydroxylase*

dehydration. Abnormal lack of water in the body

delayed orthostatic hypotension. A fall in blood pressure after prolonged standing

denervated. Lacking nerves.

denervation supersensitivity. Increased sensitivity of a process as a result of loss of delivery of a neuronal chemical messenger to its receptors that normally mediate the process

dependent variable. A measure for which the values depend on those for another measure. In a graph of distance traveled as a function of time, the distance traveled would be the dependent variable

dextro-amphetamine. The same as *d-amphetamine*

DHPR. An abbreviation for *dihydropteridine reductase*

diabetes. A disease state with an excessive volume of urination and excessive water intake. Diabetes mellitus results from the lack of insulin effects in the body. Diabetes insipidus results from lack of antidiuretic hormone (vasopressin) effects in the body.

diagnosis. A decision about the cause of a specific case of disease

dihydrocaffeic acid. A particular chemical that is a breakdown product of caffeic acid

dihydropteridine reductase (DHPR). An enzyme required for efficient production of catecholamines and some other biochemicals. DHPR deficiency causes an atypical form of PKU.

L-dihydroxyphenylalanine. Levodopa, L-DOPA

L-dihydroxyphenylserine (L-DOPS). A particular amino acid that is converted to norepinephrine by the action of L-aromatic amino-acid decarboxylase

distress. A form of stress that is consciously experienced in which the individual senses an inability to cope, attempts to avoid or escape the situation, elicits instinctively communicated signs, and has activation of the adrenal gland

DOPA decarboxylase (DDC, LAAAD). The enzyme responsible for conversion of L-DOPA to dopamine in the body

dopamine. One of the body's three catecholamines. Dopamine is converted to norepinephrine and norepinephrine to adrenaline.

dopamine-beta-hydroxylase (DBH). The enzyme responsible for conversion of dopamine to norepinephrine in the body

dysautonomia. A condition in which a change in the function of the autonomic nervous system adversely affects health

ECF. An abbreviation for *extracellular fluid*

effector. An agent of the body that helps maintain body functions, such as temperature, blood oxygen, and glucose concentrations, and delivery of blood to organs. Examples of effectors are the sympathetic nervous system, the hypothalamic-pituitary-adrenocortical system, and the renin-angiotensin-aldosterone system. The brain coordinates numerous effectors to regulate the inner world of the body.

electrolyte. A chemical that in solution is able to conduct an electric current by movement of dissociated positively and negatively charged ions to the electrodes. Potassium and sodium ions are important electrolytes of the inner world.

endocrinology. A specialty of internal medicine that concerns hormones released by glands (e.g., thyroid, parathyroid, pancreas, adrenal) into the bloodstream

enzyme. A type of protein that increases the rate of a chemical reaction in the body

ephedra. A particular natural product of the ephedra plant, the same as the Chinese herbal remedy, *ma huang*

ephedrine. A particular drug that acts in the body as a sympathomimetic amine

EPI. An abbreviation for *epinephrine*

epinephrine (adrenaline). The main hormone released from the adrenal medulla

Epogen. Brand name of *erythropoietin*

erectile impotence. Impotence from failure to have or sustain erection of the penis

ergotamine. A particular drug that constricts blood vessels

erythropoietin. A hormone that stimulates the bone marrow to produce red blood cells

ethology. The branch of zoology that deals with instinctive animal behaviors

extracellular fluid (ECF). The fluid environment surrounding the cells of the body

extravasation. Leakage of fluid from blood vessels into the surrounding tissues

fainting. Relatively rapid, temporary loss of consciousness and muscle tone

false-positive test. A positive test result when the patient does not actually have the disease

familial dysautonomia (FD). A rare inherited disease that features abnormalities in sensation and in functions of the autonomic nervous system

FBF. An abbreviation for *forearm blood flow*

FD. An abbreviation for *familial dysautonomia*

fenfluramine. A particular drug that acts in parts of the nervous system where serotonin is the chemical messenger

Florinef. Brand name for *fludrocortisone*

fludrocortisone (Florinef). A type of artificial salt-retaining steroid drug

fluorodopamine. A drug that is the catecholamine, dopamine, with a fluorine atom attached. The fluorine atom can be a type of radioactive isotope called a positron emitter. Positron-emitting fluorodopamine is used to visualize sympathetic nerves such as in the heart.

6-[^{18}F]fluorodopamine. A drug that is the catecholamine, dopamine, with a fluorine atom attached that is a radioactive isotope called a positron emitter. Positron-emitting fluorodopamine is used to visualize sympathetic nerves such as in the heart.

forearm blood flow (FBF). The rate of inflow of blood into the forearm, usually expressed in terms of blood delivery per 100 cc of tissue volume per minute

forearm vascular resistance (FVR). The extent of resistance to blood flow in the forearm blood vessels

free fatty acids. A form of breakdown products of fat released from the liver into the bloodstream

FVR. An abbreviation for *forearm vascular resistance*

galvanic skin response (GSR). An evoked change in the ability of the skin to conduct electricity because of a change in the amount of sweat

ganglia. Plural of ganglion

ganglion. A clump of cells where autonomic nerve impulses are relayed between the spinal cord and target organs such as the heart

ganglion blockade. Blockade of chemical transmission in ganglia, such as by trimethaphan or pentolinium administration

ganglion blocker. A type of drug that inhibits the transmission of nerve impulses in ganglia

gene. A sequence of genetic material that encodes the production of a particular protein. Genes are like words in the genetic encyclopedia.

general adaptation syndrome. A three-phase response to stress, as proposed by Hans Selye

globus pallidus. A part of the basal ganglia in the brain

glomerulus. A tiny tuft of blood vessels in the kidney that filters the blood

glucagons. A hormone released from the pancreas that increases blood glucose levels

glucose. One of the body's main fuels. The same as *dextrose*.

glucocorticoid. A type of steroid hormone released from the adrenal cortex that increases glucose levels

glucostat. A homeostat for regulation of the blood glucose concentration

glycogen. A storage form of glucose that is abundant in the liver and skeletal muscle. Adrenaline accelerates the breakdown of glycogen, increasing glucose levels in the bloodstream.

GSR. An abbreviation for *galvanic skin response*. A rapid increase in electrical conduction in the skin as a result of an increase in production of sweat.

gustatory. Related to tasting something

heart failure. A condition in which the heart fails to pump an adequate amount of blood for the tissues of the body, usually from a problem with heart muscle function

hemostasis. Stoppage of bleeding

homeostat. A physiological comparator, analogous to a thermostat, that senses discrepancy between a setting and information about a monitored variable, the discrepancy leading to changes in activities of effectors that tend to reduce the discrepancy

homeostatic system. A system that keeps levels of a monitored variable stable

hormone. A chemical released into the bloodstream that acts at remote sites in the body

HPA. An abbreviation for *hypothalamic-pituitary-adrenocortical*

HR. An abbreviation for *heart rate*

hydrocarbon. A chemical made up of carbon and hydrogen

hydrogen. An important chemical element that itself is a gas, but it is also part of the chemical structure of key molecules for life, such as water and glucose

hydroxyl group. A chemical structure consisting of a single oxygen and a single hydrogen atom

hyperadrenergic orthostatic intolerance. A condition in which an inability to tolerate standing up is combined with signs or symptoms of excessive levels of catecholamines such as epinephrine (adrenaline)

hyperdynamic circulation syndrome. A condition in which the rate and force of the heartbeat are abnormally increased

hyperglycemia. A condition in which there is an abnormally high blood-glucose level

hypernoradrenergic hypertension. Long-term high blood pressure associated with increased release of norepinephrine from sympathetic nerve terminals

hypertension. A condition in which the blood pressure is persistently increased

hypoglycemia. A condition in which the blood-glucose level is abnormally low

hypothalamic-pituitary-adrenocortical (HPA). A major stress effector system in which release of chemicals in the hypothalamus of the upper brainstem effects release of corticotropin (ACTH) from the pituitary gland, and the ACTH stimulates release of steroid hormones from the adrenal cortex

hypothermia. A condition in which body temperature is abnormally low
hypoxic. Lacking adequate oxygen

impotence. Inability to have an erection of the penis
inappropriate sinus tachycardia. Excessively fast heart rate because of excessively
    fast firing of the heart's pacemaker in the sinus node
incontinence. Sudden involuntary urination or bowel movement
independent variable. A variable, values for which change, resulting in changes in
    values for another variable. In a graph of distance traveled as a function of
    elapsed time, time would be the independent variable.
Inderal. Brand name of *propranolol*
indirectly acting sympathomimetic amine. A type of drug that produces effects sim-
    ilar to those of stimulating sympathetic nerves, by releasing endogenous chem-
    icals from the nerves
innervation. Nerve supply
INS. An abbreviation for *insulin*
insulin (INS). An important hormone released from the pancreas that helps to
    control the blood-glucose level
intervening variable. In psychology, an unobserved phenomenon linking stimuli
    with responses. Examples of intervening variables are emotional experiences
    and motivational states.
intravenous saline. Physiological salt-in-water solution that is given by vein
iontophoresis. A way using electricity to deliver a drug to the skin surface
isoproterenol. Isuprel
isoproterenol infusion test. A test in which isoproterenol is given by vein to see if
    this affects the ability to tolerate tilting or to measure the body's responses to
    stimulation of beta-adrenoceptors
Isuprel. Brand name of *isoproterenol*

kinky hair disease. The same as *Menkes disease*

LAAAD. An abbreviation for *L-aromatic amino-acid decarboxylase*
L-DOPA. An abbreviation for *L-dihydroxyphenylalanine*, the same as *levodopa*
L-DOPS. An abbreviation for *L-dihydroxyphenylserine*
levodopa. The same as *L-DOPA* and *L-dihydroxyphenylalanine*
limbic system. Parts of the brain arranged like a shell around the brainstem and
    in turn surrounded by the cerebral cortex
locus ceruleus. A small cluster of cells located in the pons in the brainstem. The
    locus ceruleus is the main source of norepinephrine in the brain.
lumbar puncture. A procedure in which a needle is inserted into the lower back,
    such as to sample cerebrospinal fluid

ma huang. Chinese name for an herbal remedy from the ephedra plant, the active ingredient of which is ephedrine

MAP. An abbreviation for *mean arterial pressure*

mean arterial pressure (MAP). The average blood pressure in the arteries

medulla. From the Latin word for "marrow," the medulla is an inner or core portion of an organ, in contrast with the cortex, from the Latin word for "bark," which is the outer layer. The adrenal gland has a cortex and medulla; and the innermost layer of the central nervous system, just above the top of the spinal cord, is the medulla oblongata.

Menkes disease. A rare inherited disease of copper metabolism that causes death in early childhood

^{123}I-metaiodobenzylguanidine (^{123}I-MIBG). A particular type of radioactive drug that is used to visualize sympathetic nerves such as in the heart

methyl group. Part of a chemical molecule that consists of a single carbon atom and attached hydrogen atoms

methylphenidate (Ritalin). A particular drug in the family of amphetamines

midodrine (Proamatine). A particular drug that can be taken as a pill and constricts blood vessels by way of stimulation of alpha-adrenoceptors, commonly used in the treatment of orthostatic hypotension and orthostatic intolerance

military antishock trousers (MAST) suit. A type of inflatable trousers that decreases pooling of blood in the legs

mineralocorticoid. A type of steroid released from the adrenal cortex that causes the body to retain sodium

miosis. Constriction of the pupil of the eye

monitored variable. Something that is measured or detected, where the levels or values can change and the change is sensed. An example of a monitored variable is the temperature in your home. An example of an internal monitored variable is the temperature of your blood.

monoamine. A type of biochemical that contains a component called an amine group. Serotonin and adrenaline are monoamines.

moxonidine. A particular drug that decreases blood pressure by decreasing sympathetic nerve traffic

MSA. An abbreviation for *multiple system atrophy*

multiple system atrophy (MSA). A progressive disease of the brain that includes failure of the autonomic nervous system

muscarinic receptors. One of the two types of receptors for the chemical messenger acetylcholine

mutation. A rare genetic change, like a "typo" in the genetic encyclopedia

mydriasis. Dilation of the pupil of the eye

myelin. A fatty sheath surrounding some nerves

myelinated nerve. A nerve surrounded by myelin

myocardium. Muscle tissue of the heart

NA. An abbreviation for *noradrenaline*. The same as *norepinephrine*.

NE. An abbreviation for *norepinephrine*

negative feedback. A way in which homeostatic systems keep levels of monitored variables stable. If the sensed level is too high, the system directs changes in effectors that bring the level down; if the sensed level is too low, the system directs changes bringing the level up.

nerve terminal. The end of a nerve fiber, from which chemical messengers are released

NET. An abbreviation for cell membrane *norepinephrine transporter*

NET deficiency. A rare cause of orthostatic intolerance resulting from decreased activity of the cell membrane norepinephrine transporter

neurally mediated syncope. A condition that includes sudden loss of consciousness from a change in the function of the autonomic nervous system

neurasthenia. The same as *neurocirculatory asthenia*

neurocardiogenic syncope. The same as *neurally mediated syncope*

neurocardiology. A medical discipline that focuses on disorders of regulation of the cardiovascular system by the brain

neurochemical. A chemical released from nervous tissue

neurocirculatory asthenia. A condition closely related to chronic fatigue syndrome that features exercise intolerance without identified cause, described mainly in medical literature from the former Soviet Union

neuroendocrine. A word used to describe a system that includes nerves that lead to glands that release hormones

neuroimaging tests. Tests based on visualizing the nervous system

neuropathic POTS. A form of postural tachycardia syndrome (POTS) thought to result from local or patchy loss of sympathetic nerves

neuropharmacological. A type of drug effect that acts on nervous tissue or mimics chemicals released in nervous tissue

neurotransmitter. A chemical released from nerve fibers or terminals that produces effects on other cells nearby

nicotine. A chemical in tobacco that stimulates a particular type of receptor for the chemical messenger acetylcholine

nicotinic receptor. One of the two types of receptors for the chemical messenger acetylcholine

nitric oxide. A gas that can act locally as an autocrine/paracrine substance. One prominent effect of nitric oxide is relaxation of blood vessels in the penis, resulting in penile erection.

nitroglycerine. A particular drug that relaxes walls of veins in the body nociceptor. A pain sensor

nonselective beta-adrenoceptor blockers. A type of drug that blocks all types of beta-adrenoceptors

noradrenergic nerves. Nerves that produce, store, release, and recycle norepinephrine as their chemical messenger

norepinephrine (noradrenaline). The main chemical messenger of the sympathetic nervous system, responsible for much of regulation of the cardiovascular system by the brain

normal saline. A dilute solution of sodium chloride (table salt) that has the same concentration as in the serum

NTS. An abbreviation for *nucleus of the solitary tract*

nucleus of the solitary tract (NTS). A particular cluster of nerve cells in the lower brainstem that is the site of the barostat

opioid. A chemical in the body that acts like an opiate drug such as morphine

orthostasis. Standing up

orthostatic. Referring to standing up

orthostatic hypotension. A fall in blood pressure when a person stands up

orthostatic intolerance. An inability to tolerate standing up because of a sensation of lightheadedness or dizziness

orthostatic tachycardia. An excessive increase in the heart rate when a person stands up

osmolality. The concentration of osmotically active particles in a solution. The main determinants of serum osmolality are the concentrations of sodium and chloride ions.

osmostat. A homeostat that regulates the serum osmolality

oxygen. A particular element that is a gas present in the atmosphere and a major metabolic fuel. Animals absolutely require oxygen to live.

pacemaker. A device that produces electrical impulses in the heart

PAF. An abbreviation for *pure autonomic failure*

palpitations. A symptom in which the patient notes a forceful, rapid heartbeat or a sensation of the heart "flip-flopping" in the chest

panic disorder. A condition that features a rapid buildup of fear or anxiety that the patient cannot control

parasympathetic nerve traffic. The rate of traffic in parasympathetic nerves

parasympathetic nervous system (PNS). One of the main components of the autonomic nervous system, responsible for many "vegetative" functions such as gastrointestinal movements after a meal

parasympathetic neurocirculatory failure. Failure to regulate the heart rate appropriately, such as during normal breathing or in response to the Valsalva maneuver

Parkinson disease. A progressive nervous system disease that produces slow movements, a form of limb rigidity called "cogwheel rigidity," and a "pill-roll" tremor that is present when the patient is at rest and decreases with intentional movement. Other features of Parkinson disease include a masklike facial expression, stooped posture, difficulty initiating or stopping movements, small handwriting, and improvement of the movement disorder by treatment with levodopa.

Parkinson disease with orthostatic hypotension. Parkinson disease with a fall in blood pressure when the patient stands up

parkinsonian. Having one or more features of Parkinson disease

parkinsonian form of MSA. A form of multiple system atrophy that includes one or more features of Parkinson disease

partial dysautonomia. The same as *neuropathic POTS*

pentolinium. A type of ganglion blocker drug

peptide. A short chain of amino acids

peristalsis. Gastrointestinal movements such as after a meal that move digested material

PET scanning. An abbreviation for *positron emission tomographic scanning*

Phen-Fen. Two drugs, phentermine and fenfluramine, prescribed together to decrease appetite and promote weight loss

phentermine. A particular drug that acts in the body as a sympathomimetic amine

phenylalanine. A particular amino acid

phenylephrine (Neo-Synephrine). A particular drug that constricts blood vessels by stimulating alpha-1 adrenoceptors

phenylethanolamine-N-methyltransferase (PNMT). The enzyme for conversion of norepinephrine to adrenaline

phenylketonuria (PKU). A disease of children that results from lack of activity of a particular enzyme, phenylalanine hydroxylase, resulting in a toxic buildup of phenylalanine in the body

phenylpropanolamine (PPE). A particular drug that acts in the body as a sympathomimetic amine

pheo. Slang for *pheochromocytoma*

pheochromocytoma. An abnormal growth that produces the catecholamines norepinephrine (noradrenaline) or epinephrine (adrenaline)

physiological. Referring to a body function, as opposed to a body part

piloerection. Hair standing out, as in distress

PKU. An abbreviation for *phenylketonuria*

plasma. The part of the blood that is left after anticoagulated blood settles

plasma epinephrine level. The concentration of epinephrine (adrenaline) in the plasma

plasma norepinephrine level. The concentration of norepinephrine (noradrenaline) in the plasma

platelets. Particles in the bloodstream that are fragments of particular cells made in the bone marrow. Platelets tend to clump into plugs. Adrenaline promotes this plugging.

PNS. An abbreviation for *parasympathetic nervous system*

polymorphism. A genetic change that is not as rare as a mutation but not so common as to be considered normal

pons. A level of the brainstem just above the medulla and below the midbrain

positive feedback. A form of feedback in a homeostatic system where a high level of the monitored variable leads to changes in effectors that further increase that level, and where a low level of the variables leads to further decreases in that level. Positive feedback loops therefore are inherently destabilizing.

positron emission tomographic scanning (PET scanning). A type of nuclear medicine scan where a positron-emitting form of a drug is injected and particular parts of the body become radioactive, with the radioactivity detected by a special type of scanner called a PET scanner

positron emitter. A chemical that releases a special type of radioactivity called positrons

postganglionic nerves. Nerves from the ganglia that deliver signals to nerve terminals in target tissues such as the heart

postprandial hypotension. An abnormal fall in blood pressure after eating

postural tachycardia syndrome (POTS). A condition in which the patient has a long-term inability to tolerate standing up, along with an excessive increase in pulse rate in response to standing

potassium. An important element found in all cells of the body

POTS. An abbreviation for *postural tachycardia syndrome*

power spectral analysis of heart rate variability. A special type of physiological test based on changes in the heart rate over time

PPE. An abbreviation for *phenylpropanolamine*

preganglionic nerves. Nerves of the autonomic nervous system that come from cell bodies in the spinal cord and pass through the ganglia

presyncope. A feeling of near-fainting

Proamatine. Brand name of *midodrine*

Procrit. Brand name of *erythropoietin*

progressive supranuclear palsy. A type of progressive neurological disease with particular abnormalities of gaze

propranolol (Inderal). A drug that is the classical nonselective beta-adrenoceptor blocker

provocative test. A test designed to evoke an abnormal response of the body

pseudephedrine (Sudafed). A particular drug that acts in the body as a sympatho-mimetic amine

pure autonomic failure (PAF). A form of long-term failure of the autonomic nervous system in which there are no signs or symptoms of degeneration of the brain

QSART. An abbreviation for *quantitative sudomotor axon reflex test*

quantitative sudomotor axon reflex test (QSART). A type of test of autonomic nervous system function based on the ability of drugs to evoke sweating

radial artery. An artery in the wrist that carries blood to the hand. When you have your pulse taken, it is the radial artery that the examiner compresses.

radiofrequency ablation. Destruction of a tissue by applying radiofrequency energy, which burns the tissue

RAS. An abbreviation for *renin-angiotensin-aldosterone system*

receptors. Special proteins in the walls of cells that bind chemical messengers such as hormones and neurotransmitters

reductionism. An approach to acquiring knowledge where one dissects a problem into component parts, with the assumption that reassembling the parts would then solve the problem

reflex sympathetic dystrophy (RSD). A chronic pain syndrome initiated by trauma to a limb, where the pain spreads to areas that were not traumatized. RSD is the same as complex regional pain syndrome, type I.

renin-angiotensin-aldosterone system (RAS). A system that plays an important role in maintaining the correct amount of blood volume and sodium in the body

respiratory sinus arrhythmia. The normal changes in pulse rate that occur with breathing

Ritalin. Brand name of *methylphenidate*. A particular drug that resembles amphetamine.

salivary glands. Glands responsible for releasing saliva

salivation. Formation of spit

scientific integrative medicine. A medical discipline that uses concepts about interacting, feedback-regulated systems to explain diseases

serotonin. A chemical messenger in a family called monoamines. Catecholamines such as adrenaline are also monoamines.

serum. The straw-colored fluid left after blood clots

shared effectors. The same effectors used by different homeostats

Shy-Drager syndrome (multiple system atrophy with orthostatic hypotension). A form of progressive nervous system disease in which different pathways of the brain degenerate and the patient has a fall in blood pressure during standing because of failure of the sympathetic nervous system

Sinemet. Brand name of *levodopa* or *L-DOPA*, combined with carbidopa

sinus node. The pacemaker area of the heart that normally generates the electrical impulses resulting in a coordinated heartbeat

sinus node ablation. Destruction of the sinus node in the heart, usually as a treatment for excessively rapid heart rate

skin sympathetic test (SST). A type of test of the sympathetic nervous system based on the ability of various drugs or environmental manipulations to increase secretion of sweat

smooth muscle cells. The type of muscle cells in the heart, blood vessel walls, gastrointestinal tract, and glands

SNS. An abbreviation for the *sympathetic nervous system*

sodium. An important chemical element found in all body fluids

somatic nerves. Nerves to the externally observable parts of the body, as opposed to the inner organs

somatic nervous system. The somatic nervous system is the main way the body deals with the "outside world," by way of its main target organ, skeletal muscle

SSRI. An abbreviation for *selective serotonin reuptake inhibitor*. SSRIs block one of the main ways of inactivating and recycling the chemical messenger, serotonin. This increases delivery of serotonin to its receptors in the brain. SSRIs are used to treat depression, anxiety, and other psychiatric or emotional problems.

SST. An abbreviation for *skin sympathetic test*

stereoisomer. A mirror image structure of a chemical

steroid. A particular type of chemical structure. Hormones such as cortisol and estrogen are steroids.

strain gauge. A testing device that sensitively measures stretch

stress. A condition in which the organism senses a challenge to physical or mental stability that leads to altered activities of body systems to meet that challenge

striatonigral degeneration. A form of nervous system disease in which the patient seems to have Parkinson disease but does not respond well to treatment with levodopa

stroke volume. The amount of blood pumped by the heart in one heartbeat

Sudafed. Brand name of *pseudephedrine*

sympathetic adrenergic system. Synonymous with adrenomedullary hormonal system, a component of the sympathetic nervous system in which adrenaline is the chemical messenger released from the adrenal gland

sympathetic cholinergic system. A component of the sympathetic nervous system where acetylcholine is the chemical messenger released from the nerves. The sympathetic cholinergic system is a major determinant of reflexive sweating.

sympathetic innervation. The supply of nerve fibers and terminals in a tissue or organ

sympathetic nerves. Nerves of the sympathetic nervous system

sympathetic nerve terminals. Endings of sympathetic nerves, from which the chemical messenger, norepinephrine (noradrenaline) is released

sympathetic nerve traffic. Nerve impulses in sympathetic nerve fibers

sympathetic nervous system. One of the main components of the autonomic nervous system, responsible for many "automatic" functions such as constriction of blood vessels when a person stands up

sympathetic neurocirculatory failure. Failure of regulation of the heart and blood vessels by the sympathetic nervous system

sympathetic neuroimaging. Visualization of the sympathetic nerves in the body

sympathetic noradrenergic system. A component of the sympathetic nervous system in which norepinephrine is the chemical messenger released from the nerves. The sympathetic noradrenergic system is a major determinant of reflexive cardiovascular responses.

sympathetic vasoconstrictor tone. The status of constriction of blood vessels as a result of traffic in sympathetic nerves

sympathoadrenal imbalance. A condition in which levels of adrenaline in the bloodstream increase to a greater extent than do levels of norepinephrine. Sympathoadrenal imbalance accompanies episodes of fainting.

sympathoadrenal system (also called sympathicoadrenal system or sympathoadrenomedullary system). A name for the sympathetic nervous system and adrenomedullary hormonal system acting as a unit

sympathomimetic amine. A type of drug that acts in the body like stimulation of the sympathetic nervous system

sympathotonic orthostatic intolerance. Inability to tolerate standing up that is associated with excessive activity of the sympathetic nervous system

syncope. Sudden loss of consciousness because of a decreased flow of blood to the brain

syndrome. A set of clinical symptoms and signs that occur together

systolic blood pressure. The peak blood pressure while the heart is pumping out blood

tachycardia. Fast heart rate

teleology. The doctrine that an overall design or purpose determines natural phenomena

TH. An abbreviation for *tyrosine hydroxylase*

thermoregulatory sweat test (TST). A test based on the ability of the patient to produce sweat in response to an increase in environmental temperature thymus. A gland in the front of the chest cavity that produces particular types of immune cells. The gland gets smaller as people age.

tilt-table testing. A test in which the patient is tilted on a platform to assess the ability of the patient to tolerate and respond appropriately to standing up

tomographic scans. A type of scan by which the body is visualized in slices

total peripheral resistance. The total amount of resistance to blood flow

tremor. Involuntary shaking

trimethaphan (Arfonad). A particular type of drug that blocks chemical transmission in ganglia

trimethaphan infusion test. A test in which trimethaphan is given by vein to assess the effects on blood pressure

tyramine. A chemical found in red wine and hard cheese that, in the body, works as an indirectly acting sympathomimetic amine

tyrosine hydroxylase (TH). An important enzyme required for production of the catecholamines dopamine, norepinephrine (noradrenaline), and epinephrine (adrenaline) in the body

uptake-1. Uptake of norepinephrine and related chemicals by way of the cell membrane norepinephrine transporter, such as uptake into sympathetic nerves

vagal parasympathetic outflow. Traffic in the vagus nerve, a main nerve of the parasympathetic nervous system

vagus nerve. A major nerve of the parasympathetic nervous system that travels from the brainstem to various organs including the heart

Valsalva maneuver. A type of maneuver in which the person blows against a resistance or strains with a closed glottis as if trying to have a bowel movement, resulting in an increase in pressure in the chest and a decrease in the return of venous blood to the heart

vascular resistance. Resistance to blood flow

vasoconstriction. Tightening of blood vessel walls

vasodepressor syncope. The same as *neurocardiogenic syncope* and *neurally mediated syncope*

vasopressin. The same as *antidiuretic hormone*. A hormone released from the pituitary gland at the base of the brain that stimulates retention of water by the kidneys and increases blood pressure by constricting blood vessels

vein. A blood vessel that carries blood from an organ toward the heart. (An exception is a type of vein called a portal vein, which runs between two organs, such as the spleen and liver.)

venous return. Return of blood to the heart by the veins

ventricles. The main pumping chambers of the heart. The right ventricle contains blood pumped by the heart to the lungs. The left ventricle contains blood pumped by the heart to the rest of the body. The left ventricular myocardium is the main pumping muscle of the heart.

ventricular fibrillation. The most common cause of sudden cardiac death. In ventricular fibrillation, the heart muscle fibers contract independently of each other, and the heart ceases to pump blood.

vesicles. Bubble-like organelles inside cells. In cells that store chemical messengers, the messengers are concentrated in vesicles.

vesicular monoamine transporter (VMAT). A particular type of protein in the walls of storage vesicles that transports chemicals such as norepinephrine into the vesicles

vitalism. A view that life processes contain a vital essence that is beyond understanding by physical or chemical laws

VMAT. An abbreviation for *vesicular monoamine transporter*

volustat. A homeostat that regulates blood volume

yohimbe bark. A naturally occurring form of yohimbine that is available as an over-the-counter herbal remedy

yohimbine. A particular drug that blocks alpha-2 adrenoceptors in the brain, in blood vessel walls, and on sympathetic nerve terminals

yohimbine challenge test. A test in which yohimbine is administered and the effects on blood pressure and plasma levels of chemicals such as norepinephrine (noradrenaline) are measured

References

Bernard C. 1957. *An Introduction to the Study of Experimental Medicine.* New York: Dover (originally published in English in 1927 by MacMillan & Co., Ltd.).

Cannon WB. 1929. *Bodily Changes in Pain, Hunger, Fear and Rage.* New York: D. Appleton and Co.

———. 1939. *The Wisdom of the Body.* New York: W. W. Norton & Co.

———. 1993. *The Way of an Investigator.* New York: W. W. Norton & Co.

Chuncai Z, Yazhou H. 1997. *The Illustrated Yellow Emperor's Canon of Medicine.* Beijing: Dolphin Books.

Clarke AC. 1968. *2001: A Space Odyssey.* Norwalk, CT: Easton Press.

Damasio AR. 1994. *Descartes' Error.* New York: Avon Books.

Darwin C. 1958. *The Autobiography of Charles Darwin.* New York: W. W. Norton & Co.

———. 1965. *The Expression of the Emotions in Man and Animals.* Rev. ed. Chicago: University of Chicago Press. (Orig. pub. 1872.)

Dawkins R. 1976. *The Selfish Gene.* New York: Oxford University Press.

Goldstein DS. 2001. *The Autonomic Nervous System in Health and Disease.* New York: Marcel Dekker.

Hardman JG, Limbird LE, eds. 2001. *Goodman & Gilman's The Pharmacological Basis of Therapeutics.* New York: McGraw-Hill.

Harvey W. 1628. *Exercitatio Anatomica de Motu Cordus et Sanguinis in Animalibus.*

Iversen LL. 1967. *The Uptake and Storage of Noradrenaline in Sympathetic Nerves.* Cambridge: Cambridge University Press.

Langley JN. 1921. *The Autonomic Nervous System.* Cambridge: W. Heffer and Sons, Ltd.

Lorenz K. 1952. *King Solomon's Ring.* New York: Thomas Y. Crowell Co.

———. 1966. *On Aggression.* New York: Bantam Books.

McWhirter N, McWhirter R. 1975. *Guinness Book of World Records 1976.* New York: Sterling Publishing Company.

Nesse RM, Williams GC. 1994. *Why We Get Sick.* New York: Times Books.

Olmsted JMD, Olmsted EH. 1952. *Claude Bernard and the Experimental Method in Medicine.* New York: Schuman.

Selye H. 1950. *The Physiology and Pathology of Exposure to Stress. A Treatise Based on the Concepts of the General-Adaptation Syndrome and the Diseases of Adaptation.* Montreal, Canada: Acta, Inc.

————. 1956. *The Stress of Life.* New York: McGraw-Hill.

————. 1974. *Stress Without Distress.* New York: New American Library.

Index

Page numbers followed by *f* indicate figures, and those followed by *t* indicate tables.

David S. Goldstein, M.D., Ph.D. directs the Clinical Neurocardiology Section of the National Institute of Neurological Disorders and Stroke (NINDS) at the NIH. He graduated from Yale College and received an M.D.-Ph.D. in Behavioral Sciences from Johns Hopkins. In 1978 he joined the National Heart, Lung, and Blood Institute, obtaining tenure in 1984. In 1990 he transferred to the NINDS to head the Clinical Neurochemistry Section and since 1999 has led the Clinical Neurocardiology Section, an independent section in the NINDS. He has received Yale's Angier Prize for Research in Psychology, the Laufberger Medal of the Czech Academy of Sciences, an NIH Merit Award for excellence in patient-oriented clinical research, the Presidential Executive Director's Award of the National Dysautonomia Research Foundation, and the NIH Distinguished Clinical Teacher Award. He has published more than 400 papers, two single-authored treatises, and a handbook for dysautonomia patients. His research focuses on disorders of the autonomic nervous system, catecholamines, and scientific integrative medicine.